The Making of a Yoga Master

Dear Debbie,
with love
Suhas

The Making of a Yoga Master

A Seeker's Transformation

SUHAS TAMBE

HOHM PRESS
Chino Valley, Arizona

Cover Design: Adi Zuccarello

Interior Design and Layout: Kubera Graphics, Prescott, Arizona

Library of Congress Cataloging in Publication Data:

Patañjali.
[Yogasutra. English & Sanskrit]
The making of a yoga master : a seeker's transformation / Suhas Tambe.
p. cm.
Sutras in Sanskrit with English translations.
Includes bibliographical references and index.
ISBN 978-1-935387-24-4 (trade paper : alk. paper)
1. Yoga--Early works to 1800. 2. Patañjali. Yogasutra. I. Tambe, Suhas, 1950-
II. Title.
B132.Y6P24313 2012
181'.452--dc23
2011039467

Hohm Press
P.O. Box 4410
Chino Valley, AZ 86323
800-381-2700
http://www.hohmpress.com

This book was printed in the U.S.A. on recycled, acid-free paper using soy ink.

Lovingly dedicated

at the feet of my guru,

Late Shri S. N. Tavaria

And also to his daughter of past life,

Vibha, my dear wife

Contents

Saṃskṛt Pronunciation Chart

Vowels

अ a   आ ā   इ i   ई ī   उ u   ऊ ū   कृ kṛ   ऌ lṛ

ए e   ऐ ai   ओ o   औ au   ṁ/ṃ (anusvāra)   ḥ (visarga)

Consonants

क ka   ख kha   ग ga   घ gha   ङ ṅa

च cha   छ ċha   ज ja   झ za   ञ ña

ट ṭa   ठ ṭha   ड ḍa   ढ ḍha   ण ṇa

त ta   थ tha   द da   ध dha   न na

प pa   फ pha   ब ba   भ bha   म ma

य ya   र ra   ल la   व va

श śa   ष ṣa   स sa   ह ha

(Adapted from http://www.sanskrit.org/Sanskrit/SanskritPronunc.htm)

The Sequence of Sūtras

Throughout this book the sūtras are referred to by numbers, in two styles, like 1.3 or IV.15, etc. as "Chapter # dot sutra serial #." Roman numerals, like I or II, indicate chapter numbers from a conventional book; while numerals, like 1 or 2 indicate chapter numbers of the new sequence as presented in this book. At the end of each chapter, the relevant sūtras are quoted by giving both the new and the old reference numbers side by side.

Foreword

by Chip Hartranft

Yoga is one of the most widely practiced disciplines in the world today, and its popularity has increased in the last three decades at an unprecedented rate. In the U.S. alone, a 2003 Harris poll indicated that over 15 million people had attended a yoga class in the previous year, and some estimates place the current figure close to 30 million. Yet among all these practitioners, could any be described as a "yoga master"? In order to answer this question, one would first have to ask what yoga is, what "mastery" could possibly mean, and how a person should go about achieving it. Indeed, the single most important question of all might be: why would one want to master yoga in the first place?

The motivations that draw human beings to yoga are deeply embedded in our consciousness, and wholly related to the nature of yoga's mastery. Expressed most simply, we practice yoga to arrive at happiness and fulfillment. The reason yoga is called a "practice" has to do with the fact that as we cultivate ourselves through yoga, it unfolds by degrees, penetrating and carrying us beyond what we might have thought would gratify us physically, intellectually, and emotionally. The deepest sort of happiness that yoga can bring depends, in fact, on how completely one can let go of the desires, fears, and identity that have conveyed one to the present, and can meet the reality of this moment afresh.

It is this moment, and one's connection to it, after all, that are the only truly workable elements in one's lived life—everything else is simply a memory, imagining, or other sort of mental fabrication. In its essence, the word "yoga" means *connection.* As a practice, yoga means cultivating the skill to connect so deeply with what is before one, or within, that any mental or physical pressures inhibiting the free flow of being can completely subside. As a realization, yoga means the utter cessation of resistance to life, allowing the recognition of our ultimate identity to arise: unalloyed knowing. As such, yoga completes us.

If this doesn't exactly sound like the reason that brings you from time to time to your neighborhood yoga studio, take heart: even for many of its most devoted and accomplished adherents, "doing yoga" primarily means applying the energies of body and breath to a series of invigorating physical postures. Few are aware that this dynamic movement art was probably developed for the most part in the last millennium, and is the still-evolving "baby" in the yoga family. Its 10th century creators called it hatha yoga—meaning "forceful" or "energy" yoga—to distinguish it from the "royal" or "highest" path, rāja yoga: the cultivation of bodily and mental "collectedness" (samādhi) described by Patañjali nearly 1000 years earlier in the classic Yoga Sūtra. The oldest surviving hatha yoga text, dating from the 15th century, insists that these two approaches were complementary and meant to be practiced side-by-side. When they are, it becomes evident that they are related, and in fact form a single path with many portals.

This becomes clear not only at the deep end of the yoga pool, but also in the shallows where most of us first dip a toe or two. Yoga does promise and can quickly deliver a smorgasbord of self-enhancements: to flexibility, strength, health, and beauty. However it is the peaceful sense of presence one is sure to feel even after one's very first yoga class that may bring one back. That ineffable sense of clarity and contentment can awaken us to the possibility of something far greater, like a trickle of oil bubbling up out of the ground from a vast subterranean reservoir. What may have sprung from the desire to enhance oneself can be transmuted over time into a quest for what lies beyond the self and its desires. It is then that a yoga practitioner begins to tap the ancient, meditative roots and seek to draw upon their enormous stores of knowledge, of which the Patañjali's Yoga Sūtra is the definitive non-Buddhist compendium.

The Yoga Sūtra is one of the most enlightening spiritual teachings to survive ancient times. Although probably edited into its final form in the early centuries of the 1st millennium CE, its instructions are largely based on oral traditions that harken back to a time perhaps a millennium earlier and concern the contemplative practices prevalent both before and after the Buddha. The focus of the early forms of yoga was on freeing oneself from suffering—specifically, the inherent pain of being identified with one's sensations, thoughts, and feelings instead of seeing them as mere conditions, like waves rising and settling on the current of life. In a general sense, the entire project of yoga has to do with learning to voluntarily still those waves long enough to experience the transparency and lucidity that are the hallmarks of our intrinsic awareness when it is undisturbed by the varied turbulences of wanting and not wanting.

Though this is an ancient pursuit, it has lost none of its urgency or relevance. Human beings today are, if anything, more severely crimped by identification than ever before, and deeply in need of real connection. Like Mr. Duffy, the protagonist of James Joyce's story *A Painful Case*, we "live at a little distance from our bodies," and even further from the actual, conditioned nature of body and mind, in whose fabricated byways we are ever wandering. As Patañjali makes clear, though, a deeper connection can be cultivated in every domain of a lived life: in our relationship to beings and objects; within the sphere of our own personhood; throughout the physical body; at the level of our life energy or "aliveness," prāṇa; and at the deepest strata of cognition. When a person becomes completely stabilized or "yoked" in the midst of life's flow, then the possibility arises of instantaneously seeing past the everyday illusion of experience itself, and even beyond the subliminally fashioned notion of any ultimate "experience" as well. From this direct, untrammelled knowing springs the greatest happiness a person can know: the innate freedom of awareness that is always with us, waiting to be recognized.

There is no better guidebook or roadmap to the summit of yogic attainment than the Yoga Sūtra. It explains both how a person might master yoga, and how it cuts to the heart of the human dilemma. Although a mere 196 lines, the work is unrivaled for its penetrating insight into the nature of consciousness and liberation. Indeed, it is this very concision that has inspired, if not necessitated, so very many commentaries both ancient and contemporary, including my own (Shambhala, 2003). It is not possible, however, to find an explication of this foundational yogic praxis more detailed, far-reaching, or richly elaborated than the book you have now before you. Without getting entangled in the endless vines of esoterica that have sprouted about the path since the early days, Suhas Tambe has delineated the connections that tie ancient knowledge to modern revelations about the universe, both around us and within the inconceivable microcosm of each brain and mind. There is much to learn here, to assimilate, and connect to our contemporary understandings of how we know what we know.

What is most valuable in the pages that lie ahead, however, is the fact that they issue from an understanding of yoga that is essential to any true realization: yoga is above all a *path*, not merely a philosophical perspective. As such, it cannot truly be known from a distance, but must be gone down. As such, its mastery is freely available to all, and practice will perfectly reward each practitioner in direct proportion to his or her sincerity and diligence. Although it would be most accurate to call this observation a practical and realistic view, it is also grounds for a deep and abiding optimism that each of us may yet understand and achieve fulfillment in this very life.

Preface

Yoga is defined as "union" or "enlightenment," or as "abiding in pure consciousness." Does that make any sense to you? Is it realistic, or too arcane? Does it sound close to what you are thinking right now? Or is yoga for fitness all that matters? Is spirituality aligned with *your* goals, even remotely?

It wasn't for me for so many years.

For me it started with curiosity; some interest. Friends and well-wishers made many suggestions for exploring my new spirituality, and with a sigh of relief remarked, "Thank god he is finally there!" To be honest with you I don't remember *when* my curiosity turned into seeking, though I did not know for quite some time what exactly I was seeking. In *āśrams* there was alluring peace, but also the annoying scent of a "business of spirituality." I tried to meet some enlightened people; but they appeared to keep a guarded distance. Visits to shrines and temples of various deities drew me into a whirlpool of incensed devotees and the manipulative priests. I did learn some rituals and tried to read a few books. Though seeking was alive in my guts, any spiritual journey itself looked hazy because I could connect with none of these things.

Then I met my guru who brought a fresh breeze into my spiritual quest with his awesome smile, easy accessibility and very gentle conversations about deep philosophy. Connecting to him brought spiritual aspects right into my "normal" life and seamlessly blended the two. He introduced me to Sage Pātañjali's *Yoga-Sūtra* and gave me a wonderful gift—the real sequence of the sūtras, available nowhere else. Since then I have been reading that masterpiece and assimilating its contents *to make Yoga my life*. Perhaps my initial encounter with those spiritual celebrities, the rituals and the paraphernalia was only to invite me onboard. But once I was there, that showcase did not help any further in the spiritual journey. I learned that the quest and the spiritual realization have to anchor in your own self and not be scattered all around. Nothing outside, howsoever authoritative, is of any use if you cannot absorb it as a part of your own transformation.

Over the years, this process of transformation has also continuously morphed my goals and expanded horizons to make the once completely alien goal of enlightenment real; and in fact, now, the only one for me. To my utter amazement, all help and guidance that I always looked for elsewhere is right here in the *Yoga-Sūtra*. One only has to follow it correctly and tirelessly.

Yoga-Sūtra

A masterpiece of Vedic times, the *Yoga-Sūtra* of Sage Pātañjali is a collection of 196 aphorisms or statements in *Saṃskṛt*. It is the most authoritative and instructive document about Yoga, and one that practitioners consider fundamental. But, as a beginner on this path, it is not easy to embrace Yoga just by giving it *some* space in your life while living a material existence otherwise. Soon you experience a change within; your habits, your choices, likes and dislikes, the thinking, the world-view and the self-view—everything starts changing. The more you try to visit your earlier lifestyle the more you are faced with increasingly profound and quite contrary questions about life as you once knew it, pushing you to seek the truth, the ultimate truth, if possible. At this point, seeking looks fuzzy and the means too rigorous; but this is the time when you can lean on something as authentic as *Yoga-Sūtra* to get you there.

However, *Yoga-Sūtra's* first-read, especially with the traditional sequence of aphorisms, appears to present more philosophy than practice guidelines. At times, the out-of-sequence statements confuse and create impressions of a lofty and vague philosophy, giving fodder to intellectual differences of opinion.

Now, here is the secret—despite its seeming complexity, *Yoga-Sūtra* is, in fact, written as a practitioner's instruction manual that shows clear signposts along the path to enlightenment. But you will still need to witness, at appropriate places, how the philosophy of Yoga and its practice interchange smoothly, thus proving its truth and vitality.

To discover that Yoga is not about physical exercises alone is an insightful experience; a true revelation and one that may be hard to reconcile, given the popular perception of the practice. Yoga, in fact, undeniably puts you in touch with your inner self, and that invites you to the ultimate truth in a way that is neither religious nor intellectual, but is experiential and intimate.

Why This Book

When we already have in print many translations and freelance interpretations of *Yoga Sūtra* by some of the most respected and accomplished yogis, what is the need for this one? What authority, value addition or even novelty does this presentation bring in?

Yoga Sūtra is one of those scriptures whose birth is dated but whose message is not. Though the message is forever contemporary, its ancient language, terse construction and use of cryptic symbols have required many contributors to bring to light a full spectrum of its import. This book unveils a magnificent new dimension of the sūtras—a re-arrangement by a new sequence that will only enhance and enrich other interpretations.

The author derived this hitherto unknown sequence from his guru, and believes that its time has come only now, for reasons much beyond his grasp. The author's humble presentation is based on his personal experience, fortified by the enlightened words of his guru, a Yoga Master himself.

There is another reason for this book. At the time when Sage Pātañjali authored *Yoga-Sūtra*, Yoga was widely practiced by many.

He compiled this book as a compendium of Yoga to standardize the diverse practices and to codify the disparate strands of philosophy.

Ironically, today we are in a similar situation in which the technique of body postures (*āsana*) has become mainstream Yoga, and burgeoning schools and competing styles are creating confusion among aspiring Yogis about what Yoga really is. The problem is not just that the diverse interpretations and opinions are all laying claim to authenticity, but that the physicality of practices and the intellectualization of philosophy is eclipsing the spiritual essence of Yoga to which many seekers want to return. This book attempts to present *Yoga-Sūtra* as a spiritual manual written for present-day seekers.

Sequence

In colloquial usage, the word "sūtra" is more associated with "aphorism," meaning "a terse saying embodying a general truth, or astute observation." The real meaning of sūtra however goes beyond that as "a thread or line that holds things together" or "that the words carry an underlying continuous thought." Thus, interpretation of a single sūtra is as important as the *right connection between the sūtras*; what goes before and what comes after. True Yoga has always been instructed verbally. *Yoga-Sūtra* is the first written and authoritative documentation that captured its essence thousands of years ago. In those days, scrambling the sequence was one mode of encryption, to preserve the sanctity of the precious teachings. The real sequence was then handed down by a guru only to an eligible disciple.

Framework

Yoga-Sūtra owes its philosophical origin to certain basic concepts realized by the practicing Yoga masters of Vedic times. These concepts earned acceptance not through dogmatic veneration but through first-hand experience. The correctly "threaded" concepts together form a framework of Yoga that applies to each sūtra consistently for its authentic interpretation. This basic conceptual framework of Yoga is presented here in Chapter Zero (Foundation) for a systematic validation by subsequent self-experience throughout the Yoga practice.

Milestones

At the heart of this "right framework" within *Yoga-Sūtra* is a progression in the inner evolution of a Yogi, which occurs in distinct stages, and has never before been authentically documented as intended in that masterpiece.

> *In the Yoga Sutras there are embodied for us the laws of that becoming, the rules, methods, and means . . . Step by step there is unfolded for us a graded system of development, leading a man from the stage of average good man, through those of aspirant, initiate and master on to that exalted point.*—Alice Bailey, 1927, xiii.

These milestones on the path are laid out in this book, as:

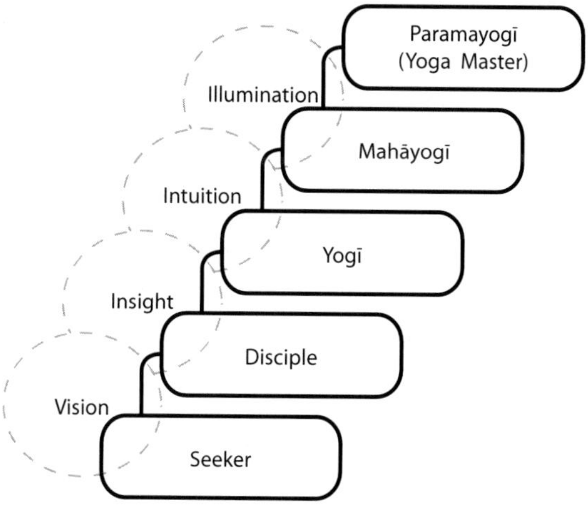

Figure 1: Milestones in Yoga

- **Chapter 1** describes how an inquisitive person turns inward, understands why mind and the thinking process are pivotal in search of truth, and feels inspired to seek the ultimate truth.

- **Chapter 2** introduces the Yoga methods and practices with which a spiritual expedition is launched, culminating into a *seeker* becoming a *disciple* with a vision.
- **Chapter 3** lays out discipleship of rigorous Yoga practice that helps develop emotional intelligence and deep insight on the way to becoming a *yogī.*
- **Chapter 4** demonstrates how a soul connection and advanced Yoga practices lead to spiritual intelligence and how a *yogī* becomes a *mahāyogī*, using intuitive powers.
- **Chapter 5** reveals how a *mahāyogī* is tested intensely and groomed for knowing the essence of consciousness, and thus becomes a Master who is in a sustained spiritual state.
- The **Afterword** revisits some complex Yoga concepts.
- **Appendices** explain *chakrās*, rhythmic breathing, upgrading of awareness, the refining exercises, the grueling process of the Master's grooming, and the illustrated progressive bio-physical changes in the seeker on the way to becoming a Yoga Master.

At each milestone, a new hypothesis is presented to the practitioner. The *sūtras* are presented both in *Saṃskṛit* and with iEnglish translation, and also with an index of the new and the corresponding old sequence, for those with an academic interest.

Neither creative imagination nor liberal interpretation can add to the profound wisdom of *Yoga-Sūtra.* My guru called himself just a scribe, thus I am no more than a courier, who has re-packaged the contents and lovingly delivered them here to inspire *you* as they did me. In Yoga, there is authority only in your experience and towards that may this book prove worthy.

Making of This Book

Many friends, well-wishers and serendipitous acquaintances have made this book possible. I remain immensely indebted to John Dobson whose writings provided a major breakthrough in my understanding of duality and non-duality; to Chip Hartranft, an accomplished Yoga author himself, for his pat on the back that meant a lot to me; to Christy Brown whose knowledge of Yoga and efficient expression helped in shaping Chapter Zero.

Prof AY Joshi's reasoned critique and initial frustration inspired a complete overhaul to the book. Angelina Calafiore provided encouragement when it was needed the most, and offered useful tips. Lori Brucato, an accomplished Yoga teacher, provided lots of input and warm encouragement. Anupama Buzruk, also a Yoga teacher, pointed out many deatils begging for lucid examples. Greg Swanson, Deborah Stensvaag, Rob Ransom, John Comperda, and Kapil Dixit formed a small, but dedicated meet-up group to review and keenly discuss the manuscript. This gave me a valuable taste of my future audience. I am grateful for their time and devotion.

Richa Prakash Asthana did professional editing while preserving my individual signature. Bonnie Granat and Jennifer Paine initially provided order to my chaotic grammar. I was lucky to get support and encouragement at the workplace from colleagues like Sadananda Mitra and many others. Ashutosh and Chaitanya, my sons, used their "payback time" seriously, and happily provided candid reviews. My spiritual journey was triggered by *The Autobiography of a Yogi* and by a dear friend Raju Nadgauda who gave it to me.

I remain deeply grateful to the team at Hohm Press (particularly Dasya Zuccarello, Bala Zuccarello and Regina Sara Ryan) for the vision they hold, expressed in their confidence in my work and willingness to see this book birthed elegantly and made available to a larger audience. Finally, if my words are readable, presentable and devoid of inconsistencies it is because of the diligence, patience, experience and insight into the subject-matter of my editor, Regina Sara Ryan. Sincere thanks.

About the Author

In 1993, Suhas Tambe (b. 1950) met with the late S. N. Tavaria, a Yoga master, who introduced him to Pātañjali's *Yoga-Sūtra*. Sri Tavariaji (1919–1994) was a master of many disciplines, most notable among which were his insights in the study of Yoga, the human body, and the many aspects of spirituality.

Sri Tavariaji met his master, known only as Sri Rama, at the tender age of seven years. Over the next twelve years, he learned the practices of a highly secret Yoga system from him, one that was passed from master to disciples in guru-disciple tradition, originating from Sage Pātañjali, the author of *Yoga-Sūtra*.

Sri Tavariaji is no longer living, but his presence is evidenced in the timely help that arrives in the spiritual pursuits of many disciples. "Enlightened" was his steady state radiating from the kindness in his deep eyes, a perpetual reassuring smile, the ease with which he would explain life's challenges in words so simple yet profound, a total absence of "I" or any scent of "holier than thou," his carrying himself through the material obligations of a family and a high-profile job, his effortless walking the talk, the utterly uncommon simplicity in his demeanour, his loving and caring discourses and the totality of his absorption in his guru.

For the last ten years, the author has studied Tavariaji's unpublished writings, researched extensively in order to understand many unexplained concepts, painstakingly avoided any apparently religious connotations, and constructed a contemporary presentation for today's readers.

The author has been a devout practitioner of these Yoga exercises himself since 1993. Tavariaji emphasized that the essence of life was in correct breathing, the purpose of which was to refine the body-brain system and to upgrade awareness.

Prior to this transformation, however, for most of his early life the author remained spiritually challenged, making him believe now that if *he* could seek and walk on the *yogīk* path anybody could! Today, the author splits his time between practicing Yoga and earning a living from a traditional career in finance and information technology. Now an "empty nester" he lives in Chicago with his wife Vibha, an attorney.

Chapter Zero[1]: The Foundation

We live life in pursuit of happiness. Sometimes when that happiness appears transient we stop and think. Personal truth then looks more like relative truth. That keeps pushing us ahead in pursuit of the absolute truth; which is where Yoga begins. But the truth *outside* is seen only to the extent that the same is realized *within*. In this inner journey one has to grow and to change.

Practicing body postures and doing breathing exercises is not all that Yoga is. The Yoga of *Yoga-Sūtra* is a process of complete transformation, of which postures and breathing are a part. Transformation implies change, and a change is never easy—even if initially it only means changing your habits. If a book makes you wiser just by reading it, that wisdom may prove too fragile in the face of real adverse circumstances. However, when the same wisdom is earned though persevered trials and tribulations, and by staying the course come what may, it becomes life-altering. Yoga brings you that kind of ingrained wisdom.

Yoga belongs to a genre of disciplines that when practiced correctly works on every cell in your body and brings about a change

---

[1] *This unconventional chapter number is intended to highlight the nature of Yoga philosophy that sees the whole Universe of matter emerging from "nothingness" and constantly yearning to re-merge back into that nothingness. Number "zero" best symbolizes that "potent nothingness" which is not some sterile void. It is no coincidence that "zero" is another gift to the world from India, as is Yoga.*

in the subtlest parts within you. Yoga works on the cause; health, happiness, and/or enlightenment are only the effects. It being so, at the high point in Yoga exercises, you would deal with the primary cause, the all-abiding energy itself.

Reading the sūtras, however, will be your first challenge.

The sūtras are not only in Saṃskṛt but are also very terse aphorisms or statements. Their apparent literal meaning is sometimes too simple and even misleading to the untrained mind. That is not all. You will soon find that by using the conventional sequence for interpretation, the sūtras keep a large part of their import hidden. In that sequence, you may find two unrelated sūtras sitting next to each other and presenting a deceptively ordinary context causing you to miss a truly potent interpretation. You may even feel obliged to connect those two sūtras somehow by attempting to derive some esoteric context, but this will help no practitioner. (A classic example is from Book II—Sādhanā Pāda, sūtras 50 and 51. While sūtra II-50 gives a detailed technique of controlling prāṇa, sūtra II-51 teaches an extremely advanced technique of motionless breath when prāṇa is directly controlled. While the first is meant for a disciple, only a ParamaYogī can practice the other). Therefore knowing the right sequence of the sūtras is critical for a practitioner. This book reveals the correct sequence of the sūtras to bring out the real and timeless essence of Yoga-Sūtra for you.

Connecting with the sūtras will be your next challenge.

A mere translation, literal or otherwise, would not take you very far. In Yoga, practice is the key and philosophy only ensures that your body-mind assimilates the essence of Yoga to make that practice a willed response and not a perfunctory effort.

But without knowing its roots, how could you put your arms around a discipline that is a few thousand years old and born in the East? So many incorrect notions surround it. Ironically, not knowing anything at all may perhaps be a blessing in disguise. Yoga is understood best when you carry no baggage. If Yoga has to change every cell in your body it should first become as intimate as the earth you walk on and the air you breathe. The sūtras should come out to you with no religious strings attached, because there are none. The sūtras should speak a universal language of humankind, because that is what they are.

While the practitioner in you learns the methods and practices, the student in you will approach the Yoga philosophy. Sage Pātañjali's uniqueness lies in his advice to rely entirely on self-realization and guidance from within, without overwhelming yourself by the theoretical knowledge dispensed either by books (including this) or by the external gurus. On your path to true enlightenment and self-discovery, it is imperative that your own experience should be the only testimony to the understanding and practice of the Yoga philosophy.

Experiencing Yoga will remain your continued challenge.

The *yogīk* path is an alien terrain. You land there with unfamiliar tools of inquiry and your own self as a reluctant target. Given our natural lethargy, it is easier to follow the dogmas. *Yoga-Sūtra* does not dispense any dogmas, but proposes hypotheses for self-experiencing. It shows the signposts, and teaches you how to reach the next milestone on this path. But you have to walk your walk. When you validate each hypothesis, your practice is more energized and you start constructing the Yoga philosophy in a way that remains uniquely yours.

Now, **where do you begin**?

This chapter lays a conceptual foundation for you to make a beginning. Please do not rush to embrace or defeat the ideas. Just give them a patient reading and leave the testing to a later date.

We will discuss the following topics here:

- Yoga Is Not a Religion
- A Complete Map of Yoga
- Is It Just a Technique?
- Basic Concepts
- The Yogīk Path

Yoga Is Not a Religion

When one looks at the purpose and the architecture of *Yoga-Sūtra*, it is easy to see that Yoga is not a religion. Though Sage Pātañjali compiled *Yoga-Sūtra* in 300 BC (or even earlier, according to some scholars) no single individual founded Yoga. He presents Yoga philosophy as the shared wisdom of enlightened Yoga masters, and prescribes authentic practices existing for several centuries. *Yoga-Sūtra* itself predates the oldest religions of the world. Over a period of time, different religions seem to have drawn upon the enormous wealth of *yogīk* knowledge, Hinduism being the most prominent, making many experts believe that "Yoga is *in* religion; religion is not in Yoga."

The sūtras serve both as instructions and as a contextual framework. Sage Pātañjali is extremely rational in his approach—not taking any dogmatic position of a theist, an atheist or a moral priest. Let us respect that matter-of-fact disposition when we approach *Yoga Sūtra*. Any inference that does not belong in the scheme of a Yoga framework has been eliminated from this work.

Religions for the most part promote belief in and worship of entities that exist outside of the self. The core of Yoga's philosophy, however, is that everything is present within the individual. A driving quest for the ultimate truth, the tools of such inquiry, and the grueling process of the actual discovery itself, all reside within. Thus, in Yoga there is no dependence on an external entity, either in the sense of a person or a god figure, or any organization.

There is also a flip side to this consideration. Being such a personal and intimate experience, each practitioner considers Yoga a personal asset. Some even consider this personal nature of Yoga as giving them liberty to innovate. All kinds of styles and Yoga brands emerge from this, all valid in their own limited way but collectively so diverse that a beginner remains confused about what Yoga really is. That is where *Yoga-Sūtra* comes in—to help as an authoritative reference book—providing a meta-map, equipping you with the wherewithal, and showing the signposts, but leaving you to traverse the path by yourself.

A Complete Map of Yoga

You need to know the terrain before traversing. The main reason for showing a complete map of Yoga here is for you to see a synthesized whole that Yoga concepts collectively configure. In a way, this map lays out a total territory—which you will eventually cover as a seeker—one step at a time. Initially, each concept is presented only as a hypothesis to facilitate a focused beginning and to serve as a reference point during your navigation. But the concepts are not at all intended to be understood merely intellectually, or worse, accepted blindly. They may require repeated visits to the book for a fuller, more holistic grasp. In fact, concurrent to the practice, the sūtras will be understood best on the subsequent visits, if approached with an introspective and absorbent mindset.

Yoga, a journey in search of the ultimate truth, is evolutionary. The transformation takes place within a practitioner through refinement of the body and empowerment of the mind. Yoga's methods and practices facilitate this, though by themselves they bring nothing if there is no transformation.

(At this stage do not worry about some of the Yoga terms used below. These are adequately dealt with later.)

A complete picture of the ***yogīk* path** is this:

- As a beginner, you first master the methods (rhythmic breathing, upgrading awareness, and refining exercises). When you are fairly regular, commence the first four practices ("limbs" of Yoga) *yama, niyama, āsana, prāṇāyāma* concurrently. They are the preparatory and Secondary Means of Yoga. Then non-attachment, *pratyāhāra*, is achieved as a breakthrough from the cumulative success of the first four limbs.
- After pratyāhāra, the three advanced limbs—concentration that leads to dhāraṇā, meditation that leads to dhyāna, and contemplation that leads to samādhī—become Primary Means of Yoga. While the Secondary Means are

practiced concurrently, the Primary Means occur linearly, in a steady progression. Pratyāhāra enables dwelling in the inner domain, to deal with the mind and the thought process directly. By spacing the thoughts, a window is created for envisioning Īśvara for further training into the subtle domains. Thus Yoga practice is no more restricted in time or space and slowly extends over all wakeful life.

- Achieving samādhī is not the end of the path. Through even more rigorous practice you master saṃyama—a state of dhāraṇā, dhyāna, and samādhī occurring at once and not linearly. Finally, even a desire for samādhī is given up to simply remain in a non-dual state through the dissolution of the primary duality. That is the state of enlightenment, total absorption.

And this is the path of Yoga as laid out in *Yoga-Sūtra*.

Is It Just a Technique?

Apparently, practice (*sādhanā*) is the key in Yoga.

Does that make Yoga a mere technique? Rather than serve a mere academic, philosophical or intellectual quest, *Yoga-Sūtra* touches one's very core of living. It tells us the secret of our mind by unfolding the human thinking process. It shows how the wholesome consciousness abiding all over the Universe (Universal Mind) gets fragmented, obscured, and disconnected, into its dwarfed version of an individualized "mind." Yoga practice brings about a reconnection and re-merging of this mind into universal consciousness, and that is the "union" we seek as the goal of Yoga. In a way, Yoga is a transformation process, taking us back to our celestial home. This process removes the obstacles and hindrances that the individual mind invites unto itself in the course of living. You use methods and techniques as part of the process that results in body-mind purification, to let the individual mind regain its status as the universal consciousness. This makes Yoga not only a technique but a process, as well as a goal.

Basic Concepts

As a process, Yoga is built on a few basic concepts. Of course, there is no need to accept these concepts as a prerequisite; this is not a belief system. Yoga practice provides enough ways and means to validate the concepts first. But just knowing about them here will make it easier for you to take the first steps on the path.

The pursuit of truth should rightfully begin with the concept of "truth." We generally rely on two sources of truth: one, undisputed science, and two, our own sensing. However, the history of science easily reveals the evolutionary nature of scientific truth. Yesterday's truth quickly becomes today's "outdated" theory.

As to the use of our senses to perceive truth, the old maxim "seeing is believing" does not point to our ability to "sense" a foolproof truth. Our five senses have limitations. Our eyes, for example, need brightness to see but cannot look at the sun. We cannot see the full spectrum of colors either. We sense the world with a limited range of wavelengths to hear, a small band of chemicals and molecules to be able to taste or smell, and touch so weak that we cannot feel the mosquito squatting on our skin until it sucks our blood. To add to that, our eyeballs are located such that, unless we pivot the head, we can only take in less than a 120^0 view of 3-dimensional space.

So what *is* real? What you see, taste, smell, hear, and touch are simply *interpretations* of sense impulses (electrical signals) that are translated by the brain to assure your survival within the physical world. The world we see around us is not what we perceive with our physical senses. In fact, today's science is struggling to accept "the quantum level of reality"—meaning that, at the smallest level of our physical universe, all matter is nothing more than a phased wave potential, but never in an actual physical state of reality as we experience it.

- Your world, your reality that you experience, is all around you. Where else can Yoga begin? Surrounded by myriad objects, you are an object yourself. Your whole thinking, dominated by objects (that includes other people), remains ceaselessly oriented towards connecting and dealing with these. Your reality is what you know; yet not only is your source (limited sensing) defective, but you rarely know *how* you know. Engrossed in the appearances, you never realize that you don't know the whole truth; that there are more subtle aspects to these objects than what meets your eyes. **If perceived rightly, all objects are multilayered (layers of gross to subtle).**

- But why are you not able to perceive objects as multilayered? Why do you remain captivated by the gross appearance alone and miss the subtlety? Your thinking process is responsible for that, since it allows mind a free hand to bring all its baggage of pre-formed ideas. The mind puts us in a bind that manipulates knowledge with our ego's unique emotional signature, conditioning it with what is already known. Thus, **the thinking process colors the perception.**
- Even if it is colored, perception is the only way you can connect with the outside world of objects. In the perceived world, objects appear to be separated by a void. When you presume the unseen subtle layers, the void that otherwise appears to be separating the objects appears filled up with this unseen subtle substance. Then it is easier to see the connection. Your own subtle desire to perceive an object that projects itself through the senses and, riding over many subtle layers, touches the subtle energy of the perceived object. In return, this contact generates sensory signals as raw material to the thinking process. This subtle energy, called *guṇa*, is alive when perceived, but otherwise dormant in all objects. Guna supplies the qualitative data we can use for knowing. **Perception activates *guṇa* and causes its cognition.**
- Dwelling in the world of subtle energy a question would naturally arise: What is the subtlest of all? But questions like this take us into a world so deep and unknown that words stop making any sense and simple answers are impossible. Until fully grasped by a capable mind cultivated through years of practice, we can only imagine the subtle

concepts. For instance, imagine an ever-extending stick with the grossest substance at your end, and the subtlest at the other. If a perceivable world is at this end, then the other end must be imperceptible. If the energy exists as excitable *guṇa* here, then at that other end, it must be by itself with no *guṇa* in attendance. For the sake of easy reference, *Yoga-Sūtra* calls such a phenomenon "at the other end" as **Īśvara, who dwells in each object but remains without *guṇa***.

By themselves, these concepts may be easy on the intellect, but when you hit the "Apply" button a considerable challenge is posed. For example, it is easy to see the world as part tangible and part intangible, but seeing yourself like that or even trying to experience your own self as an "object" is quite challenging.

The same holds true for your thinking process. The mechanism of thought generation is easy to understand theoretically, but trying to dissect your own thought process on those lines is tough when thinking itself is your dissecting tool.

Guṇa and *Īśvara* are unique concepts too. We deal with the phenomenon of *guṇa* in our individual perception continuously; in fact, we are captive to the appearances created by *guṇa*. So total is its integration with perception that to perceive *guṇa* separately as a phenomenon while in the process of perception is tough. It is like asking a ballplayer to be a commentator, simultaneously requiring that he play the game and analyze it at the same time. The concept of *Īśvara* also usually invokes pre-formed ideas of "god" or "almighty," which thwart any efforts to see it with a clean slate.

Multilayered Objects

To be able to get mired in *guṇa*, the mind has to be matter. Thus, the world of matter is a huge continuum stretching from the grossest—the most inert mass, to the subtlest—the Cosmic or Universal Mind. The gross appearance and the subtle aspects of an object make it multilayered, and that is Yoga's foundational concept. The layers span from gross (the tangible, the functioning aspects) to subtle (the intangible, the behind-the-scenes forces and energies) in a continuous gradation. However, no object is "born" multilayered, but becomes so. An object evolves in a definite order. The subtlest aspect comes first and conceives and produces the relatively gross, giving the object a graded body (as shown in *Figure 0.1*), comprising three bands—**physical**, the gross (the outermost), **astral**, the subtle (the enclosed) and **causal**, the subtler (the innermost). The causal body encases the spiritual Self, the source of life, the subtlest (distinguished as "Self," with a capital "**S**"). Mind, the mother of a material body, is independent of it and is instrumental in creating awareness of the body.

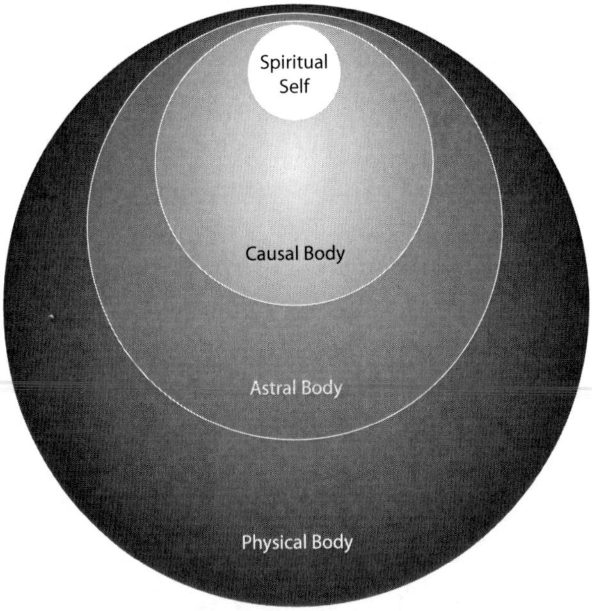

Figure 0.1: *Multilayered object*

The layers are also defined sometimes as five *koshās* or sheaths:

1. *Annamaya* sheath (physique), sustains on food,
2. *Prāṇamaya* sheath (vital energy), sustains on *prāṇa*
3. *Manomaya* sheath (psyche), sustains on sensory impressions
4. *Vijnanamaya* sheath (intellect), sustains on thoughts
5. *Anandamaya* sheath (bliss, an emotion).

Like any other object in the universe, a human being is multilayered too (see *Figure 0.2*). The concept of *kośas* is slightly different, but some common aspects are these: The human **physical body** is cellular *annamaya kośa*. The **astral/molecular body** appears to correspond with three *kośas*, at the base level with the energy sheath (*prāṇamaya kośa*), at the lower level with the psyche (*manomaya kośa*) and at the higher level with the intellect (*vidjānamaya kośa*). The **causal/electronic body** is *ānandamaya kośa* that brings the experience of bliss. Beyond these bodies is the *soul*, the divine fragment that is pure bliss, considered a fourth state beyond physical, astral and causal.[2] The Universe, also an object by itself, has three similar virtual planes: Physical Universe, Astral Universe and Causal Universe.

Mind, Matter and Thought

All matter is energy. All energy is one; everything moves, everything vibrates. The energy that puts everything in motion is consciousness. If there was no consciousness in the universe would it even exist at all? Since perception brings to us the energy of the universe as actual matter, the world as we know it would not be here without consciousness.

Every single element of matter has its own mind, consciousness or memory to exist in that state, and has its corresponding properties programmed within that arranges the cells, molecules or atomic and subatomic particles in a particular manner. Thus matter, energy, consciousness and perception are the same things in different contexts. Matter appears to be both waves of potential non-physical energy (the unseen world of mind) and small solid basic building blocks, called particles (the seen physical world.) Hence, the key to the physical world lies in the mind that moves everything

---

[2] *Take a moment. When describing the multiple sheaths that make an object, we have to use some conventional terms. For instance, we have to say, the astral body is "inside" the physical, or the causal body envelops the soul. You need to understand that in the process of getting a radically different view of the world, even these terms need to be challenged. The two bodies may remain tied together, but if the astral body is more subtle than the physical, why should it stay "inside" it? It would rightfully interpenetrate it, be inside as well as outside. What is important is to understand the relative gross- or subtleness and not be bogged down by words.*

through thoughts. We may "think" of thoughts as non-material or non-physical form, but they are actual and even physical in nature. Thoughts are matter too and they exist.

Thoughts create awareness that "we have the body," and this awareness makes humans unique. That self-awareness results from the body's cognition, produced by the thinking process. It also makes the body, its awareness and the thinking process, all independent of each other.

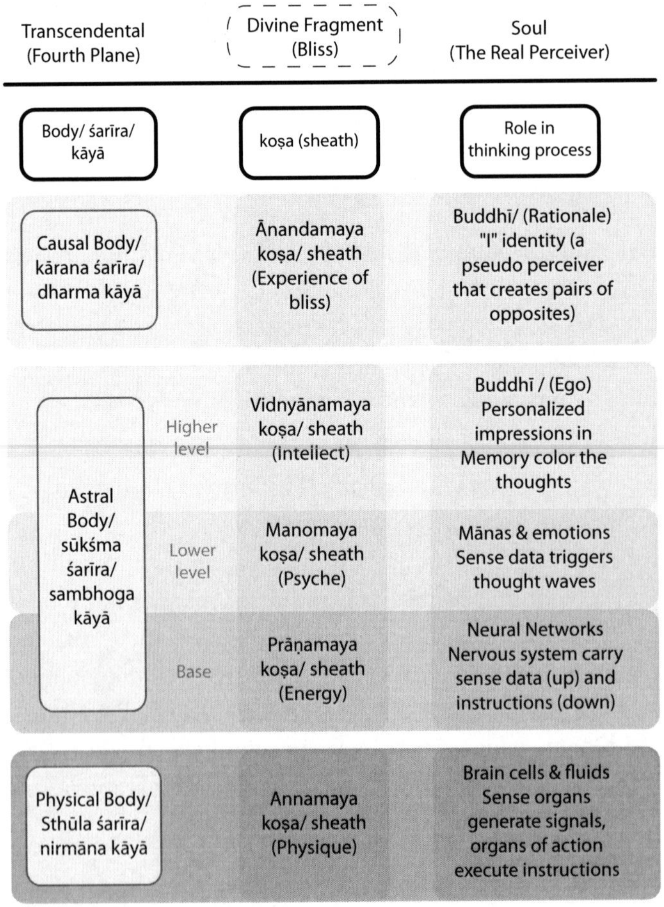
Transcendental (Fourth Plane)
Divine Fragment (Bliss)
Soul (The Real Perceiver)
Body/ śarīra/ kāyā
koṣa (sheath)
Role in thinking process
Causal Body/ kārana śarīra/ dharma kāyā
Ānandamaya koṣa/ sheath (Experience of bliss)
Buddhī/ (Rationale) "I" identity (a pseudo perceiver that creates pairs of opposites)
Astral Body/ sūkśma śarīra/ sambhoga kāyā
Higher level
Vidnyānamaya koṣa/ sheath (intellect)
Buddhī / (Ego) Personalized impressions in Memory color the thoughts
Lower level
Manomaya koṣa/ sheath (Psyche)
Mānas & emotions Sense data triggers thought waves
Base
Prāṇamaya koṣa/ sheath (Energy)
Neural Networks Nervous system carry sense data (up) and instructions (down)
Physical Body/ Sthūla śarīra/ nirmāna kāyā
Annamaya koṣa/ sheath (Physique)
Brain cells & fluids Sense organs generate signals, organs of action execute instructions

Figure 0.2: Multilayered human being and thinking

Thinking Process

Technically, "thoughts" are caused by neural electrical pulses from within the brain. Thought is like a domino actuator in the sense that there are processes that must take place for that thought to come to fruition—proceeding from the point of sensual perception, to experiential recognition, memory and emotional response, to cognition, and then to actualization.

Yoga-Sūtra presents a unique concept of a "thinking process." It is based on the same understanding of multiple layers but, interestingly, considers the thinking process as a function of mind energy and distinguishes it from the thinking apparatus, like the brain.

In fact, the thinking apparatus is also multilayered, comprised of brain, *mānas* and *buddhi* as the respective counterparts of physical, astral and causal bodies. But the thinking apparatus is only a tool, a processor, with no intelligence of its own. The intelligence comes from the mind that collaborates with and provides energy to the thinking apparatus to initiate a thinking process.

If you look at the anatomy of the thinking process (in *Figure 0.2*) there is a notable absence of the "mind." The reason is simple; mind is independent of both the thinking process and the thinking apparatus. Mind is not an organ and it doesn't have any particular location in the body. Then, what is mind? Yoga holds a view that a human mind is an abridged version of Universal Mind. That the extremely subtle Universal Mind can and does interpenetrate all objects and flow through the body too. That instead of remaining a catalyst for sharing universal knowledge, a part of the free-flowing Universal Mind gets dragged into the thinking process and is enslaved by ego. This "resident" mind tries to create its own *personalized* knowledge.

Now what is this **ego** which enslaves Mind?

The sense organs bring home signals as raw material for thoughts. When the signals reach the thinking apparatus, a thought results as a composite of physical, astral and causal elements; processed respectively by the brain, *mānas* and *buddhi*. The intensity of such thought composition and the emotional energy embedded in a thought together create an impression or *saṃskāra*. But then, because it is stored in memory, this impression serves as "a structure of predisposition." Once established, it greets the sense data, filters and sculpts it with a personal stamp even before a thought is formed.

The accumulation of *saṃskāra* thus shapes one's emotional disposition, and personal likes and dislikes, and generates *ahamkāra* (ego). Under its influence, *buddhi* breeds duality in your thinking, based on a perceived separation between your own self and "all-that-is" outside, and develops an "I" identity, an individual personality that shows up in reflex thought processes. Awareness thus remains anchored in the physical plane and this "I" appears to be the perceiver.

But is "I" the real perceiver? Ego is both a product of and an active player in the process of perception. But, the fact that what is perceived and the perception process itself is "known" to you means *something else is the perceiver*—something that does not partake in the processing of the sense impulses; something that stands aside of it.

Guṇa

What creates the sense impulses in the first place?

Physics describes the "mass" of an object as "equivalent to its energy" (even if the potential energy of location or kinetic energy of motion may not be present.[3]) Perception brings senses in contact with this quintessential mass/energy in the perceived object. When in contact, the object radiates **electromagnetic energy** that manifests in three primary modes (sensed as attributes, qualities or constituents) called *guṇa*. The perceiver receives these electromagnetic vibrations as sense impulses. ***Sattva*** represents the inherent, illuminating and pure quality of everything in nature. ***Rajas*** stands for that which is active and moving. And, ***Tamas***

---

[3] *Present-day physics maintains that everything in the universe, in all physical states, is composed of the same vibratory or oscillatory force-field. The gross, seemingly static "objects" have a slower vibration, which gives the impression of solidity, while less solid, subtler elements have a more rapid vibration. That we cannot perceive the subtle vibrations inherent in all things is a reflection of the fundamental limitation of our sensory perception. (Please see page 339 in Afterword)*

characterizes that which is inert or immobile. Ordinarily, *tamas* conceals what the object really is, and *rajas* keeps presenting it in different forms at different times, while *sattva* makes a feeble attempt at revealing the true identity, thus in effect creating half-truth or plain deception. It is obvious that a *guṇa*-based perception would never be wholesome, complete and real. Thus, only through non-sensory, direct perception, where the duality and deception of *guṇa* are transcended, can one perceive an object in its real state.

However, to bypass thinking to have a direct perception is not easy. It is not just the *guṇa* of the perceived object that participate in perception; the *guṇa* of the perceiver play a role too. To transcend *guṇa* in the perceived object, you need to have transcended your own *guṇa.* Hence, it takes a long process of Yoga transformation to earn the ability to "perceive directly" in which your own awareness is elevated to your higher subtle states. This evolutionary process cultivates increased well-being on the physical plane, tranquility of emotions on the astral plane, and versatility of intelligence on the causal plane. With recognition and experience of the spiritual "Self" deepening, your point of reference for all experience becomes less self-oriented, as the "I" definition shifts and begins to dissolve, with Self-consciousness awakening in its place. Once this happens, you are in such a subtle state with awareness anchored so close to the soul that a need for external teachers diminishes and you are guided completely by *Īśvara*, the soul.

Īśvara

Given our *saṃskāra* it is quite tempting to think of *Īśvara* as "God," which it is not in any conventional sense of the term—personal or impersonal, male or female, one or many. The word *Īśvara* refers to the principle of fundamental intelligence, the Supreme Intelligence that permeates all life.

Purūṣa, *Īśvara* and soul are interrelated terms often wrongly used as synonyms, whose fine distinction is not easy to comprehend. It is better to just hear them now and truly understand later. Pure consciousness or the Spirit, called *Purūṣa* is the most subtle phenomenon, and hence imperceptible. *Īśvara* is a symbolic representation of *Purūṣa*; a perceivable embodiment of the imperceptible Spirit. It represents soul, the innate, divine potential within the physical self. At the pinnacle of Yoga, you would reach such a subtle and fragile inner domain that only *Īśvara,* the soul, could guide through the final stages on the *yogīk* path.

The *Yogīk* Path of Self-Realization

On the *yogīk* path, personal transformation and evolution is gradual but sure, and it traverses the physical, astral, and causal planes. In the end, the three bodies (physical, astral and causal) become one harmonized vehicle for enlightenment. On the way, at the end of each stage, a milestone is reached. A student becomes a *sādhaka* (seeker), earns a vision and becomes a *śiṣya* (disciple) of truth, develops insight to become a *yogī*, cultivates intuition to become a *mahāyogī*, and finally becomes an enlightened *paramayogī* (Yoga master).

Reaching the milestones on a genuine *yogīk* path is largely a function of the strength of inner will or fiery aspiration (*tapas*) which drives the seeker's inner evolution. At first, the seeker's neutral will of ordinary consciousness is activated during the discipleship, and a *yogī* transforms it into intellectual will. Intellectual will is guided in large part by intellectual understanding of teachings pertaining to elevation of awareness. Gradually, understanding of reality gained through direct perception of a *mahāyogī* transforms the intellectual will into the spiritual will, until finally the inner will of a *paramayogī* is the Cosmic Will itself.

Yoga is transformational and not just a small routine adjunct to your life, like grocery shopping. **Yoga *is* life**. Everything changes within. An outward makeover is relatively easier, but changing the way the mind works is a tough endeavor especially when mind itself is the change agent.

Viewed from the initial stage of "seeking," the later milestones appear irrational, almost unattainable, and the whole path, an exercise in futility. But as you travel towards a milestone, the one who reaches this is not the one who started. The milestone attains a new meaning. The difference between mere knowledge of Yoga and an insight born out of practicing Yoga is beyond imagination. The transformation that Yoga brings about would change the foundation of your reality. But, this does not happen *in* the mind but rather *to* the mind. The structures and textures change in the physical, astral, and causal bodies. Such enormous changes are continuous and extremely gradual.

From Becoming to Being

But the *yogīk* path is not one sequential progression. There are innumerable trials and errors, and the path to perfection at each stage is covered with millions of baby steps.

Yoga is devoid of any beliefs or dogmas. Sage Pātañjali wants you to invest in uninterrupted Yoga practice with fiery aspiration (*tapas*) and depend only on first-hand realization of truth. At each stage in this transformational journey, you would start with a hypothesis (see *Figure 0.3*) and then you would follow rigorous *yogīk* methods and practices to prepare ground for new realization

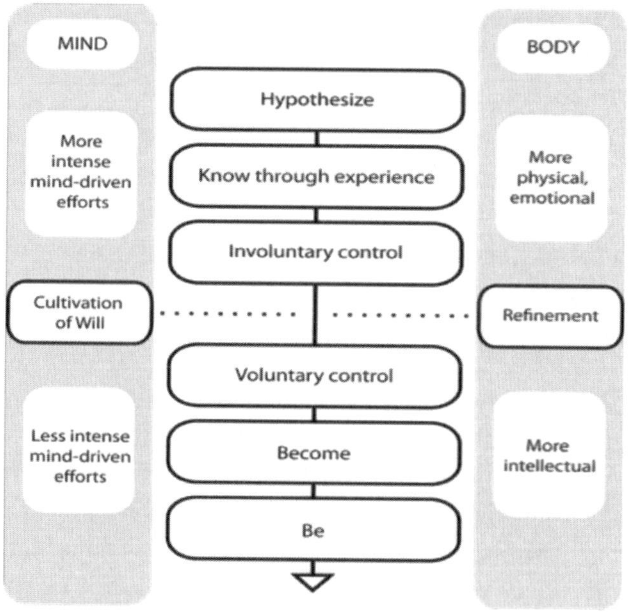

Figure 0.3: Anatomy of a Yoga milestone

or experience to occur spontaneously, by itself. But, by then you would have also understood the underlying process of reaching that experiential state which, with further efforts, you would bring under conscious voluntary control.

These efforts are twofold: bodily refinement and cultivation of will. When conscious control is gained you experience a transformation intended in that phase. But in that experience and in the process of "becoming" there is still duality. Transformation is really complete when a sense of experiencing is dissolved and the original hypothesis is now a new self-realized truth for you, altering your way of life completely.

You thus cross the thin line from "becoming" to "being."

From our mind to Universal Mind

As awareness purifies and its energetic vibration rises in frequency, the bodies—physical, astral, and the *prana* (energy) layer—have to be refined in order to properly circulate the energy up and through the energetic psychic centers called *chakras*. Higher states of awareness slowly release mind from coloration as the thinking process is clarified and the individual mind reclaims its status as a powerful catalyst by becoming as omniscient as Universal Mind.

If the individual mind knows an individual's reality, the Universal Mind must know the reality of the universe. *Yoga-Sūtra* maintains that the Universal Mind is pure awareness (consciousness), transparent and independent of all objects. It resides in and flows through the objects; and through us too. But while flowing through, it does not remain pure, transparent, and independent. *Yoga-Sūtra* shows how and why the all-knowing Universal Mind becomes the opaque and dwarfed individual mind. Because of its selective attention shaped by the predispositions and constant coloration by the thinking process, an individual's mind is an adapted version of Universal Mind. Our individual mind creates our "I" awareness; while Universal Mind creates pure awareness tinted with nothing. Yoga makes us understand our individual minds, and shows us a way of making contact with Universal Mind, the meta-mind.

From individual mind to Universal Mind is this wonderful Yoga journey! Mind is the end, mind the means. In the process, awareness locked up in the material world starts expanding and deepening, ultimately becoming pure consciousness itself. What a turn around! The brain and vehicles of perception get purified, in turn rendering themselves redundant as the source of knowledge. Instead, they become a storehouse of spiritual knowledge and its efficient users. Colored perception is replaced by a direct perception. A direct perception ushers a vision that guides and progressively leads into spiritual states where ultimately only consciousness prevails. It happens in stages and we are now going to see how.

Take a moment . . .

However, before we examine the milestones, take a moment to reflect—you are about to participate in the most incisive inquiry of life and one of the most grueling experiments with yourself. Patience will not just be a virtue but an essential tool to exercise the mind. Yet, never stop questioning. Yoga welcomes a thorough test for each of its concepts. Words like "consciousness" or "spiritual states" should acquire unambiguous meaning in your reality before they become a part of your vocabulary.

Your *yogik* path is going to be unique for reasons you will learn soon. But it helps to remember that the Yoga framework and the reference points belong to a precious legacy of several millions who have traveled their paths ahead of you. That legacy stands compiled and codified here. If you are a self-starter you can take off right away. But if your walk stalls owing to doubts, confusion or lack of peer support, just look around. Through the words of *Yoga-Sūtra,* these innumerable previous travelers will lovingly guide you.

As you advance on the eight-fold path of *Yoga-Sūtra,* you will appreciate the worth of this sequence of sutras for the amazing new dimensions it brings to the world of Yoga. May *Īśvara* bless your Yoga journey.

Chapter One: *Sādhaka* (Seeker) and Inspiration

1st Milestone

Though our first breath is excruciatingly painful, we are born happy within, and we live our whole life in pursuit of happiness. While acquiring new skills of survival we gradually connect with the outside world, and a never-ending succession of objects, people, and situations engulf us. Some things bring pleasure and some pain, and that shapes our likes and dislikes, loving and hating, the predispositions that define our personalities. But, what happens to that happy life within? Our awareness of that very life slips away. Now absorbed in an externalized life, we get disconnected from our natural state of happiness within.

People, objects, and situations are only transient sources of happiness, but we still want to hold on to them. In such an externalized life, happiness comes and goes. But we don't know how else to live and claim our innate happiness; our birthright!

We not only live life and have experiences, we are also aware that we do so. We remember our experiences. That creates for us our own personal version of reality, which is constantly rearranged, moment to moment. But neither pleasure nor pain is an object. We cannot hoard pleasure or eliminate pain. At times, our reality appears limited and uncertain in answering profound questions about life; and that makes us restless. Knowing more does not always mean knowing better. Then, in some unguarded moments, we question "knowing" itself, as a process. How do we see? How do we perceive? How do we think? We seek answers. And that brings us back home—within! A reconnection to life within is Yoga, call it what you will.

Yoga begins with the realization that you are not the physical body alone. The inner "you" wears the body as the body wears clothes. Your true self resides in it. Somewhere inside of you are the ideas, aspirations, and thoughts that collectively drive you. But even they do not appear to be the real ones. Is soul hiding behind them? How can such a vague thing as soul be real? Where is this soul? Is searching for soul spiritual? This calls for experiencing and exploring to one's very core. That's why the first Yoga hypothesis to be tested is that *the spiritual Self exists within you.* When you seek to validate this, you first stumble upon and understand your thinking process that seems to have denied this spiritual side of you all along.

Awareness appears completely conditioned by thoughts and muffled by predispositions. Take a hard look and you will see your thinking to be mostly "reflexive," utterly predictable and not "reflective." You feel that bondage, and have an inner urge to unshackle the tyranny of compulsive automated thinking.

In turning inward, you learn to separate **thinking** from **awareness of the physical body**. Experience-based awareness gently lifts from the physical dimensions of the world. And you feel inspired by the possibility of what may be beyond it.

At the first milestone on the *yogīk* path that "something beyond" is what you start seeking.

In this phase: from a Curious Inquirer to a Seeker

Yoga hypothesis	Spiritual Self exists
Know through experience	How to direct awareness inward; be conceptually aware of the subtle bodies
Involuntary control	Thinking process under scrutiny of thoughts
Achieve voluntary control	Reflex thinking arrested at will
Become	An advanced student
Be	Sādhaka, a seeker

New words used in this chapter

Mānas	The subtle thinking instrument of the astral body.
Buddhi	Even subtler thinking instrument of the causal body. It interpenetrates mānas.
nāḍīs	Subtle channels for the mind to flow through the gross-to-subtle bodies.
prāṇa	The cosmic force that the human bodies take in as energy to sustain. Prāṇa creates a sheath to envelope the astral body and energize it.
Īśvara	The principle of fundamental intelligence, the Supreme Intelligence that permeates Life.
guṇa	Energy inherent in an object that we perceive as parameters and qualities, or collectively—a form. There are three categories of guṇa.
Sattva	—that which reveals
Rajas	—that which projects or is mobile
Tamas	—that which conceals or is inert
Avidyā	Absence of proper knowledge.
vṛttis	Activities of the mind prompted by a conscious link between the senses and the object sensed.
yama	Abstentions of behavior.
Niyama	Observances.

Āsana	Postures of the three bodies.
Prāṇayāma	Regulated breathing of prāṇa.
Pratyāhāra	Non-attachment.
saṁskāra	Structure of predisposition; the likes and dislikes.
Karma	A cause of action that ends only when redeemed.

The Unseen World

> *So the reality is that at this very time there is an upheaval. People are looking for new answers, and what we are discovering reveals something totally different about life. For example, a biology predicated on Newtonian physics, which is mechanical and physical, looks to something physical—that is, chemicals and drugs—to understand disease and healing. But a new scientific reality, quantum physics, says that everything is made out of energy. It is primal to matter and shapes matter. Another myth of material science is that genes control biology, making us victims of our heredity. The new science of epigenetics, however, says that genes do not control our life; our perceptions, emotions, beliefs, and attitudes actually rewrite our genetic code. Through our perceptions, we can modify every gene in our body and create thirty thousand variations from every gene just by the way we respond to life. In short, we are leaving behind a reality of victimization (by our genes) and moving into the reality that our mind—***our consciousness, the immaterial realm****—influences our experience and potential.*—Bruce Lipton and Steve Bhaerman, *Spontaneous Evolution: Our Positive Future and a Way to Get There from Here* (Hay House, 2010).

It is amazing how such a contemporary scientific observation becomes a perfect preface to Sage Pātañjali's timeless work. As *humanity,* we are evolving now as a super organism, and seem to have evolved physically and matured intelligently. But as long as our seeking is limited to the physical pleasures, emotional comforts or the intellectual accolades, we keep moving in circles, without ever being aware of the unseen world, *our consciousness, or the immaterial realm;* leave aside exploring it. But the unseen is our promise, our next frontier, an inner evolution—a biological and spiritual evolution. Sage Pātañjali has endowed a true seeker with a carefully compiled wealth of knowledge in *Yoga-Sūtra*, for correct Yoga study and practice to make that inner evolution possible.

> *Pātañjali codified the sūtras which contain or verbalize the truth that was experienced by those who lived before him. Pātañjali codified [and] systematized Yoga as a science of psychophysical purification.*—Vimala Thakar, 3.

Yoga is universal in nature and transcends all the boundaries of gender, faith, color or nationality. But precisely for the same reasons, its ownership gets usurped by anyone with an agenda, and Yoga often gets mired in religious beliefs, vested interests or mere intellectual debates. Yoga is much more than its most visible and shrewdly peddled "fitness" version. It touches and unveils the core divinity in you. True to its vitality, Yoga is as valid today as it was hundreds (or thousands) of years ago. As a methodology, it is timeless. You can go back to these "ancient" basics and yet discover a very contemporary path as if Yoga was invented yesterday. With the right tools of interpretation, and with self-experienced truth alone as the authority, Sage Pātañjali is assuring the seeker that "you are 'now' ready to learn Yoga." This exposition of Yoga, "the union," is a compilation of its processes and hypotheses.

Yoga, a Science of Union

"Union" the literal meaning of the *Sanskṛt* root of Yoga, is a core theme throughout the sūtras. **Now, we shall begin the revised and complete instructions in the science of Union** (Sūtra 1.1/I.1).

But why do we need to talk about Yoga, the union? Take a look at the layers again (*Figure 1.1*). A multilayered human has a gross physical body on the outside that envelopes the subtle astral body, which in turn envelopes the subtler causal body, with the subtlest soul, the spiritual Self, in the core. Self is pure consciousness, our true self, the ultimate truth. But our mind locks us in the physical body and creates *faux* awareness of who we are. Thus, the layers remain disjointed and create a wall of ignorance preventing us from realizing the truth. Once you start seeking the truth, you discover the subtler bodies as the clandestine operators inside your own self, as well as in other objects. That discovery charts out a spiritual path that brings about merging or union among all fragmented and alienated parts of the self so that the final union reveals Self as the real self.

Thus, "a union of what" is something you continue to explore, and in doing so, discover its ever-deepening meaning. As externally oriented as we always are, we realize the transience of the physical union, and sometimes we desperately seek a union of minds, or better still, fantasize a union of souls; a vague, but alluring idea.

In Yoga, a world without is no different from the world within. And perception is our first rudimentary "union" or connection with other objects. Yoga naturally begins with this union until one realizes how flitting the perception process is, and how it distorts the truth.

The impermanence of an external union returns you within. But there you find no awareness of the inner bodies, and even when you know them, they appear disjointed. For reaching to the core you need all the bodies as one coherent vehicle. Thus, you seek a union of the physical body with the astral body, and of these two together with the causal body. Once purified and united, these transient bodies finally dissolve in union with the soul, the spiritual "Self."

Ironically, even the idea of "self" is very vaguely anchored in the physical body and we fail to grasp it clearly or completely. The concept of "self" is limited to awareness of the body's outward visible form or appearance. You cannot easily comprehend the complete physical body—your own or another's. A "handsome" man or a "beautiful" woman is usually a conditioned gestalt view. Don't we recognize our own body by what we see in the mirror and exaggerate it by what we *want* to see?

We place the physical "self" at the center of the world, making everything else "not-self," outside of self. Not-self comprises an endless variety of discrete forms—objects, people, events, and the whole flora and fauna. An hypothesis of Yoga is that "all these forms—from the grossest individual body to the divine life—make one (unbroken) continuity, underlying which is the same all-permeating divine principle, the spiritual Self." When we follow the *yogīk* path, we get to validate this hypothesis with first-hand experience.

The world is only as real as what we perceive it to be since our awareness is based on our perception. Under the overwhelming influence of ego, it is difficult to see our own self as an organism or as an object, as nondescript as any other. But, if you do that, you would discover a connectedness; a certain correspondence among all objects. "Space" makes us think of something infinite, spread above and beyond the "seen" sky; but we overlook the same space right here around us, even inside us. We ordinarily look at two objects as discrete entities and the gap separating the two objects as just a void. Isn't that space too?

When you are able to perceive even that space as an object with life, of course very subtle, you also realize how space connects and does not separate. But you learn the deeper and subtler aspects of the world like space only by becoming aware of the deeper and subtler aspects of your own self. Only in this way can you connect to your inner selves and eventually solve the mystery of how they evolve together into the spiritual one. This awareness is not cosmetic and intellectual. On the *yogīk* path, a milestone is reached only when the new awareness of the subtle becomes as real to you as the normal awareness of the physical is. That is *self-realization.*

How Is Yoga Achieved?

Yoga is achieved through healing of the psyche and calming of the thinking instrument, which is restrained from taking various forms (Sūtra 1.2/I.2). One may paint mental images of subtle bodies inside and may say, "Oh, if Yoga is a union of these, is that all Yoga is?" Such a statement results from deceptive mind-games, which create a mirage of spiritual experience made even more complex in the East by established images of gods. Apparent "visitations" by one of the gods is nothing more than indulgence of a memorized image. Such impatient seekers are told in this sutra that Yoga is a process of self-realization, so that awareness, the tainted consciousness, can become pure again through healing. And that occurs with calming of the thinking instruments (a herculean task) thanks to a purified and detached mind.

The human being is a complex life form, unlike any other. And unlike other forms, a human being has self-awareness and the ability to change his or her texture of sensitivity, and the structure of personality if desired. But for this change to happen, awareness has to enrich and to elevate from gross to subtle bodies. Awareness is produced by the thinking process; but caused and sponsored by the mind.

Body, Mind and Thinking

While these terms are often used randomly in our vernacular, in *Yoga-Sūtra*, the concepts of body, mind, and the thinking process are well defined and consistently followed in the three dimensions of physical, astral and causal. This makes the *yogīk* path a spiraling journey from gross to subtle, and the cherished union happening progressively on more and more subtle planes. But what kind of a "union" is this?

The cardinal principles of union are:

- To begin with, the un-manifest (yet unborn) gross is held as a "potential" by the subtle (like a child in the womb of a mother).
- Then, once the gross is manifest, the subtle controls the gross, but there is duality.
- Eventually, with the purpose of manifestation expiring, the gross folds back into the subtle, and *that* is their union.

There are a few interesting corollaries of this concept.

- First, the gross is what meets the eyes and that is what ordinary perception is. But working directly on the gross to gain control over it is futile.

- Second, the gross is an effect and not a cause.
- Third, the gross is a manifestation of the subtle.
- Fourth, the subtle is to be recognized and understood in terms of its ability to control the gross.

On each gross or subtle plane there is a body, a part of which acts as a thinking instrument to create awareness of that body. (*Figure 1.1*)

Yoga proposes this: A multilayered human being has three distinct selves acting in tandem. A physical body exists as a consortium of functioning organs at a cellular level, with a (physical) brain as its thinking instrument. It is ordinarily this body that one identifies as "I." But that's only an outer shell. Cells are composed of molecules. At a molecular level, there is an astral body with a virtual team of subtle controllers, with *mānas* as its thinking instrument that interpenetrates the brain. Molecules comprise atoms. At an electronic or atomic level, there is a causal body with even more subtle energy sources and forces, with *buddhi* as its thinking instrument that interpenetrates *mānas*.

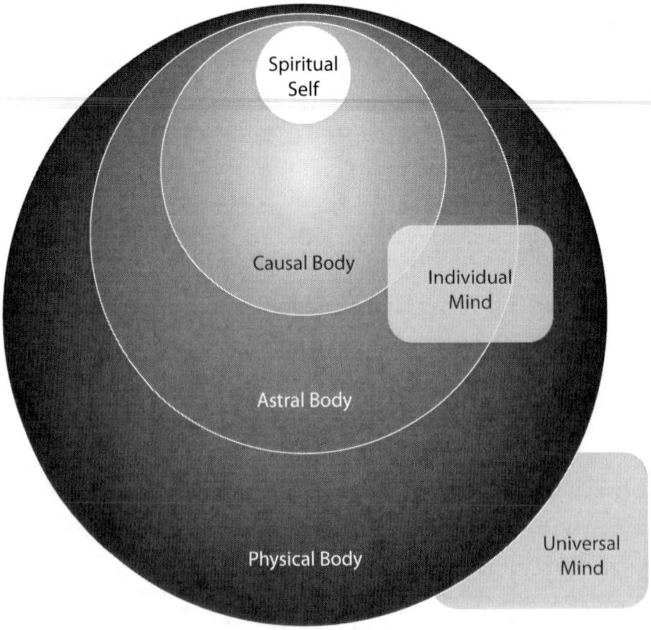

Figure 1.1: Multiple Bodies and Mind

If these are the thinking instruments, the obvious question then is, "What is the mind?"

Mind Is Independent of the Bodies

Mind on any scale, whether individual or Universal, is independent of its off-springs, the bodies or the objects. The all-pervading Universal Mind is so subtle that it is omnipresent; present in the physical brain too. Its energy activates the brain into "thinking." This indulgence robs its universality, and a part of it becomes laden with individual impressions; that part relatively less subtle and more opaque then resides in the body as an individual mind. By inducing the brain to think, the mind conjures a perceived form of any object from the sensory data. Then, it is not the object but its form or appearance that becomes a part of the personal reality.

We are aware of the existence of a network of blood vessels in our body. The physical (cellular) self also relies on a complex nervous system to carry the sensory input to the thinking instruments. Likewise, the astral (molecular) self has more subtle, invisible *nāḍīs* for the individual mind to flow through. To help you understand this concept of invisible *nāḍīs*, imagine a crude but useful analogy. We live in a wireless world, with a subtle, invisible information network. We cannot see them, but wireless radio frequency signals are subtly present all around us, undetectable until devices like a cell phone can convert these signals to a recognizable voice. This is exactly how the invisible *nāḍīs* allow the subtle mind to flow through.

We have seen that the astral/*mānas* system is far more subtle than the physical body/brain system. That is why in daily, ordinary living it gets easily bruised from the agitations of body/brain activities. Hence, the astral/*mānas* system needs healing from the hurt and that is what sūtra I.2 is referring to.

The physical system, however, cannot be forced into a calm state just by will power alone. Though we are endowed with "will" energy that can steer the physical body/brain and the astral/*mānas* systems, mostly it is not consciously cultivated and hence remains neutral.

At the heart of Yoga exercises, there is another important premise about the gross and subtle bodies and how they sustain. Human energy is constantly replenished; but our lack of understanding makes it more of a passive process rather than a deliberate or controlled one. The physical body/brain system receives its energy from food and by breathing air; likewise the astral/*mānas* system receives its energy from the incoming thought vibrations and by breathing *prāṇa*, the life-force.

The intake of food and air—eating and breathing—are known to us. They are the two basic needs of the body and, though we at least do something about food, breathing is left as a non-conscious activity; entirely an autonomous function. What Yoga does is that it makes us aware of a definite correlation between thinking and breathing. Stress causes shallow, erratic, and irregular breathing. In turn, controlled breathing can achieve calming of the thinking instruments.

However ordinarily, it is not even recognized by many that ***prāṇa*** and **thoughts** are important inputs for sustaining our subtle bodies. *Prāṇa,* the subtle life-force abounds all over in what we see as "just space or void." The astral/*mānas* system breathes *prāṇa* that has its own metabolism. Air and *prāṇa* go hand in hand, and before we develop the ability to deal with *prāṇa* directly, we take help from the breathing process. This is why you will see breathing exercises prescribed first in Yoga before moving on to controlling the *prāṇa* metabolism.

But the most significant contribution from Yoga is about the "thought vibrations" and a premise that "thoughts have subtle existence" in the form of electro-magnetic waves. (What exists is an essence of a thought, and not the desire that is its root cause or a verbalized thought that is loaded with emotional baggage).

Do you realize that you eject as well as receive an avalanche of thoughts? That others' thoughts greatly influence your behavior, thanks to a reflex thinking pattern fueled by an indulgent mind? This is one more reason why controlling the mind becomes so critical in your spiritual journey.

Awareness of subtle bodies and control over their gross-level functions is brought about by sustained Yoga practice and achieved gradually as a result of a systemic transformation of the self.

What Is Self-Realization?

In Yoga, the ultimate realization that the self is not real happens by consciously experiencing the absence of any duality between self and the Self, pure consciousness, thanks to the self's transformation. **When *this* is accomplished, the seer (self-turned-Self) abides in itself** (Sūtra 1.3/I.3). The self-to-Self metamorphosis occurs progressively, this way:

1. Yoga practices and methods purify the bodies and make breathing rhythmic …
2. Rhythmic breathing leads to breath's synchronization with the *prāṇa* respiration …
3. Conscious *prāṇa* respiration yields control over *prāṇa* that causes awareness of the inner astral and causal bodies …
4. This elevated awareness brings about identification with the inner spiritual reality and a release from the deceptive external forms…
5. And thus, spiritual consciousness is achieved.

In the above process, you become an earnest seeker and realize your real nature. There is realization that the physical self is not as primary as you always thought it to be. With growing awareness of the inner astral and causal selves, you begin to get a vague idea of an even more subtle spiritual Self that is at the very core of our being. How the spiritual Self is real, and how the outer enveloping selves are relatively unreal, is a progressive realization. In fact, this new reality does not remain just an intellectual acceptance, but it is an experienced truth totally integrated with your self-view and the world-view. Eventually, you would completely identify with the inner Self and not with any forms external to it. An absolute unity with the soul is thus the "ultimate union" contemplated in Yoga.

Yoga enables you to be consciously aware of all the three selves. You can also choose to anchor the awareness in any gross or subtle selves, depending on the need of the moment. As a seeker you would understand, accept, and yearn for a union with the soul, symbolized by *Īśvara* at whose doorstep you would stand.

> *The word Īśvara is (often) translated as "God"... that does not convey the real sense of Īśvara ... The word*

> *Īśvara refers to the principle of fundamental intelligence, the Supreme Intelligence that permeates Life. It is not referring to a god—personal or impersonal, male or female, one or many. ... In our modern language you can call it the energy of intelligence that is omnipresent, omnipotent, omniscient which has an inexhaustible potential of Creativity.*—Vimala Thakar, 29.

From self to Self

The journey from "self-awareness" to "Self-awareness" is a long one. Even awareness of the inner selves does not occur easily and by itself. Mind causes awareness. But, since mind can be known, it means we can be aware of the mind; and our awareness is distinct from the mind itself. These are difficult concepts to internalize. Mind is a "thing," a vehicle. But mind is the only vehicle of our awareness, and mind's autocracy keeps tricking us by denying any access to the truth.

Hence, up until the high-level awareness, the inner self identifies with the forms, one's own and that of others, and takes their active modifications for real (Sūtra 1.4/I.4). When we perceive an object, we perceive its outer appearance, a form. A form is a product of **that** very perception. A form is a composite image that consists of parameters like size, shape, color, smell, fluidity, warmth, and many other qualities. Each parameter has its qualitative index, with options. For example, the size is large or small, or the shape is round or conical...these perceived parameters and qualities are called *guṇa* in Yoga. Each object derives its functionality from *guṇa* energy inherent in it, and the perception of the object brings *guṇa* to life as a composite form.

The details of a form keep changing in the mind, because the mind grasps something new every time it perceives. We get drawn in by the rapidly changing forms and tend to identify ourselves with them. This results in a complete engrossment that easily mistakes the "self" as a pseudo perceiver (a sense of "I see it"), reinforces *ahamkāra* (ego) and constructs reality around the perceived forms. So overwhelming is mind's indulgence with the appearances or forms, that it "owns" them. "My house," "My family," and a series of such entitlements result.

Our ego sits in perpetual judgment about objects and people, and uses undependable yardsticks based on the ever-changing impressions of *guṇa.* Such assessments not only remain subjective but constantly change with each passing event. Thus, our understanding and description of things remains vague and swings between pairs of opposites in our effort to define them.

Mind becomes saturated with forms. Hence, to know anything about such a mind, we must first begin to stop identifying ourselves with the forms. Standing aside of our own self, we should see how a form is a product of perception, and that the real object may or may not be what we perceive it to be. This ability to "stand aside of self" becomes a stepping stone to turning inward.

Once our attention is inward-bound, a more subtle and higher dimension (the astral/*mānas* system and beyond) appears on our horizon, at least as a possibility, and beckons us to explore it further. Identification of the physical body/brain system as "I" soon turns out to be false: we begin to understand it as our basic *avidyā* (ignorance). Later, when we discover the subtle yet powerful inner self, we wonder how and why we remained engrossed in a physical body. As a human being, we only have a physical body for our inner self to express itself. But when we constantly deny even the existence of the inner self and get immersed in the ever-changing physical forms, that denial prevents the inner self from manifesting its real nature.

> *The lower forms are constantly and ceaselessly active, endlessly assuming the forms of impulsive desires or dynamic causal thought forms and it is only as this "form-taking" is controlled and the tumult of the lower nature stilled that it becomes possible for the inner ruling entity to liberate himself from thralldom and impose his vibration upon the lower modifications.*—Alice Bailey, 13.

Thus, we are slaves to the material life, not so much because of the physical body itself, but more because of the mind that keeps our awareness locked up there. That is why it is imperative that we understand mind first and foremost.

Individual Mind, the Cause

Yoga-Sūtra is all about the human mind. The mind is our greatest tool, but indulgence and ignorance keeps it abysmally deficient. Where does the mind reside? What are its characteristics? How does it work? One "knows" for sure that this invisible mind is inside the body somewhere and yet it remains an enigma. It is certainly not an organ. It appears to be subtle. As the invisible air provides proof of its existence in the wind, mind is evidenced in thinking. Thinking leads to knowing and awareness.

An individual is a superset of many organs working in tandem. In turn, each organ is formed of many cells, each cell is composed of many molecules, a molecule has atoms, and an atom has particles that bring us into a very subtle domain of force-fields and vibrations. The mind doesn't seem to be an organ, yet with its unmistakable presence appears to belong to this very subtle domain. We are told that the particles are the basic building blocks of all matter, animate or inanimate. Is mind matter or is it just a subtle process of the brain? *Yoga-Sūtra* tells us that it is possible to know what mind is. One of the Yoga hypotheses is: "What is true of an atom is true of a human being and is also true of the whole universe." If mind makes us aware of ourselves and of the objects around us, each object must have a mind in some form; there must be a mind of an atom and a Mind of the Universe. But is the invisible and inaccessible mind more important than the tangible physical body that we can see, touch, and know beyond doubt?

What is mind?

Yoga proposes that in the process of thinking, the individual mind collaborates with the brain. The brain produces thoughts as its activity, which creates waves and leaves the subtle individual mind perpetually unsettled. The human brain works continuously, except in deep sleep, and makes us believe that thoughts occur in real time, moment by moment. However, interestingly, the thinking process creates a minuscule time lag between the act of seeing and the act of perceiving. You remain disconnected from the actual moment of seeing, since during the act of perceiving, you pay attention to a ("seen") moment that is actually past.

Thus, a thinking brain works only on the images of known persons, objects, and events. The imaginative brain, on the other hand, fabricates surreal concoctions from these images. The mind-assisted thought process is memory-driven; that is, the thought process is based on past images. It is habitual, reflex thinking. The mind uses known images for fabricating fanciful thoughts to imagine things—that we call the "future." Here the brain dreams with eyes wide open. During sleep (unless it is deep sleep when the brain is not aware), it does similar acrobatics in the dream state. Brooding over the past, conjecturing the future, and dreaming the absurd are all states of fancy, because they rest upon images that by themselves have no real existence. The brain is a processing powerhouse, but it remains enslaved and conditioned by the mind.

The mind is a subtle, brittle, and malleable substance that is invisible, and interpenetrates everything. Thinking instruments (like the brain) and the mind go hand-in-hand, but they are distinct from each other. In order to move forward it is important for the seeker to first conceptualize this distinction.

The brain is a physical organ, fairly inert. The brain stores data and processes thoughts through interaction (exchange of mild electrical charge) among various parts of its functional network. The mind provides energy for this interaction when it interpenetrates the brain. The mind provides a spark that the brain's neural network makes into a wildfire by consuming the incoming impulses.

In the *yogīk* framework, the mind, the substance that flows through the brain, is the erstwhile Universal Mind, which is expected to remain only a catalyst, but instead becomes a resident of the brain, thus "individualized." This individual mind is what we have to deal with.

The mind does not belong to a body as an organ nor does it reside at a given location. It manifests itself in various ways depending on which aspect of it is at work. *Maharṣi Vyāsa*, one of the most insightful commentators on *Yoga Sūtra*, has enumerated these aspects of mind:

A. *SANSKĀRĀS*:

- **Mind, a manipulator of thoughts**: Our legacy of past incarnations with seeds of functionality that materialize as body features, susceptibility to illness, talents, actions, etc., that define a personality and the state of health. This influences the choices made in the thought-processes.
- **Mind, a pre-processor of thoughts**: Our structure of predispositions, accumulation of preferences, likes and dislikes, repressed impressions, etc., that sustain ego and trigger impulsive reflex thinking. They act as pre-processors before the thoughts are formed.

B. MEMORY:

- **Mind, a consolidator of habits:** Autonomous body functions are a legacy of human evolution that brings to us metabolism, heart-beating, breathing. etc. They convert repetitive thoughts into behavioral habits.
- **Mind, a supplier of subjective bias:** Latent impressions of past experiences unavailable to normal awareness spring up in the process of "new" cognition and in dealing with the unknown. They skew the "learning" by adding the subjective bias.

C. MIND, A DRIVER OF THOUGHTS: *Prāṇa* energy in its purest form is the Universal Mind and various grades of contaminated *prāṇa* comprise the individual mind. This energy drives the thinking process by agitating the brain, *mānas* and *buddhi*.

D. MIND, A DISTRACTOR: Universal Mind pulsates with Cosmic Rhythm; but, the individual mind loses its ability to be in tandem with that and instead, with its erratic rhythm, remains fickle and vulnerable to changes in the gross bodies. This makes the mind unstable and inherently incapable of concentration.

E. MIND, A POWER: Universal Mind is a mother and the controller of all gross matter; while the individual mind becomes subservient to the gross matter. Individual mind in its process of becoming the Universal Mind regains that control in the form of psychic powers, called *siddhīs*.

Thus, a mind that is burdened by the legacies of *sanskāra* and memory, captivated by the latent impressions, lured into the thinking process, fickle and subjugated, has to become what it originally was, Universal. That process of transformation is Yoga. And that is why we concern ourselves with annihilating *sanskāras*, bypassing memory, upgrading *prāṇa*, restraining mind modifications and investing the psychic powers in advancing these efforts. In each of these aspects there is a certain progression on the path of Yoga.

The Mind States

But as long as it remains an individualized mind, **the thinking process causes the mind modifications and leaves the mind, in concert with the brain, in any one of these states that is painful or not painful** (Sūtra 1.5/I.5):

- Wandering
- Forgetful
- Distracted
- Occasionally steady, and
- Restrained (and focused).

This is how it is brought to our attention that, though the mind modifications are responsible for creating the subliminal impressions (which in turn cause more modifications, an unceasing "chicken and egg" cycle), it is the same quality of mind that ultimately empowers the mind. The impulses bring in sensory data that is neutral and colorless. In collaboration with the thinking instruments, mind creates impressions that are painful or not-painful during the thinking process (it is important to describe it as "not painful" to differentiate it from "blissful" which it is not).

These states—let us call them "mind states"—are caused by the interplay of the mind, the brain[4], and the memory of emotions. It is not possible to be free from these states as long as we have not developed conscious control, and we are conditioned to depend on the mind-states for normal living.

Moreover, the not-so-painful states occur intermittently between the painful states. On the *yogīk* path, one learns to move from the painful to the not-so-painful mind states and then ultimately away from any mind-induced state at all! That is true bliss!

The "thinking" itself is enacted on the astral (*mānas*) and causal (*buddhi*) levels. The entire astral/*mānas* system is so subtle that it resembles a tuning fork whose arms start trembling the moment it hits something relatively gross. The three arms correspond with the three *guṇa* (qualities) present in ourselves. Calming the mind and the thinking instruments is the art and practice of bringing the agitated *guṇa* from an imbalanced into a state of balance; from trembling to stillness.

Does mind fluctuate or modify? When we say "fluctuate" there is a hint of mind coming back to normal on its own. But, the mind is such a brittle substance that, with each vibration, it modifies itself and stays that way until the next change comes along. It becomes what the thoughts are. Therefore, the calming of the mind will result only when the mind modifications [*see the next section*] are consciously stilled by deactivating their change agents, the thoughts. To do that, the awareness must be turned inward, because the five mind-states give rise to the five types of mind modifications, which in Yoga we want to eliminate in order to have a "no-mind" state.

Five Mind Modifications

So, what is a mind modification?

Any thought or action is really a *cause* for a mind modification. Mind is like clay with unlimited plasticity that can be recycled in

---

[4] *Ordinarily, the mind-states are more prominent when the awareness is low and at the physical level; which means out of the thinking instruments the brain is active, but its subtle counterparts,* mānas *and* buddhi*, are not yet active enough.*

different images, again and again. Or like a heap of fine sand that constantly changes its shape with the blowing wind. Or, if mind is pictured as a fluid like water that is ordinarily calm and still, imagine how a drop of water can cause the surface to stir. This would set in motion a chain reaction, either limited to a few ripples on the surface or to a vortex of stirring movement deep down. Once in motion, it takes a while before the surface returns to the original state of calmness. This whole episode is a mind modification, and because thoughts occur so incessantly, mind is perpetually modifying.

Each physical action (or a conscious non-action) is preceded by an "action in thought." So the process of "thinking" itself is the cause of a mind modification. In the *yogīk* framework, thought registration takes place in the frontal lobe of the brain. A modification plays itself on the physical stage, in this thought registration area. If the subtle mind is like water, the registration area is like a vessel that contains water. Thinking is normally an automatic process, and one can do nothing about it even with one's "will."

Mind modifications are in five categories (Sūtra 1.6/I.6):

- *Pramāṇa*, Valid knowledge derived by thinking (though valid, still a mind modification)
- *Viparyay,* Misconceptions or incorrect knowledge (wrong sensing and/or inference), when derived from forms alone
- *Vikalpa,* Delusion (wrong use of imaging faculty), when derived from images
- *Nidrā,* Passivity (a self-induced half trance or sleep), when derived from impressions and
- *Smṛtī,* Memory (compulsive hoarding of emotion-laden thought forms into storage) when derived from associated impressions.

VALID KNOWLEDGE

We need to realize that valid knowledge at its very best is still derived knowledge (Sūtra 1.7/I.7). Whether based on a sensory cognition or on an intelligent analogy or inference, as long as it depends on mind as a medium, knowledge is conditioned by one's *learned*, prior experiential knowledge, and is essentially dominated by forms and symbols that are personal to the perceiver. That these forms and symbols are collectively recognized and belong to a widely shared public vocabulary would not make them any less subjective. Is valid knowledge useful in daily life? Of course it is. But what is deceitful is the air of objectivity and the implied superiority that it acquires over other knowledge.

Why is even valid knowledge a mind modification? A drop of water causes a stir on the surface of still water, regardless of whether the drop is clean or unclean. (*Yoga-Sūtra* does present the concepts with no biases and without any value judgment.) That's important to remember. We need to realize that, ordinarily, mind also acts as a source of knowledge and not just as a user. Since mind operates in space and time, mind-produced knowledge is stamped with its *space-time* contexts.

Hence, valid knowledge is a truth that is relative (to space and time). Statements like "the Earth is flat" and "the Sun revolves around the Earth" were commonly held truths at one point in time. The history of science is replete with examples of how certain hypotheses became widely acknowledged as the prevailing scientific truth, only to be eventually shattered by another, newer hypothesis.

Our knowledge of an object is derived from a mind-driven process of a series of perceptions. The main players in the process are the thinking instruments and the sense data is its raw material. The sense organs constantly capture and deliver the sensed vibrations into the brain. But while the brain starts churning them, its subtle counterpart, *mānas,* pours stored pre-dispositions into the process and colors them. What results is a personalized information which the ego, product of a more subtle instrument of *buddhi,* further builds into self-serving knowledge. Knowledge consists of recognition of an object as what it is and what it is not. But, as long as the knowledge is derived through the thinking process one cannot escape the coloring and the conditioning. To use technical terminology, an object inherits generic attributes from the class or type of objects it belongs to (say, an apple as a fruit is "an edible part of a plant, usually fleshy and containing seeds") and possesses its own attributes that distinguish it from others within the same class (apple is however different from an orange, another fruit). Attributes often remain as the subtle aspects hidden behind the appearance.

Knowledge is valid when both generic and specific attributes are correctly inferred or evidenced. Obviously, the quality of the thinking process is more important than the quantum or duration of thinking; even the most valid knowledge is still an exercise in relative truth.

Simply put, valid knowledge of an object will consist of as many parameters as could be accurately grasped through observation and smart logic.

INCORRECT KNOWLEDGE

Incorrect knowledge is based upon ordinary perception (mere seeing without understanding) **of the form and not upon the state of being of the object** (Sūtra 1.8/I.8). Our everyday perception is sense-driven, conditioned by the form or the external appearance of an object. This is potentially incorrect knowledge, inasmuch as it could be proven defective by subsequent valid and correct knowledge. Incorrect knowledge usually occurs in the physical domain, while correct knowledge is usually derived in the subtle domain that involves *buddhi*. (We have just seen how data is raw in the physical domain and in the process of knowledge-creation, gets personalized in *mānas* and intellectualized in *buddhi.*)

The importance given to the brain as "a source of knowledge" is misplaced and can only lead to incorrect knowledge. In fact, the brain should not be always relied upon as a source of knowledge. It is too entangled in forms and does not reveal an object's subtle aspects. Ideally, the source of real knowledge should be more subtle, and knowledge from it should be then transmitted to the brain, which remains the best means of its storage and usage. An action based on real knowledge would thus automatically be more mature and temperate.

Now, is this easier said than done?

The subtlest knowledge really occurs in "direct perception" that takes you even beyond valid knowledge. *Yoga-Sūtra* provides a clear direction and step-by-step roadmap for achieving this ability. Through the Yoga practices, you first secure a firsthand and direct knowledge of the inner selves and learn to communicate with them. This in turn allows access to the deeper and subtle aspects of all objects. Thereafter, the Self itself guides and ensures that there is no faulty perception leading to any incorrect knowledge.

DELUSION

Delusion or fancy is akin to a dream state with eyes wide open (Sūtra 1.9/I.9). On the physical plane, one sees objects. In delusion one sees images of the objects. Perception takes place in the present, but image-processing is not about the present; it is either brooding over the past or hankering after the future.

But delusion or fancy make us understand the very process of perception. Ordinarily, when you look at an object through the lens of your eyes and perceive it, what is *seen and processed* is only an image. The image is constructed by the mind, with energy arriving from the willed attention, and the image stays in the mind only as long as the attention is not diverted to something else. Delusion is different from perception only because its energy springs from desire and not from attention.

The mind constructs the fancied images out of three things:

1. The images of the physical world that are stored in the human memory from birth
2. Self-created images that borrow bits and pieces from the former but are reconstructed with a self-serving logic disconnected from the physical world
3. Superimposed images from collective thought forms of family, peer groups, community, race, religion, or any other shared system of belief, simply mass-copied by individuals and commonly accepted as truth.

As long as the mind is the means of processing and holding images, perception of the physical world is inseparable from the process of delusion; it feeds the self-view and the world-view, a relative untruth cherished as the "only" truth.

PASSIVITY

The simplest form of passivity known to us is sleep. (Sūtra 1.10/I.10). Passivity is a mind modification because the mind appears to have withdrawn from outward sensing but remains responsive to internal memory triggers and image-processing. But the sūtra uses the word *"vṛtti,"* and that expands the whole context much wider. *"Vṛttis are those activities of the mind which eventuate in the conscious relationship between the object sensed and the sense employed in doing so"* (Alice Bailey, 21). So, apparently, in passivity, sensing does not stop. But the awareness is defused and turned away from the senses; thus, the senses remain active, but you are unaware of them.

At this point let us revisit the process of mind modification. Think again about the supposition that, if one of a series of drops of water is suspended and its falling is sufficiently delayed, the surface of the water in the vessel will get a window of opportunity to regain its calm and a steady state. "Passivity" means a presence of the sense impulses, but a delayed thought-formation resulting in a similar brief state of calmness in the thinking instrument.

Sleep, coma, or even concentration can produce periods of mind passivity, but the difference between each of these states is significant. Ordinary sleep is a kind of physical state. There is a recollection on awakening, because sleep is not exempt from fancy (dream state) in which one oscillates between the past and the future and connects persons and places in a strange manner. Only in a deep sleep does passivity really result, and one has the "quiescent state of the *vṛttis*" too. Coma is induced by some external agent or could be a result of a physical disorder. This kind of passivity is a result of total disablement of the thinking apparatus and creates no awareness at all. But this passivity is at the mercy of an external agent or a cause, and can never be under conscious control. Early efforts of concentration can also result in involuntary passivity of mind.

However, it is important to understand why passivity has been described as a mind modification and why it also needs to be restrained. The goal of Yoga is the right activity of the *conscious* mind and its correct use. Passivity results in an absent or a "blank" mind, and that is not a part of the intended process. The mind can bounce back from passivity into any other state with the right trigger.

MEMORY

Memory is as essential for normal living as is the mind (Sūtra 1.11/I.11). However, at an advanced stage, Yoga prescribes suspending our reliance on mind and memory. As seekers, you may not just be uncomfortable with such an idea, but may find it utterly fantastic. How can you not rely on your mind and memory? In the modern world, it is unimaginable to do away with these vital tools that have brought about such a phenomenal material progress. However, in our quest for truth we have to look deeper.

Yoga reminds us that memory as an accomplice of the thinking mind is only a tool, and that fact is not an easy one to grasp. Memory and thinking as aspects of mind are certainly essential for living, and the two together should be the keeper and a user of knowledge. Limitations occur, however, when the mind becomes instrumental in *sourcing* knowledge through individualized thinking. For example, someone with whom we have "nice" memories is thought to be "good." Tomorrow, if we learn about any allegations against that person, our immediate reaction is denial, without even wanting to know the facts. Thus, instead of collecting "correct knowledge" and using it, the mind "fabricates" knowledge of its own from the threads in the memory.

Likewise, memory has to play an important role in supporting the use of knowledge. But we use memory not so much for holding knowledge, but for compulsive hoarding of personalized images that are energized by emotions; and that is more of an impediment to a real experience. For example, our favorite movie that stirs our emotions, makes us completely incapable of realizing that what is seen are only images on the screen, or that the movie was actually made of millions of distinct pieces artistically sewn together. Yoga is pointing to that unnecessary emotional hoarding. *Yoga-Sūtra* defines memory as a mind modification, as a process of "holding on to that which has been."

Before we move forward, let us understand what all gets consigned to memory. When we perceive, the visual image gets bundled with a voice-over and millions of other details. Alongside the basic image of an object, mainly its form, the associated process of knowing is also stored—such as the driving desire, or a sense of gratification, how it was sensed, and so on.

Also stored is the resultant pain, pleasure, or delusion, as well as the associated thinking that was driven by the intellectual processes of classifying, connecting, judging, and observing the resultant gestalt vision. Memory consists of a package of all these add-ons and becomes a collage of impressions; not just a direct experience of an object. These add-ons need to be dropped and not held on to.

Memory is also described as "residual potency," a term that describes the power of memory. Impressions are not just stored in memory. They sit there like live landmines waiting for the sense impulses to activate them. Don't we experience sudden arousal of childhood memories that we thought had vanished forever? Or how often some innocuous happening triggers memory of a long-forgotten song? In the case of human beings, besides the brain memory, there is organic memory percolating down to each cell. Each cell that dies is replaced by a cell having the same memory. Such an organic memory, drawn from successive experiences moment-by-moment, even birth after birth, cannot be destroyed easily. Change at the cell-level, if any, takes place so imperceptibly that it takes many reincarnations before manifesting.

Memory is also a residue from each mind modification, and creates a multiplier effect. The stored images have energy and they create internal triggers for a "mind chatter" even when the outward triggers are quiet. This creates vicious spirals of brooding to give extra spin to the other mind states and creates more mind modifications. This is why it is best to release "memory" to remain in the present and not be weighed down by "excess baggage" of the past.

How to Calm the Mind Modifications?

The calming (for eventual control) of these mind modifications is to be brought about through tireless endeavor and through non-attachment (Sūtra 1.12/I.12).

For calming the mind, any direct effort either to stop the thought formation or to suppress mind modifications would not succeed. In fact, it may be harmful to try to do so. Mind can be compared to the blades of a windmill and the incoming sense impulses to the wind. Sage Pātañjali is not talking about *stoppage* of mind modifications but a cessation, an effortless control—a control that eventually becomes an automatic reflex.

How do you do that? It all begins with the sense impulses. We have five sense organs (ears, skin, eyes, tongue, and nose) that allow the five senses (sound, touch, sight, taste, and smell) to flow, just like a wire allows electricity to flow. An individual mind is often referred to as the sixth organ that allows the sixth sense to flow. This sixth sense is a catalytic element that throws light so that the brain can understand what is carried to it by the five senses. Unlike the brain, which exists on a physical plane, the mind exists on a more subtle plane. This is highlighted by a slightly different interpretation of mind when Sage Pātañjali calls it an "internal" organ. It is obviously not just internal to the body/brain but rather integral to it, in the sense that it enables the brain, a physical organ, to perceive.

Fundamental to this is the Yoga hypothesis that "subtle creates gross," or more specifically here, "the dense physical organs are not the principal organs, but are merely tangible sprouts of the subtle organs." Like all objects in the universe, even an organ has been first a functional concept or an idea from which a subtle organ emerges and eventually a physical organ. Thus, mind comes first, and *buddhi, mānas* and the brain with its processes of perception follow in succession to fulfill mind's need to perceive. Again, refer to the earlier parallel between the water surface and the falling drop. Water, the mind, is *contained* in the thought-registration area of the brain. We need to conceptualize this "containing" really as "interpenetrating."

Making the mind modifications subside, leading to their eventual control, has to be a *tireless endeavor*. Any lapse in it will result in the drops falling one after another and disturbing the calmness of the mind. If thoughts cause mind modifications and thoughts are continuously formed without any possible direct restraint, then the calming effort also has to be tireless and never-ending.

When you make a passionate and tireless endeavor, you can liberate yourself from the tyranny of perception-induced *guṇa.* Only thus, you will wake up from *guṇa's* captivity and be free to explore your innate spirituality. However, before validating Yoga through a marathon practice regime, the "inner spiritual Self" is to be initially understood intellectually as a concept. But identification with the spiritual Self is not an easy process; neither is it solely intellectual. To go beyond the physical, one has to first recognize and identify oneself with the astral and the causal selves within. While this happens, the spiritual Self becomes your cherished dream and *an object sufficiently valued.* There would eventually be a stage when one has no longing for any worldly object. When such non-attachment is continuously and perfectly practiced, having repeatedly done it over and over again, it results in an *exact* knowledge or experience of the innate spirituality, a breakthrough moment for the seeker.

Incidentally, this knowledge would be "exact" as opposed to "correct." Correct knowledge is derived; always an outcome of form-based and subjective thinking, regardless of how correct logically it may be. In contrast, exact knowledge just shines forth from a non-indulgent, now empowered mind; it is like experiencing something as it truly is in its essence.

Thus, Sage Pātañjali is prescribing a four-fold solution for calming the mind modifications:

- First and foremost he insists on *yatnobhyāsaḥ*, **making tireless endeavor**, since mind modifications are occurring continuously.
- To ensure continuity in the face of repeated failures, the goal of Yoga is to be *satkārāsevito*, **valued sufficiently** and methods and practices to be *nairantarya*, **followed persistently** with passion.

- It is essential to **practice** *vairāgyam*, **non-attachment,** as only freedom from longing can bring about real freedom from objects.
- And finally, one has to *guṇavaitṛṣṇyam,* **liberate from *guṇa,*** because only that will ensure form-free perception that does not feed into the thinking process thus eliminating mind modifications.[5]

MAKE TIRELESS ENDEAVOR

Given the flitting nature of mind, awareness can be steadily anchored in the subtle bodies only when the intended change of any kind is in the core. What makes such inner evolution a long and difficult process is its dependence on a structural change at the cellular level. Such a change is internal and requires *turning of awareness inward* as the first step. Being internal, the change can be brought about only by the individual herself/himself. This can be done only by practicing, and no amount of philosophizing would help. Change does not come without stiff resistance from your own self, and that results in repeated failures, which can lead to a sense of guilt and frustration.

Hence, fiery passion and tireless endeavor is thus required at each stage of the evolution. **Tireless endeavor is the constant effort of the will to restrain the modifications of the thinking instrument** (Sūtra 1.13/I.13); so that, when the material self willingly accepts the spiritual identity, the latter can become the teacher. You move on to reap the fruits of evolution in the form of abilities to concentrate, meditate, and contemplate. The rewards are powerful, and one is easily tempted to use the powers in the objective world for material gain. It is the internal teacher that helps and

---

[5] *There is apparently a simple way out. Thoughts and the resultant mind modifications have an uncanny relationship with breathing. The rate and the depth of a mind modification seem to bring about a distinct change in the rhythm and depth of the breath. Breathing is the only body activity that can be left autonomous or done consciously, as one desires. The direct one-to-one relationship between mind modifications and breathing can be used to reverse the process of creating mind modifications. By applying the will to make the breath even and rhythmic, the mind modifications can be arrested. Using this method is also the only way to make a true tireless effort possible, because breathing is a continuous, ceaseless activity! (But more about that later).*

guides how not to get trapped in these powers and not to stall the evolutionary momentum.

As we will see later, sense impulses, the raw material for the thinking process, travel via the short-term and long-term memory pools at the hind brain, en route to the brain's frontal lobe. Sitting in the long-term memory is a structure of predispositions that compels the impulses to selectively pick up stored impressions closely resembling them. Hence, thought that forms ("the drop of water that falls") and agitates the calm mind in the thinking instrument comprises:

- Incoming sense impulses, and
- The near-identical patterns stored in memory as impressions.

The stored impressions have intellectual-emotional-sexual and movement triggers[6], and when the impulses and the memory patterns enter the registration area, a thought gets registered in the thinking instrument and creates a modification in the process.

Once a tuning fork is struck, the vibrations are fast and furious for some time, and then slowly die down. If hard metal takes so long to return to stillness, can you imagine how much faster the sensitive and subtle mind would agitate and how much longer it would take for that agitation to subside? And given our naturally outbound awareness, the sense organs are constantly active, and sense impulses continuously barge in to make it almost impossible to restore the calm. Therefore, we are in a state of perpetual and compulsive mind modifications.

Yoga-Sūtra leads us later to a technique that enables non-registration of the sense impulses so that the mind remains free from modifications. Such a period of calm is initially for a moment

---

[6] *Intellectual-emotional-sexual triggers arise respectively from* buddhi *(causal),* mānas *(astral) and the brain (physical), while the movement trigger is a combined effect of the three in altering or creating new impressions in the memory. My guru used to give it a ratio based on their relative dominance over the thinking process. A seeker would initially have a ratio of 2:4:8:2 where the physicality is dominant and eventually a yogi would have that transformed into 5:2:2:1 where the spirituality is dominant. A* mahayogī *learns to bypass thinking in direct perception so the ratio becomes redundant. See diagrams at the end of the book.*

only, and, over a period of time, would progress into the states of *dhāraṇā*, *dhyāna*, and *samādhī*. But you have to keep in mind that in Yoga such calm is maintained consciously and is not a passive state of trance or a daze.

Non-attachment of mind is also to be understood in this sense—as soon as any thought registers, one experiences an attachment (or an aversion, which is simply the other side of the coin) to the impressions. To enable a real perception of things, one must be free from both:

- Registration of thought, and
- Attachment to the impressions.

A truly tireless endeavor is needed to achieve this. The later sūtras explain why and how proper breathing takes center stage in this endeavor. Breathing is the only constant and automatic body function that we can bring under conscious control at will.

"The right use of the will is the steady effort to stand in one's spiritual being" (Charles Johnston as quoted by Alice Bailey, 27). The will has energy that is slowly directed, first to make the awareness turn inward, and then to create and to prolong the gap between thought formation. This way, your spiritual Self makes a constant effort to restrain the mind modifications and to still live a normal life on the physical plane.

VALUE SUFFICIENTLY AND FOLLOW PERSISTENTLY

When the object to be gained is sufficiently valued, efforts toward its attainment are persistently followed without intermission. Only in this way is the steadiness of the thinking instrument (restraint of the *vṛttis*) secured. (Sūtra 1.14/I.14)

No human endeavor is ever possible without passion. That the goal or object is *sufficiently valued* is a highly critical prerequisite for such efforts with which the *steadiness of the thinking instrument* is obtained, whatever the object may be. The student has to be devoted to the path first, purely from passion; and the steadiness of the thinking instrument has to be as desperately and completely sought as a dying person seeking life.

Two moments are extremely important on the *yogīk* path:

- when you turn the awareness inward
- when you experience a gap between two thoughts.

When your awareness turns inward it is a launching point and a critical junction in your journey. But what is "turning inward?" When you close your eyes, the thoughts still keep projecting outward. It takes time even with the closed eyes to trust our familiar immediate surroundings and to keep the inward attention rooted "safely." But, while the thoughts remain inside, what images do you see? Can you see your own self as a skeleton of bones and flesh with functioning organs? Perhaps not. We are so enamored even with our own appearance witnessed in a mirror and in the eyes of others that our own "not-so-sweet" anatomical images are hard to emerge. Can you see your body as the nonstop food-churning and waste-disposal plant that it really is? The answer is probably another "no."

However, with practice, as you would slowly get accustomed to visualizing the solids, the liquids and the gasses that make up the inside of your body, you would get ready to understand it further. The first sign of any progress comes when you become aware of your "act of visualizing," and in the separation of awareness from that act of visualizing, you would experience a new misty lightness to yourself.

The second important moment, a real turning point, comes when you experience a gap between two successive thoughts. That gap yields a thrilling direct perception unaided by mind. That is an unforgettable moment of joy, a moment signifying that your inner self is activated.

This moment brings you face to face, for the first time, with that which you want to gain, and then it is not difficult to sufficiently value it. Labeling that experience becomes pointless. We only want this priceless experience to repeat; we want to hold on to it forever. That desire leads us to unending efforts.

It is true that passion and desire eventually become a drag on rarefied states. But, in the initial stages you need them to push yourself out of the physical body inertia.

PRACTICE NON-ATTACHMENT

Non-attachment is perhaps the least understood concept of Yoga.

But first, what is "attachment?" It is an intrinsic quality of the mind to be attached to an object via its image. But the mind's attachment results from an invisible connection. In perceiving an object, the mind sends out its subtle sensors and practically connects itself to the object in order to induce perception. But, while the mind, the sixth sense, enables perception, it does not just stand aside and throw light so that the brain can "see." Instead, during the same process, mind indulges itself by elaborating on and coloring the sense data obtained by the five senses. If the mind did not stay attached to the perception of the object, the sense data would flow into the mind and then out, as it is, and no mind modifications would occur. **Non-attachment is the freedom from craving for all objects of desire, either experienced or known** (Sūtra 1.15/I.15).

A superficial definition of non-attachment implies physically staying away from objects. For some people, a path of renunciation facilitates this. But perception is not possible unless the senses engage with the objects. So apparently, sensory contact is not the main culprit. The control of mind modifications has to occur *during* the process of perception. A mind has to remain a catalyst and remain non-attached to the sense data arriving from the objects. That is the fundamental non-attachment in Yoga.

Keep in mind that you are not going to get there—to non-attachment—tomorrow, and there is no need to rush either. Not indulging itself in such a fashion is possible only to a purified mind, and only *after* the thinking instruments have changed their roles by becoming effective users of spiritual knowledge. Consequentially, a prerequisite to non-attachment is cleansing and purification of the mind, and that warrants tireless and ceaseless practice over a fairly long period of time.

Sage Pātañjali elaborates on the state of non-attachment. It is not limited only to *freedom from objects*, because if there is no *freedom from longing*, mere seclusion and renunciation are futile.

And conversely, a freedom from longing for the objects of desire renders it immaterial, whether you are a *sanyāsī* (a recluse) or live a secular life.[7] **Hence, to calm the mind modifications, non-attachment of mind is the key.**

Thus, the secret of real freedom is to detach the mind at will in order not to meddle with the brain. If only the objects of matter were to blame, total seclusion from all objects could bring about the desired non-attachment of mind. But one needs to work on the mind and not on the objects. Hence, Yoga-Sūtra provides a path that appears to support a normal householder's life, with its attendant duties and obligations, and yet helps achieve non-attachment. Reconnecting with one's spiritual self, with its innate happiness, requires a willed disconnection from the outside world.

Renunciation is a state of mind and can be achieved even in the householder's role. Let our mind and the conscious brain understand that going after external objects in the course of our obligations and duties is neither wrong nor harmful, as long as we are careful about the means and the methods we use. The *yogīk* path in *Yoga-Sūtra* is a two-lane highway, not a road with two mutually exclusive pathways of either renunciation or living in the world.

Why is it important to live life and yet be non-attached? *Karma* requires that each cause seeded by our past actions must come to fruition in an effect that needs to be lived out. There is no short-cut because, in living out the effects, we discover the symbiotic relationship between the effect (gross) and its cause (subtle), and that prevents the effect from becoming a new cause. When we learn this truth, without rushing a reflex reaction, the cause stands redeemed and its repeated occurrence is not needed anymore. *Karma* is not fatalistic. We can choose to keep mind non-attached

---

[7] *Some scholars draw an interesting parallel. Gravitation and electromagnetic force in the Universe, the macrocosm, are mimicked as love and hate in a human being. Both emanate from attachment, but one attracts while the other repels. The state of non-attachment (*vairāgya*) is the take-off force (or the escape velocity) required to counter the gravitational force and inertia. Realization and actualization of this force is a moment of grace. It is a turning point in one's inner evolution, as mentioned earlier.*

and thus create no new *karma*. We can redeem past *karma*, stop creating new *karma*, and thus liberate ourselves.[8]

But, even after keeping mind away from the thinking process, the *guṇa*-charged impulses continue to feed in and generate thoughts. So, for a complete stoppage of the mind modifications, you will have to work on *guṇa*.

LIBERATE FROM GUṆA

When you perceive an object, philosophically speaking, the object is *born* at that moment in your individual, subjective world. "Born" should not be construed as "created," because even if the object is perceived by someone else, it does not exist for you unless you perceive it yourself. What we perceive is what we describe the object as, in terms of *guṇa;* its qualities, features, or attributes.

Let us review here. *Sattva guṇa* represents the revealing aspect, *rajas* represents mobility or action, and *tamas* represents inertia. The *guṇa* results from the energy entrapped in the object independent of what form it takes during perception. When we perceive an object, the connection results in *guṇa* resonating in our senses to create a form. In non-attachment, you would liberate from all *guṇa*, perceive no form, trigger no thought and thus avoid a mind modification. It is important to remember that in the end one needs to liberate from all *guṇa*, including *sattva*, which also brings about a mind modification.

The crucial point is that *guṇa* do not enter our senses uninvited. Rather, our desire-driven perception invites them. So, you can liberate from the captivity of *guṇa* in other objects only by that same liberation first happening within you. Liberating from your own *guṇa* is as challenging as getting rid of your own shadow; but there is no other way to be truly free. This ability would bring you closer to your own spiritual Self.

---

[8] *An experiential knowledge of Yoga is a prerequisite to properly understanding it, just as a description of the world viewed from the top of Mt. Everest, howsoever vivid, will remain fanciful and untrue for one who stays put at sea level. It may not be even known how much is not known. Another underlying fact is that every aspect of Yoga is for practice and self-verification, and Yoga cannot be fathomed simply as an intellectual exercise of a bystander.*

In the end, un-attached, free from the *guṇa*, released from form-creation, you would enter a new state of awareness of extreme subtlety that would be consciousness itself. **When non-attachment becomes a way of life, one is liberated from the qualities of *guṇa* and possesses knowledge of the spiritual being that one is** (Sūtra 1.16/I.16). To reach this point from the stage of seeking is the complete Yoga road map. Until it happens you can only speculate about that state of consciousness.

Yogīk Path: The External Obstacles

Having charted the *yogīk* path, it is essential now to see what obstacles will confront us. This path is unique in the sense that it progressively transforms the seeker into a disciple, a *yogī*, a *mahāyogī*, and finally a master, each almost a reincarnation. The milestones on the path morph the very definitions at the core of your world-view and self-view. The next milestone is always hidden behind a curve on the path. But even when we get a glimpse of what to expect, the path is not often easy. Ironically, **the same mind that takes us to new states of spiritual awareness also creates obstacles; nine of them** (Sūtra 1.17/I.30).

The Obstacles

A state of spiritual awareness is the first major milestone. But to move from the first momentary occurrence of that awareness to the state of being able to hold onto it requires a long journey, and *Yoga-Sūtra* is repeatedly exhorting you to be a good student willing to make tireless efforts. This exhortation is needed because no milestone guarantees that you would not slip back or would not feel complacent and then stagnate.

Let us now take a look at the obstacles created by the mind.[9] The obstacles are given in the order of their relative power over a

[9] The following description is substantially based on a commentary by Alice Bailey, pages 62-71.

seeker. Typically, harmful or inappropriate thoughts produce most of these obstacles.

BODILY DISABILITY

Rising to a new level of awareness is not done by rejecting or ignoring physical awareness. In fact, even with an elevated level of awareness, the world would still be experienced only via the physical body. It is for this reason that the first obstacle is physical. You have to tune up the physical vehicle in order to withstand the demands later to be made upon it. This tuning up requires three actions:

- Eradicating present diseases
- Refining and purifying it with a view to rebuild it eventually
- Protecting it from any future attack.

In Yoga, a disease at the physical level is regarded as a pronounced symptom of a disequilibrium in the rhythm and balance in the energy flows. It is first experienced in the *chakras* and the brain, and then passed on to the body. When the body is purified, the natural immune system runs a self-diagnostic check and warns of any impending "dis-ease."

The forces and the fires a student eventually passes his body through on the *yogīk* path presuppose that the body is as ready as the rest of the being. *Yama*, the five abstentions, *niyama*, the five rules, and *āsana*, the posture, all of which are discussed later, are therefore the first three means of Yoga that help overcome the obstacle of bodily disability (Solution is in Sūtra 1.20/I.33).

MENTAL INERTIA

Some individuals are resigned to the status quo. They take happy and sad moments nonchalantly. It looks deceptively like equipoise, but is in fact indulgence because it does not emerge from any understanding of the world around them. It emerges instead from a resignation to the fact that what exists at any given point in time is the inevitable state of things. Riding on the waves and being joyful or sad in turn, they live in their emotions and refuse to think of anything beyond them. The inability to think clearly about the need for spiritual attainment generates insufficient momentum in their efforts. It is further coupled with a failure to appreciate the real magnitude of the reasons for which one is seeking a spiritual solution. At its extreme, this inertia can lead to a disinclination to apply your mind, or to lethargy of the mind (Solution is in Sūtra 2.1/I.34).

DOUBT

Right and proper questioning is essential for a seeker to move ahead. However, wrong questioning would cause stagnation and make you go round and round. Constant doubting is often based on a weak perception, the trivialities of the senses, and identification of the self with the physical body. A weakness of wrong questioning may continue even when the identification with the astral or causal bodies is achieved. When the questioner's ego protrudes through the question or masquerades as pious curiosity, it is generally a wrong question.

Right questioning is often an earnest enquiry. To be able to ask intelligently and properly, you must first free yourself from all the traditions, dogmas (religious or scientific), and any imposed authorities. The role of a teacher is to induce proper questions in your mind and then to leave you to find your own answers (Solution is in Sūtra 2.2/I.35).

PROCRASTINATION/CARELESSNESS

Procrastination/carelessness is a light-mindedness that breeds upon the mind's intrinsic versatility and makes it difficult to sharp-focus and to sustain attention. Consumed by the thinking instrument's natural tendency to flit from one object to another, the mind does not pay sufficient heed to the aids of contemplation. Such mind-wandering may run the risk of information overload as the student is drawn to anything and everything. Many times the sheer weight of information creates a false sense of intellectual achievements that lead nowhere, complacency creeps in and that actually stalls the progress on the *yogīk* path.

Empty punditry takes you nowhere on the *yogīk* path. Firsthand knowledge is more important than a lot of knowledge *about* things. However, even more important is the transforming nature of such knowledge that a mere hoarder of knowledge cannot experience (Solution is in Sūtra 5.1.4/I.36).

LAZINESS OR LETHARGY

Laziness or lethargy perpetuates a gap between a seeker's aspiration and performance. A strong will is needed. But in the initial phases on the *yogīk* path, unrefined will is neutral. Ironically, in such a situation, sharp perception may help intellectually recognize what to do. But you just don't measure up to your own aspirations. You glimpse the ideal, are aware of the obstacles, know exactly what steps you have to take, but there is no connection between the knowledge and the action. Drowned in a lack of vitality, you allow time to slip by and do nothing.

Two things are usually missing in such an individual: awareness of a limited life span and appreciation of the worth of a human life as a vehicle to spiritual consciousness (Solution is in Sūtra 2.3/I.37).

CRAVING/LACK OF DISPASSION

Addiction to objects results from desires for material and sensuous gratification. Strong cravings from sense perceptions and an attraction for all objects puts such a seeker on a never-ending roller-coaster of repeated occurrence of temptations on the physical plane. This leads to entanglement in the forms and the associated attachment. Strong cravings are habit-forming, and the seeker needs a strategy to disengage from their grip. A dispassion for objects needs to be carefully cultivated (Solution is in Sūtra 4.9/I.38).

ERRONEOUS PERCEPTION

The inability to perceive correctly and to envision things as they really are is the natural outcome of the previous six obstacles. As long as you identify with the form, as long as the objects and persons enticing the mind can hold you in thrall, and as long as you refuse to disassociate from the material aspects of objects and people, your perception remains erroneous.

Erroneous perception is also volatile. There is a constant movement in the self-view and the world-view as appearances of objects change, and instead of realizing the basic error in perception, you may get enticed by the dynamics of the appearance itself. For some individuals, new interpretations are intellectually stimulating, new teachers and new styles always look more promising, and newer appearances are taken as the new reality, simply because of their newness (Solution is in Sūtra 4.10/I.39).

INABILITY TO ACHIEVE CONCENTRATION

Old mind habits are hard to break. The thinking patterns calcify and that makes concentration difficult to achieve because impulses generate predictable reflex thoughts that fly in all directions. The mind needs to focus on what lies ahead and to meditate on what has been known so far. In Yoga, the mind needs to understand the mind. Hence, observing the drift of one's thoughts is an essential effort. But as long as the habitual predispositions afflict thinking, there is no room for concentration to bring you to the doorstep of your spiritual Self for guidance on the path. (Solution is in Sūtra 4.19/III.2)

FAILURE TO HOLD THE MEDITATIVE ATTITUDE

Even when concentration is achieved after much effort, the aspirant is lured away again and again, which results in lack of meditation. The truth is, as long as you cannot hold on to a meditative state, the meditative attitude cannot take root. It is apparent that obstacles occur not just in the beginning but all along the path as well.

This last obstacle is the most difficult one to overcome. In the Bhagavad Gita III (36), Arjuna asks, "My lord, tell me what is it that drives a man to sin, even against his will and as if by compulsion?" The answer that arrives is, "O Arjuna, the mind of him who is trying to conquer it is forcibly carried away, in spite of his efforts, by his tumultuous senses." (In other words, wrong methods and forcible use of the will fail; the animal cells triumph). In living with a false vision and concentrating on the objects of matter, which at the time are "valued sufficiently," all sorts of means are used to achieve the ends, and in doing so, countless types of emotions and motives are allowed to run riot. The result is pain, despair, and faulty breathing.[10] (Solution is in Sūtra 4.20/III.3)

Results of the Obstacles

The obstacles affect the lower psychic nature of the astral body/*mānas* system, making it difficult to take care of emotions and *prāṇa* circulation unless these obstacles are first taken care of. No philosophies, morals, or religions are otherwise of any avail.

Obstacles are varied but their cumulative effect—**pain, despair, misplaced bodily activity, and unrhythmic breathing**—always makes the *yogīk* path more challenging (Sūtra 1.18/I.31).

PAIN

The obstacles keep an aspirant heavily immersed in the physical environment. This results in a wrong polarization of emotions that gets *mānas* constantly dragged by pairs of opposites. It indicates a lack of equilibrium. Senses bring in discordant and conflicting signals that mind reads as pain.

DESPAIR

As an aspirant, you have a perception of where to go on the *yogīk* path, but the obstacles are still an overwhelming deterrent. This makes you constantly conscious of failure, and this awareness engenders a condition of remorse, disgust, despair, and despondency.

---

[10] *Emotional swings affect a seeker's the lower psychic nature and create many* granthī *(knots in the flow of energy) in the body/brain system. Unless these* granthī *are dissolved and the lower psychic nature is refined, no progress is possible. A natural rhythmic breathing, which one is born with, is disturbed. In the rhythmic breathing, we are simply reverting to and reestablishing this original correct breathing. At this stage, a large-scale mutation of animal cells is taking place. These cells have yet to be cultured, tamed, and civilized.*

MISPLACED BODILY ACTIVITY

The inner condition works out on the physical plane as an intense activity, a violent seeking for solutions or solace and a constant running hither and thither in search of peace. Formal education and other intellectual activities today are designed to stimulate the mental faculties. Yet people's awareness and conscious control remain on the physical plane. This circumstance results in a physical overdrive and an aggressive intensity of endeavor in all areas of life. To be silent, to be still, and to be at peace with oneself is not a part of any educational curriculum. All parameters of achievement are defined solely in material terms, and there is an ingrained sense of winning or losing in every action.

WRONG DIRECTIONS OF LIFE CURRENT

This inner turmoil resulting from misplaced bodily activity in turn affects both of the following:

- The life breath or *prāṇa* (energy of the psychic body)
- The life force or the fires of the body (energy of the physical body).

Prāṇa ordinarily directs a proper functioning of the glands, the immune system, and the sympathetic nervous system. Any misuse or wrong utilization of *prāṇa* is a likely cause of most of our present physical ailments.[11]

How to Overcome the Obstacles

Yoga is all about practice. Knowledge takes you only so far as long as it is not insightful or intuitive knowing. Our structure of predisposition keeps us confined to reflexive thinking that finds

---

[11] Prāṇa *is pivotal to bodily health and that makes* prānāyāma *so important. Though the* prāṇa *breath cannot be directly regulated, you can learn to synchronize normal breath with* prāṇa *breath in a rhythmic manner and thus put normal breath in rhythm and balance. Doing this will help in making the astral/mānas system primary and the physical body/brain system secondary, which marks the beginning of the inner evolution. Eventually,* prāṇa *in rhythm and balance will reverse the ill effects of the inner turmoil.*

ways of skirting around the obstacles rather than dealing with them. Hence, to overcome the obstacles you must persevere.

1. **Do Yoga *abhyāsa* (discipline): To overcome the obstacles, an intense application of the will to the truth and the principle is required** (Sūtra 1.19/ I.32)**.** Yoga is a path of self-realization.

   Naturally what is prescribed here concerns your "self." The three main threads of Yoga *abhyāsa* are:

   - Self-study (self-examination)
   - Self-restraint
   - Self-surrender to *Īśvara.*

   This discipline is the first tool that extends Yoga's role and value in your life. "Yoga is life" sounds good to hear, but Yoga *abhyāsa* makes it happen. Since the obstacles are present as long as you are awake, an effort to overcome them has to be equally unceasing. There is no need for you to sit in meditation and close your eyes all the time, if that is your idea of Yoga. Using your thinking process as a scalpel to dissect, analyze, understand and control your thinking is Yoga too. In fact, this way you will directly face the mind that you intend to keep unattached to thinking, and target it for eventual transformation into Universal Mind. In this effort, proper breathing will help and *Īśvara* will guide.

   Self-study enables you to watch the mind-drifts and to avoid the most repetitive drifts through corrective exercises. Self-restraint occurs in the form of rhythmic breathing with which the wrong flow of life current is arrested. The misplaced bodily activity that draws us towards external objects is now herded towards *Īśvara* through self-surrender.

   In our vocabulary, "surrender" is "giving oneself up"; prostrating before the mighty. It is important to understand the concept of *Īśvara* as not being a human-made "god;" it is equally important to understand what is loving self-surrender. This surrender is more of immersion, of setting aside the ego, an attitude of recognizing the all-permeating principle called *Īśvara.*

> *Surrender is not giving up your efforts; surrender is not becoming a slave to it . . . To me an elegant, magnificent, majestic humility is the content of surrender—praṇidhāna. Ego does not know humility. Ego is assertive, aggressive, acquisitive, competitive.*
>
> —Vimala Thakar, 37-3.

To set aside the ego, however, we should be able to know it when it manifests, since it is really difficult to separate ego from self-awareness. Self-identity and self-preservation are sometimes such daunting survival mechanisms that self-assertion gets ingrained into our reflex behavior. Ego is usually operating in unwarranted self-assertion, and thus requires careful watching. A hardened ego is never ready for the dissolution of self-awareness into any kind of surrender, loving or otherwise.

2. **Apply will intensely:** Please look at sūtra 1.13/I.13: **Tireless endeavor is an intense effort of [the] will to restrain the modifications of the thinking instrument.**(One has to be careful here. Some translations suggest application of the will to "some" truth. Such generality and vagueness is inconsistent with Yoga-Sūtra. Some others interpret that one truth as the "one and only one" implying the ultimate truth; that becomes a repetition of other sūtras, which also is uncharacteristic of Yoga-Sūtra. It cannot even be referring merely to concentration, which will be discussed later as a Primary Means of Yoga*)*.

   It is important to reiterate the sūtra here, as the intended emphasis appears to be more on the *intense* application of the will and the objective of overcoming the specific obstacles. Later, specific cures for specific obstacles will be discussed. But Sage Pātañjali subtly points out here that a mere theoretical understanding of the obstacles and their cure is of no consequence unless constant, steady, and enduring effort of the will is present as a practice.

   Again, it is not just *any* truth that is learned here, but rather a *principle* about the truth. We know that the nature of the perceived truth; even at its best, is relative. When the obstacles wither away, the truth unfolds gradually. Once the intense application of the will is directed to one truth on the given plane, the realization of that truth itself leads an aspirant to seek the next level of truth on a higher plane.

Then a day arrives when the soul is seen as the ultimate truth, and it is realized that the soul that keeps projecting itself through the relative truths on the various lower planes. That is the principle. Understanding relativity and duality on the lower planes as a means to realizing non-duality is the purpose. And that duality is only a deceptive perception of non-duality is the revelation.

Truth is realized only in stages, but it always exists as a single phenomenon. Lower level truth is not independent of the higher-level subtle truth. Like yogurt, buttermilk and butter are all potentially present in a pot of milk; it is one's ability to perceive that makes milk a reality for some and butter for a few. A seeker becomes aware of this underlying principle about truth itself and that is the purpose of this sūtra. Pursuit of truth is to be consciously undertaken and achieved through an intense application of the will.

There is another way of looking at this sūtra. Though there is only one ultimate truth, there are several paths leading to its realization. Sage Pātañjali is exhorting the seeker to choose any one path, but to apply the will intensely, without intermission. Instead of studying or practicing a little of this and a little of that and thus "digging many shallow wells," as Sage Rāmakṛṣna Paramhansajī says, "it is necessary to dig one well deep enough to find water."

3. **A four-way practice: The peace of mind (and the thinking instruments) can be brought about through the practice of sympathy, tenderness, steadiness of purpose, and indifference with regard to happiness, misery, virtue, and vice** respectively (Sūtra 1.20/I.33). This is the first and the foremost of the solutions aimed at overcoming bodily disability. Disabilities that one is born with, or that one incurs as a result of

genetic disorders or accidents, are to be seen as a legacy of past *karma*. They need to be lived out. But many other disabilities caused by diseases are here at our own invitation, resulting from bad choices in this life. Before such diseases manifest on the physical level, they first appear potentially on the causal and astral levels and are followed by an imbalance in the person's health as a whole. Bad choices are often compulsions of the thinking instruments that resist behavioral change.

Since the mind and the thinking instruments primarily engage in perceiving the world to be able to relate with it, the recommended change is in the perception of and behavior toward physical objects. The change is fourfold: sympathy, tenderness, steadfast joy, and dispassion.

- **Sympathy** concerns all living beings engaged in the joy of living. You have to be helpful to them with a sincere understanding of the principle "live and let live." We need to avoid double standards. For example, we may love pets while we may eat other animals at the same time. Genuine spiritual insight would let you see the life-force present at the core of all beings.
- **Tenderness** is your relationship with the animal kingdom and toward people who suffer. In today's competitive world, you have to run fast to stay put, leaving little room for any concern for others, let alone for animals or people who suffer. Besides, many people consider tenderness of any kind as a weakness, and we need to get over that to really connect to other beings.
- **Steadfast joy** is in lauding the virtuous. Today, the news-greedy media has planted a belief in the collective psyche that anything virtuous is listless, nothing to write home about. You have to rise above that influence and place things in relation to the purpose of life. When the virtues shine, higher and enlarged vision inevitability follows.
- **Dispassion** is an unattached distance from the vicious. A major part of human response appears driven by hatred for vice instead of by dispassion. But hate is still an

engagement of the lower personal self. Hate leads to anger, and anger ignites a host of physical appetites. With a view to bringing discipline to all the physical appetites, the vicious needs to be consciously ignored.

With these behavioral changes, the individual mind becomes transparent; devoid of reflex reactions, the brain becomes more conducive to clear focus, and this state eventually leads to a completely calm and quiet mind. However, a sustainable change in behavior does not occur by itself. It needs to be preceded and supplemented by the refining processes that are primarily based on proper breathing techniques on the physical plane.[12]

But dealing with the obstacles is only a part of the story. There are hindrances to remove. And that is even tougher because hindrances get built into us.

Yogīk Path: *Avidyā* and Other Hindrances

While external objects cause the obstacles, the hindrances emerge from within. In addition, the obstacles shape the inner *structure of predispositions*, and are in a way unique to an individual. Hindrances are generic to humanity and relate to the very process of human perception.

In our discussion so far what we have touched upon are the ***causes*** of the hindrances—the unseen, behind-the-scene mind tendencies, such as impulse/reaction, habits, drifts, brooding, and daydreaming. The resultant hindrances are now explained.

Obstacles bear a stamp of individual weakness, but hindrances are seen as a sign of weakness in the entire human species. Many so-called spiritual celebrities are no exception—those who talk

---

[12] *The advanced student may find it interesting that the solutions prescribed by Sage Pātanjali for calming the mind modifications also correspond with the* chakras. Sutra *1.20 is the first in a series that relates to the* manipūra chakra *(the solar plexus). The other solutions appear in this text wherever the development of a specific* chakra *is needed. Please see* Sūtra *2.1, 2.2, 2.3, 4.9, 4.10, and 5-1.4.*

wisely on spiritual subjects may still be afflicted by the hindrances and fail to "walk their talk." Sage Pātañjali tells us loudly and clearly that some of the hindrances are present even in the wise who know only how to camouflage them in the public eye.

The Hindrances

The internal hindrances—*Avidyā* (ignorance), the "I"-sense (personality), desire, hate, and the sense of attachment— appear on all the three layers (Sūtra 1.21/II.3).

Ignorance (*Avidyā*) and the sense of personality originate on the physical plane; hate and attachment are products of egoism belonging to the astral plane; while desire belongs to the causal plane. They produce the seeds for difficulties in the threefold personality of a person, and they flourish to hinder and obstruct the self-realization process. To make it worse, they feed off each other. For instance, ignorance breeds desire and desire sustains ignorance. So also, actions fortify afflictions and vice versa.

The cumulative effect of these hindrances is to keep your awareness locked up in the lower physical/psychic nature. Our "I" awareness hypnotizes us, making our physical and emotional habits more stubborn. You need to free yourself from these shackles to realize your true potential and to seek the soul connection. Elevating awareness from physical to spiritual is one of the objectives of Yoga.

In fact, when awareness is lifted as a result of destruction of the seeds of hindrances, three things would happen:

- Karma *would be redeemed.*
- *Liberation would be achieved.*
- *Vision of the soul would be awakened and perfected.*

—Alice Bailey, 128.

Avidyā is the main hindrance that keeps most people locked up in the low levels of awareness. Unaware of your spiritual Self, the self-view and the world-view remain tainted with a **sense of egoistic personality**. Thinking is skewed in favor of external objects and your experience of them keeps you enthralled.

Experiencing objects is addictive. **Desires** spread like a wildfire engulfing and obscuring your perception. Some unfulfilled desires breed **hate**. When an effort is made to elevate awareness, hate and desire are arrested and ego is progressively dissolved. Eventually, you become acutely aware of a **desire for** your very **existence,** deep inside, and that becomes the last hindrance to overcome.

AVIDYĀ

Avidyā (ignorance) is in terms of low awareness that is not elevated to any subtle level. Ignorance has little to do with the level of formal education. (Besides, the way it is designed and delivered, the bulk of school education today has little to do with human awareness.) Low awareness comes from a lack of understanding of what the real nature of the universe is and how you are related to the universe. *Avidyā* comprehensively describes the condition of every human being, from the savage to the sage and everyone in between. Since our normal awareness is form-based, the root of ignorance lies in the limitations of form itself.

Yoga views each entity, from an atom to the entire universe, as composed of both the elements of life (form) and the elements of spirituality (core). Spirituality gets attracted toward the form-less, but it remains feeble and veiled against the overpowering manifestation of life, which in turn does not allow us to be aware of our own spiritual side. This is *Avidyā* or low awareness.

***Avidyā* remains in seed form in memory (whether the seeds be latent, in the process of elimination, overcome, or in full operation), as a potential cause of all the other hindrances** (Sūtra 1.22/II.4).

That's why it can remain **dormant** and become manifest during the act of perception, when it comes face to face with objects having predominantly *rajas* and *tamas* qualities hiding or distorting their true nature. At times, *Avidyā* can appear **attenuated** or weakened when an opposite thought overshadows this affliction. It can also remain temporarily **repressed** while something else is active in the body/mind at a given point in time. For instance, when you feel love, anger is repressed and not felt. Similarly, when you are attached to one object, there is no awareness of another object.

But *Avidyā* doesn't go away. In time and with stimuli, the dormant, attenuated, or repressed low awareness can be kindled and can become **active**. This results in repeated failure to overcome low awareness, which is the hallmark of the process of elimination of *Avidyā* on the *yogīk* path.

So, *Avidyā* remains present in all the afflictions and this explains why at certain times, even when you appear not affected by certain affliction, you are not necessarily free from it. At no stage, however advanced, can you afford to be off your guard. (As we will see later, only a meditative attitude and continuous rhythmic breathing can ensure that you remain truly free from any afflictions. Eternal vigilance is the price of even spiritual liberty!)

We are overwhelmed with our self-view. It holds our perceived appearance—a collage of role-models, fantasies, feedback, self-esteem, and self-projections—as true. We are aware only of the form that meets the eye, and remain engulfed in the consciousness of self and the physical environment. Desire-driven contacts with other forms reinforce this physical awareness into a *personalized* knowledge of our self. This knowledge becomes a self-serving limited reality. But we need to break away from it and that can be done only by questioning the purpose of our life, which lies latent in our personality.

Once the out-flowing awareness gradually turns inward, awareness of higher vibrations occurs and connects you with objects and persons without relating to their forms. This shift in awareness becomes a process of learning that leads you to wisdom, where eventually the spiritual Self takes over and awareness rises above the forms. This is how the inner evolution is fostered.

We have already seen that *Avidyā* is the cause of all afflictions; now let us see what *Avidyā* really is. It is obviously not valid knowledge, and it is not a complete lack of knowledge, either. *Avidyā* is any knowledge that has not been validated through a direct experience. ***Avidyā* is the condition of confusing the permanent** (the pure, the blissful, and the Self) **with that which is**

impermanent, impure, painful, and intellectually understandable (Sūtra 1.23/II.5).

Avidyā has four types:

- Taking the transient (such as even the earth, moon, and stars) to be permanent
- Seeing the impure (such as a human body that needs constant cleansing) as pure and beautiful
- Overlooking the eventual pain (such as after-effects or contradictions) in taking material things as blissful because of the momentary pleasure they provide; and
- Mistaking the physical (such as external adjuncts, both animate and inanimate) to be the real self.

On a philosophical level, *"... [The] spiritual self is born blind and senseless*" (Alice Bailey, 132), which can be taken to mean that the spiritual Self is "free from sense perception" at birth. However, while experiencing the world, the spiritual Self becomes aware only through the senses, using the physical body as its vehicle to manifest, and in turn creating a pseudo-perceiver "I" that gets attached to a form in the process. Sensory perception is mistaken for reality, and the fact that sensory perception was meant to be only a vehicle of manifestation is forgotten. As a result, the physical body is declared as self, "I"'s sovereignty.

The basic mistake then becomes that we take for granted the external physical self and ignore the spiritual Self within. But merely understanding this tendency philosophically does not dispel the ignorance. Practice is needed to get connected with the spiritual Self and to elevate the awareness. *Avidyā* lures you into thinking and acting in a wrong manner at every step. Here, right or wrong is not a moral precept. The "right" here is the relative truth at a point in time, and the "wrong" is anything that is otherwise; both however, do change over time.

Only earnest and sustained practice can eliminate *Avidyā*, and along with it, other obstacles and hindrances. However, caution is essential. Though the human physical body/brain system is impure, that does not mean it should either be looked down upon or abandoned. It still remains the only vehicle for the soul's unfolding and it can be made pure with constant effort. Then, the indwelling spiritual Self can show us how to go even beyond the purified body/brain system.

Yoga is a path of this earned knowledge.

SENSE OF PERSONALITY

Avidyā places the physical brain on a high pedestal instead of venerating the inner spiritual Self. This misplaced reverence, like a small shift in snow on a mountaintop, rolls and creates an avalanche of wrong acts, ultimately suffocating and burying the seeker deep in it. The conscious brain usurps the place of a real knower, and a false "I," a faux personality, is enthroned.

The sense of personality is due to the identification of the knower with the instruments of knowing (Sūtra 1.24/II.6). It is rarely realized that the human brain has neither intelligence nor awareness of its own. It merely stores and acts upon the intelligence and awareness reflected by the mind. An individual mind reflects because it is contaminated and opaque, and no longer as luminous and transparent as Universal Mind.

However, the spiritual Self is the real knower, and its manifestation and experiencing brings into action the instruments of knowing. These thinking instruments, brain, *mānas* and *buddhi*, take three different forms on the three planes.

Mind, as a catalyst, collaborates on all three planes with the respective thinking instruments. On the physical plane, the brain receives information from the five senses (sound, touch, sight, taste, and smell) that is provided by the five external sense organs (ears, skin, eyes, tongue, and nose). Energy for the thinking process comes partly from the experiencing knower (the soul) and from the mind that experiences objects via the five sense channels. However, the very process of experiencing through the body creates a bind (a "ring-pass-not," a self-created hypothetical boundary made insurmountable by ignorance) and these two distinct energies are taken to be one. What is known (*guṇa* of the objects) is equated with the knower (soul). Thus, the true soul identity gets obliterated as a series of experiences conjure a sense of personality that is external, object-centric, and ultimately erroneous.

That is why the first breakthrough on the *yogīk* path occurs when you identify the knower, the spiritual Self, as separate from both the experience (in the brain) and the objects of experience. As the mind turns inward and awareness gets elevated, its identification shifts to *mānas*, and that starts conveying its thoughts, wishes, and will to the brain. Eventually, *buddhi* takes over in a similar way.

On the path of Yoga, as will be seen later, the first five means of Yoga (*Yama*, *niyama*, *āsana*, *prānāyāma*, and *pratyāhāra)* bring about the first conveyance of thoughts of the spiritual Self to the brain. Consequently, the erroneous sense of personality starts fading away. Finally, the remaining three means of Yoga (*dhāraṇā*, *dhyāna*, and *samādhī*) bring about *soul visioning*. Soul-visioning results in pure perception and in the separation of the real knower from the objects of experience, thus eliminating the reliance on bodily experience as the only means of knowing.

DESIRE

Desire is a generic term for the tendency of the Spirit to move outward via the bodies towards the life forms. **Desire is attachment to the objects of pleasure** (Sūtra 1.25/II.7). Though the Spirit remains unattached, an object of pleasure sensed by the respective thinking instrument results in attachment for the bodies. There is no qualitative difference in attachment on the different planes.

A savage's desire for food is as much an attachment as a sage's desire for God's blessings. The *guṇa* latent in various objects create a sense of pleasure and an attachment for the perceiver. Even when the more chaotic *tāmasik guṇa* give way to the *sāttvik*, and the concepts of pleasure are more refined and holier, an attachment is nevertheless caused. All attachments ultimately result in pain.

The soul's outbound manifestation causes desire. But desire causes you to remain engaged with the vehicle of the bodies that seem to be moving from one attachment to another, until your awareness is only spiritual, where there is no attachment and no desire.

HATE

Hate arises from an initial experience of pain but still results in attachment, because one remains immersed in it. **Hate is aversion for any object of pain** (Sūtra 1.26/II.8). Hate or aversion is also based on the form, and results from ignorance of anything else that the form reveals. The root of hate can be found in the base instincts resulting from the physical personality that is further aggravated by ignorance. Hate repels you from the physical object, but in that reflex reaction the mind remains attached to the object nonetheless.

Hate is particularly contrary to Yoga. Yoga is all about unity and oneness; hate separates and fragments. Hate creates a negative energy that destroys. Hate is the opposite of love, and the seeker has to resist being swayed by either.

INTENSE DESIRE FOR EXISTENCE

An intense desire to live is natural, and universal. The desire is pronounced in the attachment to worldly objects, since that provides a context and a reason for living. The intense desire for sentient existence is attachment. **This is inherent in every form, is self-perpetuating, and is experienced even by the very wise** (Sūtra 1.27/II.9). In Yoga, this desire serves as a great outbound urge that pushes the subtle into more and more gross manifestations. This desire causes all beings to stay attached to the gross and to bear the resultant pain. Thus, low awareness keeps one confined to the gross until death brings an end to it.[13]

Since this attachment to life is inherent in every form, it cannot be restricted only to humans; the animal and plant kingdoms are no exception. The desire to live is intense and self-perpetuating. It is so innate that we don't even recognize it as a desire. Unlike some low-level desires, this desire cannot be easily given up because

[13] *Fear of death is a strong argument in favor of the theory of reincarnation. If all actions are preceded by thoughts, if thoughts breed on the preceding reason, if reason is only a degenerated experience—it follows that such a fear can only come from previous painful experience of death. It also means that some seeds of experience like this are carried across lifetimes.*

it has become a part of the roots and *saṃskāra*, the structure of predispositions. Sage Pātañjali emphatically says that **"this desire is experienced even by the very wise"** regardless of how one may pretend otherwise. This is another terse and clinically correct statement implying that mere knowing is of no use unless it is internalized by practice.

But there is an even a deeper meaning to this sutra. The three planes of the universe (gross to subtle) have a hereditary structure. Having such a structure means that the physical plane has a shorter life-span (from form-creation to form-destruction) than the astral one, and the astral has a shorter life-span than the causal plane. Thus, death on the physical plane does not coincide with death on the astral plane. The astral self continues to live after the physical death. So, when your awareness is raised from the physical plane to the astral, it can be carried beyond the physical death. Likewise, raising awareness beyond the astral will enable you to survive death on the astral plane. Yoga teaches how to elevate awareness that remains unbroken by death.

Giving up the desire to live appears fundamentally flawed. Only if we step outside of our compulsive, conditioned thinking can we understand the real meaning of this concept. Sage Pātañjali is pointing out that a desire to live is still a desire, and brings its natural painful consequences. Yet it is not suggested that this desire needs to be given up tomorrow. The *yogīk* path is a long journey that brings about a metamorphosis of sorts. The desire to live is the last threshold to cross. Just as we don't die the moment we sign a living will, getting rid of this desire in no way entails ending one's life. The one who would travel to that advanced threshold wouldn't be the same "you" that finds it absurd to live with no desire to live.

Dealing with Hindrances

Ironically, the mind itself is the initial tool on the *yogīk* path that recognizes the mind's hindrances, a recognition that Sage Pātañjali calls *discrimination*. Mind makes the brain a conscious organ and no one has ever won against this devil of a conscious brain with conscious efforts and the will alone. You cannot reach the end by being at war with the very means. The control has to be achieved through an almost effortless practice. Hence, in Yoga, exercises and practices are crucial, and the only way to bring about a permanent change in the individual's structures. **For dealing with these five hindrances** (Sūtra 1.28/II.10)

- **know them subtly**
- **create an opposing mental attitude.**

KNOW THE HINDRANCES SUBTLY

Implied here is that you may know the five hindrances on the overt physical plane but may not be able to overcome them on that plane as they will continue to exist on the subtler planes and will continue to fructify like seeds. Elevating your awareness is, however, a prerequisite to knowing the hindrances subtly.

Their gross activities (of the hindrances) **are to be done away with through the meditation process** (Sūtra 1.29/II.11). A meditative attitude is recommended to substitute for the reflex behavior on the physical plane. While *saṃskāra* are being burned through right-thinking habits, the mind and the thinking instrument should be in the meditative mode to direct all behavior on the physical plane. If it is not, then as long as the physical activities induced by the hindrances continue, the incoming sense impulses, co-joined by memory patterns soaked in emotions, will continue to bombard the thinking instruments and keep compelling them to act like an android.

This bombardment happens to such a degree that most of us are completely ruled by the five hindrances. Through accumulated *saṃskāra* and the ingrained memory patterns, thinking becomes a habitual reflex action. This type of thinking does not allow any room for *thinking about the thinking process itself* or being able to burn the *saṃskāra*. The thinking process operating in the reflex mode has to be stopped consciously.

To make that happen, first the rate of thought formation has to be slowed down. The rushing torrent of impulses should be tamed into a rhythmic pattern. This paves a way for the rate to slow down so much that there is a nanosecond gap between two thoughts. Eventually, during the gaps, the thinking is suspended and pure experiencing takes place. This leads to internalized silence and provides extremely limited opportunities for the seeds of afflictions to become active.

CREATE AN OPPOSING MENTAL ATTITUDE

Knowing is fine, but of greater importance is the second part—how to overcome hindrances. *Yoga-Sūtra* prescribes creation of an *opposing mental attitude* that refers to the thinking process. The individual thinking instruments (brain, *mānas*, and *buddhi*) and the process of thinking need to be first clearly understood in order to use them this way. You have to realize, with increased firsthand awareness, how the Universal Mind flows through the senses and then through the thinking instruments while becoming an adapted and diluted individual mind.

It would slowly occur to you that the hindrances are generated out of the thinking process when the *saṃskāra* (the structure of predispositions) filters and colors the thoughts and when subjective forms are created in the process of perceiving the objects. Thus, wrong habits of thought formation and misuse of the thinking process are the real subtle seeds of hindrances that merely manifest on the gross plane.

In the East, people often differentiate good *saṃskāra* from bad. This shows limited understanding of how it works, like how good behavior results from good *saṃskāra*. But *saṃskāra* that cripple inquisitiveness and brainwash a person into an automatic reflex behavior serve no one. Such *saṃskāra* may bring good behavior as understood by a community in a given space-time context, but the same may soon become a hindrance to the inner evolution of a seeker. Similarly, moral values have a limited social and space-time context. Though they are definitely valid for the ignorant, a spiritual seeker has to rise above their constraining limitations on the *yogīk* path.

It then follows that, in the pursuit of truth, only by knowing, conquering, and ultimately destroying *saṃskāra* can the thinking process be cleansed. With the right-thinking habits cultivated to create an opposite mental attitude, the seeds of the hindrances can be burned and destroyed forever. The most valuable principle laid down by Sage Pātañjali is that the hindrances can be overcome only by burning their seeds at the subtle level when they appear stealthily in the thinking process. That principle is also a reason why the internal hindrances cannot be overcome merely through external behavioral changes. (*Yoga-Sūtra* places paramount importance on the mental postures and not just the physical, the āsanās).[14]

Seen this way, when the five afflictions are reduced to the seed form and burned, they vanish. A purified individual mind, with its task finished, evolves when the process of *individualization* of the Universal Mind (the coloring with afflictions) slows down and stops.

***Karma*, the Law of Cause and Effect**

Fear of death is a hindrance but obviously it is not the only *saṃskāra* that you carry across life or lives. If *saṃskāra* are imprints that do not dwell on the physical plane, all *saṃskāra* (structure of predispositions) must have been carried from an earlier life/lives. *Saṁskāra* leave their signature on the thought process as well as on its outcome—thoughts and/or actions. They are therefore unique to a person and form a unique personality (Sūtra II.12 to 14).

Thoughts do survive in a coded (non-verbalized) form, stripped down to the underlying desires. They wait for their fruition into effects as events on the physical plane. Billions and billions of human beings have, during trillions and trillions of life-times,

---

[14] *The original Sanskrit word in* Sūtra 1.28 *is* "pratiprasavā." Prasavā *is unfolding, or "transformation of cause into effect," or "manifestation of subtle into gross." What the* sūtra *recommends is contrary to it*—"pratiprasavā," *which is Yoga's spiritual "evolution," folding back or "resolution of effect into its cause," or "the gross dissolving into the subtle, when the purpose of gross manifestation is over."*

generated an almost infinite volume of thoughts. Because each thought has to ultimately express itself in a consequent effect, it awaits an opportune moment and a circumstance to do so. This is a fundamental cause and effect relationship and its inevitability is the *law of* karma.

But *karma* is such a multi-dimensional complex model that when, how, and why an effect follows its cause is beyond ordinary human comprehension. It may happen in an immediate context to the same person (easy to understand) or may occur in a distant future in such a manner that it will be humanly impossible to correlate the effect to its context or to the person (events which make us wonder "why me" or view the sufferers as "innocent victims").

Sage Pātañjali assures us that the cycles of *karma* do not roll infinitely and that's good news. Thoughts that carry no baggage do not create any *karma*. The reservoir of *karma* itself has its roots in the five hindrances and *karma* must come to fruition in this life or the next (Sūtra 1.30/II.12). This fact has two very important implications.

- When the five hindrances are removed, the resultant *karma* ceases to affect one's future.
- *Karma* is not a self-generating phenomenon.

So, one who understands the reason why *karma* must come to fruition can also understand how *karma* can be redeemed and how that preempts the need for its fruition.

Thus, contrary to a very popular opinion, *karma* is not a fatalistic concept. While the effect following its cause is inevitable, the nature of that effect is largely dependent upon a variety of choices you make. Besides, *karma* can be redeemed by learning and knowing, so in redemption the cause and effect chain is broken. It is important to also note that Sūtra II.12 is not talking of good *karma* against bad. It is only emphasizing that *karma* (good or bad) has to meet its appropriate consequence sooner or later. Taken to its logical conclusion, a true end to attachment can occur only when all *karma* (good and bad) ceases to exist. And the solution is twofold:

- Burn the seeds of the five hindrances.
- Redeem *karma*.

Hindrances, the Real Roots of Karma

Now we may be able to see why mind and the thinking process assume such prominence in Yoga. *Karma* may be perpetuating life, but what *causes karma* in the first place? **So long as the roots (or *Saṁskāra*) exist, their function will be birth, life, and experience that result in pleasure or pain** (Sūtra 1.31/II.13).

In *birth, death, and experiences*, the whole human life is summed up. It must be reiterated that as the cause of *karma*, the *saṃskāra* not only impact the experiences and life, but also cause the next birth and ones thereafter.

This puts *karma* in three modes:

- ***Latent*** karma***:*** *Those seeds and causes which are yet undeveloped and inactive and must work out to fruition in some part of the present or future lives.*
- ***Active*** karma***:*** *Those seeds and causes which are in the process of fruition and for which the present life is intended to provide the needed soil for their flowering forth.*
- ***New*** karma***:*** *Those seeds and causes which are being produced in this life and which must inevitably govern the circumstances of some future life.*

—Alice Bailey, 145-146.

In Yoga, you learn how active *karma* can be reduced by redeeming (or knowingly living out) its effects, and how in this way an accumulation of new *karma* can be prevented. All *karma* is rooted in the thinking process. This is why the central theme of *Yoga-Sūtra* is controlling the mind modifications. Thoughts that dance to the tune of chaotic impulses drawn from the *guṇa* manifesting in the objects need to be discerned before reining them in. A seeker has to engage in a continuous exercise of thought-watching, thought-spacing, and thought-delaying until non-attachment of mind is achieved. In a state of non-attachment, the new *karma* seeds cease to sprout.

A superficial reading of the law of *karma* may lead one to perceive human life as mechanical, automated, and fatalistic. If *karma* dictates what should happen, an individual seems to be left with little, if nothing at all, to make anything happen otherwise. This is not a correct interpretation. Let us look at the *potentiality—possibility—probability* concept.

Karma as a cause of action exists with *infinite potentialities* that form a superset. Say, one kills another individual. Such cause has millions of potential ways in which a consequence will return to the killer. But each potentiality does not result in an effect or an actual incident. Thus,from the above superset of potentialities emerges a subset of relatively *finite possibilities* depending on the finite circumstances of one's specific life. Say, the killer lives amidst political unrest. Then, the possibilities are greater that the killer actively participates in the riots. But, one goes through life and makes a variety of choices at each moment. Those choices shape up a further subset of *near-probabilities*. Say, the choices create greater probability for the consequence to arrive as death. These probabilities present fertile soil for certain seeds to come to fruition, seeds from which an *actual event* occurs when the right context is present. Say, the circumstances decide that the killer should suffer with grief and not with death, and hence, it results in the death of a near and dear one. (This example is only for explaining the concept; otherwise, it is over-simplification and subject to several questions and opinions.)

Let us remember, however, that it is still *you* who make the choices. An individual with low awareness would naturally be influenced by the experience and resulting pleasure or pain, and the choices would be made to repeat pleasure and avoid pain. As the product of thoughts and *saṃskāra*, such choices would unwittingly foster vicious cycles of new *karma*, new episodes of similar pleasure/pain experiences, and would necessitate another life in which to live that out.

As awareness increases and one realizes the true nature of *karma* and *saṃskāra*, one is naturally eager to break the chain of self-induced life after life. We are so engrossed in "living" a life that a desire to break the chain of lives appears paradoxical. We are not talking about *ending* life, either. The *yogīk* path is an ever-so-gentle lift-off from engagement with life at the physical level. It is a fully conscious process. All the seeds of desire are burned that could have pushed the subtle bodies to manifest into another physical life full of experiences of pleasure and pain. Thus, another physical life is rendered needless.

This path of inner evolution seems natural only if you possess a heightened awareness. As your purpose of life deepens, the horizon expands. Burning the seeds of *saṃskāra* and expiating *karma* appear to be a logical aspiration of life. If one must die, can it be a conscious and willing death, and a passing on peacefully to eternal freedom? Unless we are on the *yogīk* path, we can only speculate.

Life, the Effect of Karma, *the Seed*

So is the effect, as is the cause. **Birth, life, and experiences produce pleasure or pain according to their originating cause (the seeds) being good or evil** (Sūtra 1.32/II.14).

The thoughts defined and shaped by the structure of predispositions sow the seeds of *karma.*

Thoughts, like all other tangible objects, are also composed of three qualities in varying proportions. The thought qualities *sattva*, *rajas*, and *tamas* are governed by the incoming sense impulses and are soaked in emotions owing to the associated patterns of memory. When the *sattva* qualities are more predominant than the *rajas* and *tamas*, the seeds are varying grades of "tranquility." They are grades of "agitation" otherwise. But the tranquil or agitated seeds differ only in terms of the severity and depth of the mind modifications that they produce.

Thus the seeds are impregnated with the potentialities of *karma.* To the ordinary human being, for whom the sense of pleasure and pain prevails, the experience of objects brings about the fruition of *karma* in the same intensity and proportion as the seed has been tranquil or agitated. This is why, in the final effort of burning all the seeds, the first step is to reduce the agitated ones and replace them with tranquil seeds that may be easier to deal with. Ultimately, however, one would want to get rid of all such seeds—tranquil or agitated.

Guṇa, the Final Frontier

Thus, how you experience objects holds a key to *karma* redemption. But, the mother of all objects is the mind. To access and control the objects, the mind must be controlled first. We have seen how an individual mind is a wayward and dwarfed off-spring of the all-knowing Universal Mind. Experiencing lures the individual mind into attaching to the perceived objects and that attracts obstacles and hindrances. You can struggle to overcome them but their root cause is somewhere else. An experience is a sum total of cognition derived from the sensory impulses generated in the process of perception because of the excited *guṇa* in an object; and that is the root cause of mind modifications.

Hindrances Originate in Guṇa

If *karma*-seeds emerge from the hindrances, the hindrances themselves are caused by *guṇa*. **To the illumined person with discrimination, all existence (on the three planes) is painful owing to the activities of the *guṇa* over time and space** (Sūtra 1.33/ II.15).

We talked about pain and pleasure earlier. We also naturally believe that the *illumined Yogī*, who has overcome the hindrances, will have no pain when spiritual ecstasy is within reach. However, even for the illumined, everything is ultimately pain. *Purūṣa,* the Spirit, and *Prakṛtī*, the Mind, make an odd couple. They form the primary *pair of opposites*.[15] They are peaceful until united in the process of manifesting as matter. Both resist each other and create

[15] *Inherent in perception is duality that builds our personalized reality on building blocks laying somewhere between a pair of opposites rendering them inexact and subject to change. For example, hot and cold, effective and ineffective, fullness and emptiness, difference and sameness, beauty and ugliness, one and many, even, time and space. Opposites make a pair because assigning any one quality to an object also means negating or denying the other.*

friction, suffering, and pain while remaining tied up in time and space. One needs to understand this to realize why everything is pain for the illumined one.

In the context of *time*, pain is produced through:

- **After-effects (past):** The spiritual Self is in the confinement of the bodies, heredity, and surroundings formed as a result of past *karma*. Thus, some of today's pain is the result of the activity of the past.
- **Anxieties (present):** In the present, while the spiritual Self is awakening, and even otherwise, one is inflicted with anxieties and apprehensions. These cover the entire gamut of fears, including the fear of evil in suffering and the fear of losing the fruits of one's labor. Even a *Yogī* is not free from anxieties when the fear of failure in the spiritual pursuit brings doubts. Fear brings pain.
- **Subliminal impressions (future):** The forebodings of the future and the fear of the unknown, not just for oneself but also for loved ones, keep us going on with our lives and living under stress. The consequences of this stress are painful.

In the context of *space*, pain is produced through:

- **Dominance of *tamas* (inertia) on the *physical plane*:** Pleasure or aversion is experienced in the context of objects and persons on the physical plane. Such feelings are pervaded with attachment and give rise to the latent deposit of *karma* seeds. Any attachment or action leads directly or indirectly to hurt on the physical plane. Satiety that comes after sense gratification is short-lived and does not expiate the desire. This also is a source of pain.
- **Dominance of *rajas* (mobility) on the *astral plane*:** Wants, needs, attachments and aversions play on the psyche and result in wishing favor for friends and harm for others. On the astral plane, aversion and delusion result in anxiety, because we are constantly engaged in judging and discriminating, and that creates pain.

- **Dominance of *sattva* (revealing) on the *causal plane*:** The illumined becomes as sensitive as an eye. A piece of cotton may be pleasurable for the rest of the body, but it hurts when it comes in contact with the eye. Likewise, the latent impressions on the causal plane caused by actions, even if *sāttvik* and ordinarily pleasurable, in turn generate seeds (cause) for future action and perpetuate the chain, thus causing pain for the illumined.

Guṇa *Inherent in Experiencing*

The theory of *karma* tells us that the cause and effect relationship produces a wide variety of both happy and painful events across several lives. Sūtra II.15, one of the most important ones, can be correctly understood only if we take human life on this scale. Now we need to understand the intricacies of how *guṇa* work. **That which is experienced, the world of matter, has three coexisting qualities: *sattva, rajas*, and *tamas* (revealing, mobile, and inert). Experiencing consists of the five basic elements and the sense organs. Their mutual engagement produces experience and eventual liberation** (Sūtra 1.34/ II.18).

One principle hypothesis of Yoga is that what is experienced through the physical-astral-causal bodies is the "world of matter," and the one who experiences it is the Soul. Experiencing concerns external objects, persons, events, and our sense organs (which are objects too). Each element, gross or fine, is characterized by three *guṇa*. These three material factors are what each element is born with, and they are mutually dependent energy components. *Guṇa* are ever-changing vibrations and possess the qualities of uniting (through attraction) with and separating (through repulsion) from one another. They acquire a composite form through the support of one by the others, but even when one is predominant, the others do not lose their individual distinctive powers. They take different lines of manifestation of their powers in objects. This is the *knowable* world.

Perception is an engaging event between two objects. Now let us expand what we know about *guṇa*. An object is composed of the five basic elements of earth, water, fire, air, and *Ākāś* ("space" or "ether" are inadequate but close translations).[16] When one object perceives another, the two connect through *guṇa*. The manifestation of *guṇa* (in the perceived object) is caused by the attachment via sensing (by the perceiving object) with a view to experiencing the perceived object. The sense impulses, which are also vibrations, derive from the dominant *guṇa* in an element, but the other subsidiary *guṇa* are also there to jointly compose an appearance. Permutations and combinations of the three *guṇa* create an infinite variety of elements, and the changing nature of *guṇa* makes the perceived elements unique to the perceiver. Thus, the basic elements of earth, water, fire, air, and *Ākāś* play their part in building one's own forms and are incorporated in the object's very being.

Let us not forget that an individual human being is also an object. Ordinarily, in your life as an object, *tamas* (inertia) distinguishes the gross forms in infancy, while the sense organs become active one by one over time. The forms are initially so gross and heavy that many violent contacts are needed to build up awareness of the surroundings. When the second quality, *rajas* (mobility), is firmly established, the mind starts developing, and this development brings awareness of the same qualities in all objects in the surroundings as in your own being. From this awareness begins a distinction between self as the perceiver and that which is perceived, the forms.

Until you consciously try to subdue *rajas* and *tamas*, their interplay dominates your life and *sattva* remains weak. You remain engrossed in the violent love/hate relationship with forms of all sorts. On the *yogīk* path, your concept of self expands and becomes the spiritual Self when you enter the *sāttvik* state. You are

---

[16] *The concept of the element is an ancient one which developed in many different civilizations in an attempt to rationalize the variety of the world and to understand the nature of change. The four elements "earth, air, fire and water" were popularized by Greek philosophers, to which Vedic philosophers added "space." These basic elements were not generally considered to exist as the actual materials we know as earth, water, etc., but rather to represent the principles or essences that the elements conveyed to the various kinds of matter we encounter in the world: shape and inertia for the earth, viscidity and fluidity for water, heat and metabolisms for fire, velocity and subtlety for air and omnipresence for* ākāśa. *(Article: "Atom, Elements and the Nucleus" at www.chem1.com)*

increasingly harmonized within yourself and consequently with your environment. Then, *guṇa* in yourself and around you are not just in balance but are also in rhythm and harmony. They are more tranquil and at your command. There arrives a state where you are still a part of the whole yet are freed and liberated from the tyranny of the forms, of the elements, and of the senses, because now you use them and are no more being used by them.

As a person evolves, the purpose of life evolves too. Ordinarily, a seeker's default purpose is sensory experiencing. Soon the purpose changes to *seeking pleasure and not pain*, which changes to *seeking permanence and not transience*, and finally evolves into *emancipation*.

The Seed Atoms

At this stage, you may ask: If objects are multi-layered and the subtle survives the gross, what ensures continuity across bodies and across lives? All physical experiencing is coded in a seed atom located on the fourth plane. Similar seed atoms get activated—for emotional experiencing on the astral plane and spiritual experiencing on the causal—when the emotional and spiritual awareness rises.

It is quite tempting to liken the seed atoms to what modern science calls the DNA. Prior to taking a human birth, the information stored in the seed atoms goes to the drawing board of the spiritual Self when the next astral body is conceived and, in turn, that design is executed when that astral body conceives a physical body. A seed atom stores everything, including the kārmic seeds and the structures of predispositions and functionality that the grosser bodies inherit at birth. But "causal" is still a body; what happens after the causal body dies?

The Fourth Plane, beyond Guṇa

Guṇa is a fascinating concept. It really works at both ends of perception when the two sets of *guṇa* meet. The three-dimensional *guṇa* give a form to the perceived object, but in fact, the nature of that form depends on the three-*guṇa* structure of the perceiving object. Bringing that to its logical conclusion, when a *yogī*, as the perceiving object, puts his or her own *guṇa* at full rest, the perceived objects are rendered form-less. In other words, being "form-less" is a steady-state of all objects, and forms are created all the time by the restless *guṇa* of the perceiving object. That is why where some people see God, most others see just a stone!

The states of the *guṇa* are experienced on all three planes and beyond (Sūtra 1.35/II.19).

Now, *Yoga-Sūtra* introduces the fourth plane, which is *beyond* the other three—the physical, astral, and causal. Interestingly, all the four planes coexist virtually, here and now, providing the Universe with four virtual dimensions in addition to the conventional three.

On the physical plane, *tamas* (the deceptive) is predominant and carries small traces of *rajas* and *sattva* to create *differentiated and specific* forms. At the perceiving end, they correspond with the five elements of matter, five organs of action and five sense organs energized by the individual mind. The forms when experienced on this plane hide more than reveal their true nature. **This is our normal world view**—which encompasses distinct physical objects, each of which we can describe and distinguish clearly.

On the astral plane, *rajas* (the restless) is predominant and carries small traces of *sattva* and *tamas* to create *differentiated but unspecific* forms that are not so much in black and white. They are experienced by the *tanmātrās* (subtle senses) when energized by one's ego, the personality. These forms are ever-changing and mesmerizing. **This is an emotional world-view**, full of pain and pleasure, and results in love and hate. More than the objects themselves, here we deal with our emotional relation with them, which is not sharply distinguished as one from the other.

On the causal plane, *sattva* (the revealer) is predominant and carries small traces of *rajas* and *tamas* to create *undifferentiated* and *indistinct* forms that are nebulous and only indicated in a broad-brush. They are experienced as unarticulated ideas and concepts when energized by *buddhi* (intellect). They almost reveal their true nature but leave a shade of doubt or some deceit. **This is**

an intellectual world-view where beliefs, logic, and philosophies are constructed as a stepping stone to spirituality. Functionality or appearance of the objects takes a back seat, making it hard to distinguish them.

There is, however, a **fourth state** where the three *guṇa* are in such an absolute balance, harmony, and rhythm that they collapse into nonexistence, thus denying any perception, awareness or any other duality. This is a form-less state, untouchable for the world of matter. **On this plane is the soul; a fragment of the divinity that lies enveloped and veiled by the three planes.** All along, this has been the true perceiver, but the mind fools us to accept "I" as the one. This real perceiver is *Īśvara*, the ultimate teacher who guides us to the final destination on the *yogīk* path.

In Yoga, a seeker's transformation takes many forms. Definitions change. Words assume different dimensions. A seeker starts examining words which are otherwise used almost carelessly in common parlance. For instance, as we have seen earlier, if the astral is subtler than the gross and is also its cause, then to say that it resides "inside" the gross does not seem to make sense. A better term is "interpenetrates"—the astral is within as well as without. As molecules project from each cell of the physical body, the molecular/astral body appears virtually from within the physical body as its subtle counterpart, which is neither inside nor outside of it, like vapor arising from water.

Yoga refers to time and space as the products of mind. It does not imply that time and space are fictional; it does imply that they are *relative*. The seeker starts getting a new "feel" of time when he or she realizes that thought processes do not capture the real "present." The interpenetrating nature of the subtle is likewise understood by the seeker experientially. Slowly, spatial concepts like inside/outside and within/beyond appear deceptive, too. This realization is essential for moving toward a common ground between the Self (*Purusa*) and everything else (Prakriti) as one seeks eventual unity of all matter and Spirit.

This becomes a paradigm shift. You become an inspired seeker when you perceive the apparently solid dimensions of time and space as relative, and the apparent stark duality of self and not-self as fragile.

And with this refined perception you reach the first milestone on the yogīk path.

Chapter One: Rearranged Sūtras: (Numbers in the brackets are from the conventional sequence)

1.1 (I.1) अथ योगानुशासनम् ॥

atha yogānuśāsanaṁ

Now we shall begin the revised and complete instructions in the science of Union.

1.2 (I.2) योगश्चित्तवृत्तिनिरोधः ॥

yogaś citta-vṛtti-nirodhaḥ

Yoga is achieved through healing of the psyche and calming of the thinking instrument, which is restrained from taking various forms.

1.3 (I.3) तदा द्रष्टुः स्वरूपेऽवस्थानम् ॥

tadā draṣṭuḥ svarūpe'vasthānaṁ

When *this* is accomplished, the seeker knows what he or she really is.

1.4 (I.4) वृत्तिसारूप्यमितरत्र ॥

vṛtti-sārūpyam itaratra

But up until then, the inner self identifies with the forms, one's own and that of others, and takes their active modifications for real.

1.5 (I.5) वृत्तयः पञ्जतय्यः क्लिष्ट अक्लिष्टाः ॥

vṛttayaḥ pañcatayaḥ kliṣṭākliṣṭāḥ

The individual mind, in concert with the brain, has five states that are painful or not painful.

1.6 (I.6) प्रमाणविपर्ययविकल्पनिद्रास्मृतयः ॥

pramāṇa-viparyaya-vikalpa-nidrā-smṛtayaḥ

The five mind modifications (activities) are: valid knowledge, incorrect knowledge, fancy or imagination, passivity (sleep), and memory.

1.7 (I.7) प्रत्यक्षानुमानागमाः प्रमाणानि ॥

pratyakṣānumānāgamāḥ pramāṇāni

The source of valid knowledge is correct cognition (understanding), correct deduction or inference, and correct witness (or accurate testimony).

1.8 (I.8) विपर्ययो मिथ्याज्ञानमतद्रूपप्रतिष्ठम् ॥

viparyayo mithyā-jñānam atad-rūpa-pratiṣṭhaṁ

Incorrect knowledge is based upon ordinary perception (mere seeing without understanding) of the form and not upon the state of being of the object.

1.9 (I.9) शब्दज्ञानानुपाती वस्तुशून्यो विकल्पः ॥

śabda-jñānānupātī-vastu-śūnyo vikalpaḥ

Fancy is like a daydream that rests upon images and words that have no real existence.

1.10 (I.10) अभावप्रत्ययालम्बना वृत्तिर्निद्रा ॥

abhāva-pratyayālambanā vṛttir nidrā

Passivity is based upon the quiescent state of the *vṛttis*.

1.11 (I.11) अनुभूतविषयासम्प्रमोषः स्मृतिः ॥

anubhūta-viṣayāsaṁpramoṣaḥ smṛtiḥ

Memory is holding on to that which has been known.

1.12 (I.12) अभ्यासवैराग्याभ्यां तन्निरोधः ॥

abhyāsa-vairāgyābhyāṁ tan-nirodhaḥ

The calming (and eventual control) of these mind modifications is to be brought about through tireless endeavor and through non-attachment.

1.13 (I.13) तत्र स्थितौ यत्नोऽभ्यासः ॥

tatra sthitau yatno 'bhyāsaḥ

Tireless endeavor is the constant effort of the will to restrain the modifications of the thinking instrument.

1.14 (I.14) स तु दीर्घकालनैरन्तर्यसत्कारासेवितो दृढभूमिः ॥

sa tu dīrgha-kāla-nairantarya-satkārāsevito dṛḍha-bhūmiḥ

When the object to be gained is sufficiently valued, efforts toward its attainment are persistently followed without intermission. Only in this way is the steadiness of the thinking instrument (restraint of the *vṛttis*) secured.

1.15 (I.15)

दृष्टानुश्रविकविषयवितृष्णस्य वशीकारसंज्ञा वैराग्यम् ॥

dṛṣṭānuśravika-viṣaya-vitṛṣṇasya vaśīkāra-saṁjñā vairāgyaṁ

Non-attachment is the freedom from craving for all objects of desire, either experienced or known.

1.16 (I.16) तत्परं पुरुषख्यातेर्गुणवैतृष्ण्यम् ॥

tatparaṁ puruṣa-khyāter guṇavaitṛṣṇyaṁ

When non-attachment becomes a way of life, one is liberated from the qualities of *guṇa* and possesses knowledge of the spiritual being that one is.

1.17 (I.30)

व्याधिस्त्यानसंशयप्रमादालस्याविरतिभ्रांतिदर्शनालब्धभूमिकत्वानवस्थितत्वानि चित्तविक्षेपास्तेऽन्तरायाः ॥

vyādhi-styāna-saṁśaya-pramādālasyāvirati-bhrānti-darśanālabdhabhūmi-katvānavasthitatvāni citta-vikṣepās te 'ntarāyāḥ

The obstacles to soul cognition are bodily disability, mental inertia, doubt (wrong questioning), procrastination (carelessness), laziness, craving (lack of dispassion), erroneous perception, inability to achieve concentration, and failure to hold a meditative attitude when it has been achieved.

1.18 (I.31)

दुखःदौर्मनस्याङ्गमेजयत्वश्वासप्रश्वासा विक्षेपसहभुवः ॥

duḥkha-daurmanasyāṅgamejayatva-śvāsa-praśvāsā vikṣepa-sahabhuvaḥ

Pain, despair, misplaced bodily activity, and unrhythmic breathing are the results of the obstacles in the lower psychic nature.

1.19 (I.32) तत्प्रतिषेधार्थमेकतत्वाभ्यासः ॥

tat-pratiṣedhārtham eka-tattvābhyāsaḥ

To overcome the obstacles, an intense application of the will to the truth and the principle is required.

1.20 (I.33)

मैत्रीकरूणामुदितोपेक्षाणां सुखदुखःपुण्यापुण्यविषयाणां भावनातश्चित्तप्रसादनम् ॥

maitrī-karuṇā-muditopekṣāṇāṁ sukha-duḥkha-puṇyāpuṇya-viṣayāṇaṁ bhāvanātaś citta-prasādanam

The peace of mind and the thinking instruments can be brought about through the practice of sympathy, tenderness, steadiness of purpose, and indifference with regard to happiness, misery, virtue, and vice.

1.21 (II.3) अविद्यास्मितारागद्वेषाभिनिवेशाः क्लेशाः ॥

avidyāsmitā-rāga-dveṣābhiniveśāḥ kleśāḥ

These are the internal hindrances: *Avidyā* (ignorance), the "I"-sense (personality), desire, hate, and the sense of attachment.

1.22 (II.4)

अविद्या क्षेत्रमुत्तरेषां प्रसुप्ततनुविच्छिन्नोदाराणाम् ॥

avidyā kṣetram uttareṣāṁ prasupta-tanu-vicchinnodārāṇāṁ

Avidyā (ignorance) is the cause of all the other hindrances, whether they be latent, in the process of elimination, overcome, or in full operation.

1.23 (II.5)

अनित्याशुचिदुःखानात्मसु नित्यशुचिसुखात्मख्यातिरविद्या ॥

anityāśuci-duḥkhānātmasu nitya-śuci-suhkātmakhyātir avidyā

Avidyā is the condition of confusing the permanent (the pure, the blissful, and the Self) with that which is impermanent, impure, painful, and intellectually understandable.

1.24 (II.6) दृग्दर्शनशक्त्योरेकात्मतेवास्मिता ॥

dṛg-darśana-śaktyor ekātmatevāsmitā

The sense of personality is due to the identification of the knower with the instruments of knowing.

1.25 (II.7) सुखानुशयी रागः ॥

sukhānuśayī rāgaḥ

Desire is attachment to the objects of pleasure.

1.26 (II.8) दुःखानुशयी द्वेषः ॥

duḥkhānuśayī dveṣaḥ

Hate is aversion for any object of pain.

1.27 (II.9) स्वरसवाही विदुषोऽपि तथारूढोऽभिनिवेशः ॥

svarasavāhī viduṣo 'pi tathā rūḍho 'bhiniveśaḥ

The intense desire for sentient existence is attachment. This is inherent in every form, is self-perpetuating, and is experienced even by the very wise.

1.28 (II.10) ते प्रतिप्रसवहेयाः सूक्ष्माः ॥

te pratiprasava-heyāḥ sūkṣmāḥ

These five hindrances are to be subtly known and overcome by an opposing mental attitude.

1.29 (II.11) ध्यानहेयास्तद्वृत्तयः ॥

dhyāna-heyās tad-vṛttayaḥ

Their gross activities are to be done away with through the meditation process.

1.30 (II.12) क्लेशमूलः कर्माशयो दृष्टादृष्टजन्मवेदनीयः ॥

kleśa-mūlaḥ karmāśayo dṛṣṭādṛṣṭa-janma-vedanīyaḥ

This reservoir of *karma* itself has its roots in these five hindrances and must come to fruition in this life or the next.

1.31 (II.13) सतिमूले तद्विपाको जात्यायुर्भोगाः ॥

sati mūle tad-vipāko jāty-āyur-bhogāḥ

So long as the roots (or *Saṃskāra*) exist, their function will be birth, life, and experience that result in pleasure or pain.

1.32 (II.14) ते ह्लादपरितापफलाः पुण्यापुण्यहेतुत्वात् ॥

te hlāda-paritāpa-phalāḥ puṇyāpuṇya-hetutvāt

Birth, life, and experiences produce pleasure or pain according to their originating cause (the seeds) being good or evil.

1.33 (II.15)

परिणामतापसंस्कारदुःखैर्गुणवृत्तिविरोधाच्च दुःखमेव सर्वं विवेकिनः ॥

pariṇāma-tāpa-saṁskāra-duḥkhair guṇavṛtti-virodhāc ca duḥkham eva sarvam vivekinaḥ

To the illumined person with discrimination, all existence (on the three planes) is painful owing to the activities of the *guṇa* over time and space.

1.34 (II.18) प्रकाशक्रियास्थितिशीलम्भूतेन्द्रियात्मकं भोगापवगार्थं दृश्यम् ॥

prakāśa-kriyā-sthiti-śīlaṁ bhūtendriyātmakaṁ bhogāpavargārthaṁ dṛśyaṁ

That which is experienced, the world of matter, has three coexisting qualities: *sattva, rajas*, and *tamas* (revealing, mobile, and inert). Experiencing consists of the five basic elements and the sense organs. Their mutual engagement produces experience and eventual liberation.

1.35 (II.19) विशेषाविशेषलिङ्गमात्रालिङ्गानि गुणपर्वाणि ॥

viśeṣāviśeṣa-liṇgamātrāliṇgāni guṇa-parvāṇi

The states of the *guṇa* are experienced on all three planes and beyond.

Chapter Two: *Śiṣya* (Disciple) and a Vision

2nd Milestone

By knowing the thinking process you become aware of your mind. In your reflections you start recognizing the conditioning that mind brings to your thinking. Gradually, you can separate the layers of conditioning to recognize subtle aspects of things in general and the subtle corrupting forces within your body-mind, in particular. Now, you get some idea of an absolutely unblemished, condition-free, virtual universal mind, the "mother" mind that knows everything and brings to life every single space.

But the most striking discovery you make is how the subtle is instrumental in the conception and creation of everything gross. In fact, you grasp the big picture and know why the gross emerges out of the subtle. Objects do not remain inert anymore for you when their subtle antecedent is recognized and you deal with the second hypothesis that *the subtle mind progressively unfolds into grosser and grosser matter; thus mind becomes matter.*

To take one's own self as the center of the Universe and consider everything else as "not-self" is our natural response. This automated response is embedded in our perceptions. As a seeker, an unsettling realization occurs now that it is not so. In Yoga, awareness is the key. Even after embarking on the Yoga journey, it is not often clear what you are doing, and more importantly, why. The *yogīk* path appears to veer away from so-called "normal, everyday life," demanding a change in your habitual thinking and that does not come easily. It is not a smooth ride from a polarizing "I" to a coalescing whole. In normal life, there are ups and downs, pain and pleasure, but at least one is at home with it. But on a seemingly pious *yogīk* path, the mind occasionally acts in a cunning fashion, the senses repeatedly draw into a vortex of gratification and a struggle to remain on the path leads to pain. Added to that pain is the guilt for straying from the path. Any pain is perhaps an initial wake-up call from the spiritual Self. However, the pleasure-seeking brain keeps lurching outward to the objects via the senses. Since experiencing the world is possible only through a mind engaged with the brain, this outward mode prevails.

On the "home" front, the connection between physical breathing and subtle mind modifications is no more a mystery. Your understanding of the thinking process, and how the mind encounters the obstacles and hindrances, make you rely more and more upon the proper breathing processes that, in your experience, go hand in hand with a willed control of thoughts. At this opportune stage, a set of Yoga methods (refinement exercises) and practices[17] (restraints, observances, postures, and breathing exercises) are introduced to equip you for the Yoga journey.

These Yoga methods and practices, as noted above, are complementary and need to be concurrently undertaken, a necessity that is often ignored or not known. Only *together* do they bring about purification and the inner evolution. Bodies have to serve as a dependable conduit for the energy generated by the exercises. A diligent practice yields certain abilities and powers that are intended to support an advanced practice on the subtler plane.

The Yoga regimen is laid out very well in *Yoga-Sūtra*, with certain qualifying bars at each milestone. Each exercise and practice starts out as a simple activity that eventually requires an immense

---

[17] *Yama, niyama, āsana* and *prāṇāyāma.*

number of tiny steps toward its perfection. Progress is sensed subtly when a new reality dawns as a harbinger of the next milestone.

At that stage, your consciously controlled thoughts are uncluttered and even-paced, eventually allowing a gap between two thoughts. This gap provides a small window for direct perception to occur unaided by mind. When "mind" is consciously withdrawn from the thinking process, you reach a very important breakthrough that gently opens a window to the "beyond." That transforms a seeker into a disciple who passionately embraces Yoga methods and practices as a way of life.

Inner Evolution from a Seeker to a Disciple

Yoga hypothesis	The subtle mind progressively unfolds into grosser and grosser matter; thus mind becomes matter
Know through experience	Subtle-to-gross hierarchy
Involuntary control	A "pause"
Achieve Voluntary control	*Pratyāhāra*
Become	A seeker with a vision
Be	A disciple

New words used in this chapter

Granthī	A knot that hinders a smooth flow of *prāṇa* energy.
Mūlādhāra chakra	The first of the seven main chakras. It is located at the perineum. Chakras are energy centers.
Swādhisthāna chakra	The second main chakra. It is located at the base of the reproductive organ.
Chitta	The mind-stuff.
Dhāraṇā	Concentration in the subjective mode.
Dhyāna	Meditation in the subjective mode.
Samādhi	Contemplation in the subjective mode.

Saṃyama	A state of *dhāraṇā*, *dhyāna*, and *samādhi* occurring at once and not linearly.
Suṣumna	A very subtle *nadī* that serves as a channel not just for the sense impulses but also for *prāṇa* to rise.

Methods, the Preliminary Exercises

Knowing the overall Yoga map, you are becoming equipped with the tools for the expedition. The Yoga **practices** of *yama*, *niyama*, *āsana*, and *prāṇayāma*, would bring about a structural change in your body/mind constitution. Purified physical, astral, and causal bodies would become a smooth vehicle for unhindered energy flows to support elevated awareness and to restrain mind modifications. Consequently, your own three *guṇa* compositions would become more and more harmonized to deter the gratification-seeking lower-nature impulses from entering your thought process.

But even before introducing the practices, some preliminary practices, called **methods,** need to be introduced first. They consist of the basic building blocks— rhythmic breathing, upgrading awareness, and the internal purification processes.

The practices are not a cinch. Consequently, from a life of comforts and consumption, you cannot suddenly start a demanding practice routine requiring adaptability and flexibility that the body-mind is not fully ready for. The experience of a good farmer is that even if the proper rains fall and the seeds are sown in the ground at the proper time, there may be years of no harvest. And the good farmer learns the hard way that preparing the soil—digging deep and making furrows in the soil, breaking large lumps of soil, and removing all weeds (refining and upgrading)—was essential. If the soil was not prepared, the weeds would destroy the harvest. In a similar vein, Sage Pātañjali says that the practices and methods in themselves do not cause illumination, but they do remove inner impurities and obstacles like *granthī*. Like the wise and experienced farmer who prepares the soil, we too must prepare our bodies for the spiritual harvest to come.

Hence, these Yoga practices require you to be *ready* for change. The body-mind system ordinarily resists change. The practices enforce a demanding curriculum for breathing, the postures, and the behavior for which you may be *willing* but not battle-ready. Hence, the following preparatory methods are prescribed as a warm-up, stepping stones designed to support the eightfold Yoga practices. Let us see how they work.

- **Rhythmic Breathing** converts your normal breathing into the initial alignment with *prāṇa.*
- **Upgrading of Awareness Exercises** provide a glimpse of Yoga's transforming process and make your awareness more fluid.
- **Refining Exercises** purify the body-mind system and prepare it for the demands of Yoga practices.

Rhythmic Breathing

After explaining how mind modifications prevent the soul-union from happening, and how the obstacles frustrate any efforts to restrain them, the first *yogīk* method, called rhythmic breathing, is introduced, since **the peace of mind is *also* brought about by the expiration and retention of *prāṇa*** (Sūtra 2.1/ I.34). Breathing is a great tool that we are all naturally gifted with; a means for controlling *prāṇa.* But we waste this tool through sheer ignorance and abuse. Hard as it is to believe, life's fundamental solutions are apparently as simple and cheap as correct breathing. Hard . . . only because we are not ready to venture into trying it.

Prāṇa control has been used as a synonym for "breath control" almost universally. It is difficult to understand how breath—a *process* (of inhalation and exhalation)—is the same as *prāṇa*—the energy or *substance.* It makes sense and is correct to say that "regulated breathing" would bring about desired "changes in *prāṇa* energy." So, they are connected but not the same.[18]

---

[18] *"[T]he science of breath helps the student to bring* prana *under control in order to attain the higher rungs of spirituality. He who has controlled his breath and prana has also controlled his mind." Swami Rama and others.* Science of Breath, a practical guide, *Honesdale, Penn: The Himalayan Institute Press, 1979, 73.*

Commentators observe in sutra 2.1/I.34 that Patañjali uses the words "expulsion and retention" of *prāṇa*. But, as expulsion and retention are primary designations of the movements of breath, the commentators offer that the reference could be only to "breath." Since the concept of multi-layered objects tells us that *prāṇa* forms a sheath between the physical body and the astral body, is it so difficult to realize an important distinction: air is breathed by the physical body while *prāṇa* is breathed by the astral body? *Prāṇa* is the universal energy that manifests itself as motion or force in the universe and does the same in an individual. In effect, *prāṇa* is the vitality behind ordinary breath (of air).

> *Citta (the mind-stuff) is the engine which draws in prāṇa from the surroundings and manufactures from prāṇa all the vital forces in the body that run through the nervous system and keep it preserved and also other forces like thoughts and will.* —Swāmī Vivekānanda, 151.

We have observed earlier that regulated breathing can pacify mind modifications. Now let us add another dimension to it—the rate of breathing. The rate is twofold:

- Duration of inhalation in relation to exhalation, together forming one **breath cycle**
- **Number** of such breath cycles per minute.

If the physical-air breathing is made rhythmic, and that rhythm is synchronized with the rate of *prāṇa* breathing, this also regulates the vital forces in the body. Rhythmic and synchronized breathing tames the senses, regulates the flow of sense data, which in turn pacifies the erratic thought process, and helps reduce mind modifications. Then the uncluttered mind is energized and more focused. Thus, regulated breathing of air and *prāṇa* resolves the second obstacle, *mental inertia*.

The discipline of *prāṇayāma* contains various methods of regulating *prāṇa*. The latter-day commentators of *Yoga-Sūtra* and some Yoga innovators have added many improvised methods of breath/*prāṇa* control that are not mentioned here. Sage Pātañjali is highlighting the cardinal relationship between *prāṇa* breathing and peace of mind. It is vital for us to grasp this. At a deeper level and in the given context, Sage Pātañjali shows the right *prāṇayāma*.

Since the thought-chatter works unceasingly, our efforts to pacify also need to be unceasing. All the improvised methods of *prāṇayāma* involving regulated expulsion and retention of breath are deliberate and labored actions that cannot be done continuously (24/7) by a normal person. Hence, *c***onverting one's normal breathing itself into Rhythmic Breathing does that trick**. Now the question is, what should be that rhythm of breathing? The rhythm should be such that the breathing of air can *synchronize* with the breathing of *prāṇa*. That's the great secret. By doing so, one achieves significant results that are threefold in nature:

- Internal *prāṇa* is automatically regulated because it is coupled with the regulated normal air-breathing.
- Mind modifications are arrested through the regulated *prāṇa*–breathing.
- This is unceasing and done with only *slight effort,* as intended (Sūtra 2.21/II.47).

Rhythmic Breathing is to be consciously practiced during the learning phase, and eventually gets automated in the form of a reflex body function. This rhythm seems to be derived from these three phenomena:

- The **diaphragm** pulsates in rhythm for a correct physical-air breathing (mainly for the intake of oxygen),
- The **heart** pulsates in rhythm for blood circulation and purification, and
- The **perineum** (*mūlādhāra chakra*) pulsates in rhythm for the *prāṇa* interchange.

These are all linked. The physical body is joined to the astral body at the perineum. At full rest, a healthy heart pulse is 60 a minute.

To sum up, Rhythmic Breathing has to be done with the chest as well as upper abdomen (to involve the diaphragm), it should be synchronized with the perineum's pulse cycles of 3 counts (seconds) of inhalation and 2 (seconds) of exhalation, making 12 breath-cycles a minute.

However, it cannot be overemphasized that a true regulation of breathing is achieved only gradually. A human breathing apparatus (lungs, connecting muscles, and the diaphragm) is generally abused for years due to massive swings in emotions, mind modifications, residues from unhealthy food habits, and an overall anxiety-driven life-style. It is an arduous task to resist the groove. Hence, in sustaining rhythmic breathing over a good length of time one would need an accompanying Yoga life-style that is regulated (an external and internal purification of the body through *yama* and *niyama*, and *āsana*). Only that kind of body will render a breathing apparatus strong enough.

The method of **Rhythmic Breathing** is given in Appendix 1. An essence of this method has been derived from sūtras I.12, 13, 14, 31, 34; II.46, 47, 48, 49, 50.

Upgrading of Awareness

Now Sage Pātañjali introduces the core of Yoga methodology, how to upgrade and elevate awareness from gross to subtle for *higher* sense activity, so as to make the normal sensing redundant. Normal perception is driven by the five senses and is completely captivated by the *guṇa* theatrics. The mind acts as the *sixth* sense for this perception to happen. Any perception beyond *guṇa* influence is possible only if the mind remains just a catalyst, as it is intended to be. Such perception would be direct, and hence without the coloring, conditioning or complicity with *guṇa*, and bring peace to the mind. **Such perception is higher and beyond sense perception** (Sūtra 2.2/I.35).

To offer a glimpse of such a direct perception, a preliminary method of upgrading awareness is prescribed here. This method prepares the practitioner for the use of other advanced practices, which would eventually lead to direct perception as a controlled process. In fact, by themselves the five senses are only input vehicles and do not create any perception. It is when the mind is involved that normal sensory perception results. But ordinarily, as long as the mind is not under one's control, that kind of perception does not create any real knowledge. Upgrading Awareness as a preliminary method is a form of simulated concentration that lets the mind stand aside, purely as a catalyst, so that the selected object is perceived directly; and thus the level of awareness is upgraded.

Yoga is a journey into subtleness. Words of authority from the masters can only explain the true nature of things *as they are*, and you may even understand this intellectually. But if even a part of it is not imbibed through your own experience, doubts may still prevail and *wrong questioning* (an obstacle) may still result. This exercise of Upgrading Awareness is designed to provide the seeker with an experience as an answer to thousand potential questions.

Unfortunately, many writers have interpreted this Sūtra in a very crude manner.

> *[W]hen one concentrates on the tip of one's nose, one gets a sensation of supernormal smell (like perfume); attention fixed on the tip of the tongue leads to the sensation of a supernormal taste (flames); on the palate, to the sensation of supernormal sight (pictures, vision); on the middle of the tongue, sensation of a supernormal touch (vibration); and on the root of the tongue, to the supernormal hearing (sound).*—M. R. Yārdi, 140.

Some of these analogies (smell: perfume; taste: flames; sight: visions) are expressed with entirely different symbols in occult semantics.[19] But a lay reader can be justifiably fascinated by the above style of interpretation, which sounds so exotic and esoteric. Unfortunately, the crux is completely lost in the process. Interpretations such as this run the risk of creating mythical impressions about Yoga. Such impressions may also mislead an aspiring seeker to imagine that Yoga is out of step with our normal life.

A direct perception as if through the sixth sense happens in a moment (or flash) when the individual mind separates from and is not involved with the brain processes that rely entirely on the five senses. Only then can the mind perceive the object as it is. Sage Pātañjali is assuring us that once the awareness is upgraded,

---

[19] *For more details please refer to Alice Bailey, 79-80.*

such a direct perception does not remain an involuntary flash but becomes a conscious process providing mastery over the unrestrained mental states. Thus, to this extent, the mind can be trained to become steady.[20]

Once a conscious use of mind as the sixth sense is possible, then life changes dramatically. Breathing and chaotic thinking slows down enormously and is increasingly rhythmic. There is a progressive widening of gaps between two thoughts. Every time this happens *inner peace* is experienced. Your structure of predispositions changes for the better. You succumb less to the compulsive automatic reflex thoughts. A positive, upward spiral is launched in the *karma* cycles because there is less germination of pain-producing *karma* seeds. This is how **"pain which is yet to come is warded off"** (Sūtra II.16). But more about that later.

The method of **Upgrading of Awareness** is given in Appendix 2. An essence of this method has been derived from sūtras I.35, 41; II.17, 25, 53, 54, 55; III.1, 12, 15, 17.

Refining Exercises

Sage Pātañjali now introduces the refining exercises for preparing the seeker for advanced *prāṇayāma.* As we will see later, *yama*, the five abstentions, are behavioral and they tackle the external triggers of mind modifications. *Niyama*, the five observances of life, are self-regulatory and address the internal triggers. Conventionally, it is believed that one starts on the eightfold *yogīk* path with *yama* and *niyama*. But changing the behavior and self-regulation can never sustain unless your gross body is in tandem with the subtle body that holds the key. Our life-style offers a hostile environment for *yama* and *niyama*, making these initial practices

---

[20] *The seeker's learning avenues on the Yoga path are multiple and varied. While learning, it is up to the seeker to quickly synthesize the seemingly disparate threads from one's own experience and braid them into a new reality. For example, it is not a small coincidence that the roots of the five senses are found in the mouth, which is one's instrument of producing sound. And we realize that words are only a form of sound. One important understanding that eventually develops regarding this ability to create proper sound is that in this creation lies a key to all the creative processes of the world that yield a control over all that is created. Mantra and its proper chanting is hence very important.*

such a struggle that *dhāraṇā-dhyāna-samādhi* may appear almost impossible.[21]

The *prāṇa* sheath connects the gross and the subtle bodies and sustains them; hence, we work on it to achieve harmony between the two bodies. Sage Pātañjali has provided a solution for a sincere seeker in the form of Refining Exercises that purify and unclog the *prāṇa*-path of the chakras. On the face of it, the refining exercises appear to be mere body movements. But the associated breathing is used as a connector between the gross and the subtle, and that puts these exercises in a totally different genre. Together, they provide a launch-pad for *yama* and *niyama*.

The gross and the subtle bodies are ordinarily just "next to each other." These vibrant structures need to be connected and positively synchronized, too. Engrossed in the physical, we not only ignore the subtle body but also end up damaging it in the hassles of daily living. It needs healing. Most of the diseases that manifest in the physical body (the effect) really originate in the wounds and scars of the subtle body (the cause). Thus, ordinarily the subtle body remains primary only in this negative sense. Healing of the subtle body enables the gross and the subtle to work in tandem, causing a polar shift in our awareness, and makes the subtle body primary in an affirmative sense.

Awareness itself needs energy. But elevating awareness needs another kind of fine energy, that of "will," which is ordinarily uncultivated and neutral. Energies are constantly replenished. But, lack of understanding and a weak will make the replenishment

---

[21] *Sūtra II.34, 35, and 37 point to a common goal that can be achieved in different ways and should be read as one single statement. That is why it is necessary to interpret Sūtra II.37 more contextually than literally. A literal translation becomes vague and confusing because it runs along these lines: "[M]editate on the heart (of an enlightened soul) that has given up all attachment to sense-objects." It is indeed noble to respect the enlightened souls. Their lives are full of examples of rightful behavior worth emulating. But* Yoga-Sūtra *is not written in that fashion. It consistently maintains that anything external provides only limited help and that real spiritual progress arises only from self-realization. So such translations make this sūtra inconsistent with the rest. No other sūtra externalizes Yoga practice.*

Yoga is all about refinement and aims at a state that is so advanced that the seeker eventually remains virtually separate from the physical and psychic bodies, completely free of any desire for any object. The only desire left is to be one with Īśvara. *(This* sūtra *refers to the* swādhisthān chakra, *the sacral center. Control of this center is vital to becoming free of desires).*

a passive rather than a deliberate or controlled process. We have already seen how regulated breathing calms the thinking instrument; a stronger, more energized will facilitates the regulated, rhythmic breathing.

Thus, **the mind needs to be stabilized and rendered passionless as the lower (sex-dominated) nature is refined, purified and is no longer indulged in** (Sūtra 2.3/I.37). Though rhythmic breathing calms the thinking instruments, the real source of mind agitations lies elsewhere. As long as the source is not tackled, the calming effect remains temporary. The source of mind agitations is thoughts (on the astral plane) that emanate from desires (on the causal plane). You need to cultivate a conscious will to obliterate desires, and that needs subtle energy. The Refining Exercises help to:

- Create higher subtle energies by transforming the lower ones or by refining them.
- Provide energies to reactivate the *chakras*, the energy centers in the subtle body.
- Remove obstacles to synchronization of the subtle and the physical bodies.
- Prepare ground for inner communication with soul for guidance in fortifying the practice of *yama* and *niyama.*

The method of **Refining Exercises** is given in Appendix 3. An essence of this method has been derived from sūtras I.2, 15, 16; II.35, 36, 37, 38, 39, 40, 41, 42, 43.

Secondary Means of Yoga

Why do we call Yoga transformational? In Yoga, as you reach a certain milestone, a new one appears on the horizon. But the journey is not just from one stage to another. On the way, almost as a precondition, everything about you changes. You are transforming in every nanosecond. The cell-level changes alter your personality, which manifests itself in profound changes in your self-view and the world-view. The world of matter is seen as the world of mind, and when even the mind is transcended, the self is realized as nothing else but Self, the soul. How do we reach spiritual enlightenment, the pinnacle of Yoga? In realization that it is the Universal Mind that has rolled out—across eternity—a subtle-to-gross universe of matter that surrounds us in the form of objects, persons, and events.

The en*light*enment is literally so.

> *First seen by the mind's eye as a spark, it steadily grows into a flame. To a human being composed of three layers, this light is like the physical sun in the solar system and it grows in effulgence, eventually becoming a blaze of glory.*
> —Excerpt from Alice Bailey, 179-80.

Referring back to the inner evolution, it must be remembered that Yoga practices cause change on the cellular, molecular, and electronic planes in the brain, *mānas,* and *buddhi* as well as in the body structures respectively. **When the eightfold Yoga has been steadily practiced and when impurity has been overcome, spiritual enlightenment culminates into full illumination** (Sūtra 2.4/II.28). And of course, this does not happen overnight or accidentally; the culmination is a steady progression consciously brought about by the deliberate following and perseverance of Yoga practices (of this or in previous birth/s).[22] So, what is the eight-fold *yogīk* path?

The Eightfold Yogīk *Path*

The path leading to self-realization is *aṣṭānga* eightfold. How does the self-realization occur?

The eightfold Yoga practices ultimately eliminate the causes for the five states of mind modifications, making all the soul-eclipsing inner impurities wither away. Even correct knowledge, a long-cherished goal of successful living, is now seen as limited, and instead, true knowledge is seen manifesting unhindered from direct perception. To shake off your anchor in derived/correct knowl-

---

[22] *As one approaches illumination, as explained in Chapter Five, the vital airs and forces are reorganized and act directly on the pineal and pituitary glands. The illumination is experienced in the form of light in the region around the pineal gland (referred to by many as the third eye and the eighth* chakra*).*

edge you need courage that comes only from first-hand experience of the potency of true knowledge.

The effulgence of knowledge grows as impurities vanish, making an individual mind as omniscient as the Universal Mind. Finally, a state of illumination occurs when discriminating knowledge that creates an artificial and relatively untrue difference between your "self and not-self (the rest of the world)" makes way for discerning knowledge.

The discerning knowledge dissects each object (including your own self) with an awareness of Self as distinct from not-Self, the Spirit distinct from matter. You witness with this raised awareness an amazing connectivity in all objects, with the inherent Self as the common link. This knowledge is discerning—neither theoretical nor dogmatic, but experiential—and it would steer you successfully through the worldly activities since your "I" stance dissolves in the process.

Yoga philosophy is inclusive. As mentioned again and again in the *Yoga-Sūtra*, the elevation of awareness is not accomplished by abandoning the lower self even when subtle bodies are discovered, purified and aligned. Instead, awareness expands and brings you face to face with the mystery of subtle life. A practitioner should realize that a causal body is as conscious an experience for a *yogī* as a normal physical body is for a seeker. Patience is needed until that actually happens. And however gross it is, a seeker needs a physical body for the eight-fold practices.

The eight limbs of Yoga are: (Sūtra 2.5/II.29)

1. The five abstentions (*yama*)
2. The five observances (*niyama*)
3. The posture (*āsana*)
4. Right control of *prāṇa,* the life-force (*prāṇayāma*)
5. The abstraction (*pratyāhāra*)
6. Concentration (leading to *dhāraṇā*)
7. Meditation (leading to *dhyāna*)
8. Contemplation (leading to *samādhi*)

Sage Pātañjali has chosen to introduce the eightfold *yogīk* path only now, after you have sufficiently tilled the ground and made it fertile with the refining exercises. Otherwise, even *yama* and *niyama* that apparently need no "learning," may seem, in their truest sense, difficult to follow and adopt as a way of life. That's the reason why so much effort has been invested in the first chapter in preparing the conceptual foundation, and now, in describing methods leading to this vision of Yoga.

Please see the complete picture of the *yogīk* path carefully (*Figure 2.1*) as it radically departs from its conventional version:

- The first four limbs *yama, niyama, āsana, prāṇayāma* are for a concurrent practice until *pratyāhāra*—the breakthrough; after which *dhāraṇā, dhyāna, samādhi* follow linearly.
- Concentration leads to *dhāraṇā*, meditation leads to *dhyāna*, and contemplation leads to *samādhi;* they are not pairs of synonyms.

The continuous rhythmic breathing creates a red carpet over which the practices accelerate the spiritual progress. A beginner is well advised to first master the methods (rhythmic breathing, upgrading awareness, and refining exercises). When you are fairly regular, you can commence the first four limbs of Yoga concurrently. They are preparatory and secondary means of Yoga. They are complementary as real success accrues only as their cumulative result. This is why one can go only so far in the practice of popular Yoga, the "fitness" version of *āsana* and *prāṇayāma*, while long-lasting peace and happiness may remain elusive unless the practice is supported by *yama* and *niyama*, which incidentally are not some vague directives. These behavioral instructions comprehensively sum up all those events and experiences that can obstruct a process of purification of the bodies and support the huge, real and permanent change Yoga brings to your life.

On this eightfold path, the importance of non-attachment in *pratyāhāra* is enormous. It is a breakthrough point after the cumulative success of the first four limbs. The fundamental non-attachment between the mind and the brain occurs here when the mind remains a catalyst and does not attach itself to the thinking process. Our normal thinking process, driven as it is by myriad incoming impulses, is indispensable on the physical plane. Only a trained and tuned mind can be gradually willed to stay non-attached. These moments of non-attachment pave the way for a steady vision of the spiritual Self. Eventually, one loses any desire for object-induced gratification and there is a physical non-attachment toward objects, in the form of relaxed indifference.

After *pratyāhāra*, the three remaining limbs represent advanced states and processes. These three limbs are, in a sense, the Primary Means of Yoga. While the secondary means are practiced concurrently, the primary means occur linearly. Many authors use the word "concentration" to mean *dhāraṇā*. But, there is a differ-

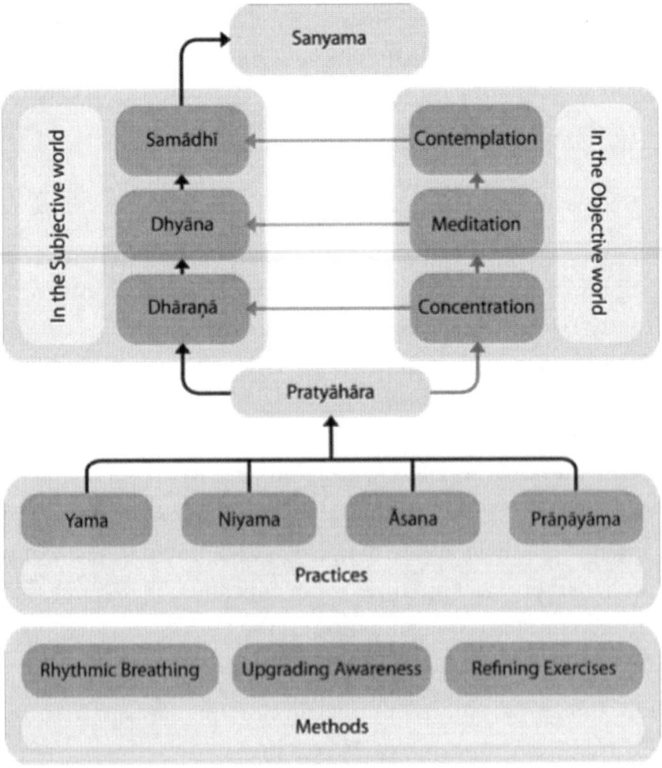

Figure 2.1: The Yoga Schematic (Path)

ence between concentration that occurs in the objective context and *dhāraṇā* that happens in a direct perception mode. The same applies to the other two stages of *dhyāna* and *samādhi*. This important point is often lost in translation.

Pratyāhāra is a take-off experience that suspends the object-dominated reflex thinking and enables direct perception to yield intuitive knowledge not ordinarily accessible. Physical, emotional, intellectual response and even *objective thinking* are still mind-assisted processes. So even when the skills of concentration, meditation, and contemplation are honed in the objective domain, the *pratyāhāra* take-off is needed, eventually, to launch the same skills as *dhāraṇā, dhyāna*, and *samādhi* in the direct perception mode. The latter three are substantially different and much harder to achieve.

However, achieving *samādhi* is not the end of the path. While becoming a *yogī* and *mahāyogī* you will have to continue with the rigorous practice of *saṃyama*—a state of *dhāraṇā*, *dhyāna*, and *samādhi* occurring at once and not linearly. The initial experiences of *samādhi* are prompted by a desire to remain in the *Īsvara* consciousness. That is still a *desire*. Finally, you have to give up even that last desire and just await a state of *samādhi*, the ultimate Union, a state of spiritual enlightenment, illumination, or total absorption.

If the description above creates a picture of a regimented exercise routine that promises to deliver such and such results in a certain timeframe, it is a misconception. It needs to be understood that on the yogic path *you will undergo* a transformation. *Yama-Niyama*, for example, though deliberate efforts initially, should change into effortless restraints and reflex observances. Only in this way do you really master them. In fact, as Sathya Sai Baba always says, in true *yama,* restraints would hardly leave traces of deprivation; in fact, one would abide in the consciousness that needs no restraint, and observances would rather become offerings of love to *Īsvara* whose characteristics are inherent in true *niyama.* **The eightfold path itself is an embodiment of Yoga's basic premise: what appear as eight different "limbs" are ultimately One in essence**!

So, on this Yoga path let us look at the first "limb."

Yama

***Yama*, the five abstentions** (Sūtra 2.6/II.30) are:

- *Ahimsā*, abstention from harming
- *Satya*, abstention from untruth
- *Asteya*, abstention from theft
- *Brahmacrya*, abstention from indulgence
- *Aparigraḥ*, abstention from avarice.

These abstentions imply a change in behavior. In ordinary parlance, these are simply general canons of external good behavior, nothing great about them. But what makes these harder in Yoga is their intended absoluteness in compliance, which is often contrary to the hesitation and favoritism we use in judging our own actions. External changes are temporary and cosmetic unless backed by a change in the thinking that promotes behavior. Moreover, since ordinary thinking is mostly reactive, for such behavior to be spontaneous the real change has to be in the very structure of your predispositions.

Though the abstentions invite generous interpretations, what is prescribed in *Yoga-Sūtra* is not vague, but rather calls for *total compliance*. Harmlessness, for example, has to be in deed as well as in thought, and has to be complete. Achieving this will require an expansive concept and strict adherence, stopping short of nothing. While putting such a concept in practice, there may be apparent conflicts with the other abstentions. In order to save someone from harm, you may be required to speak a little untruth. Here is a classic example in the Indian context: "You are threatened by a gang of robbers. They ask you which way a marriage procession has just passed. The completely truthful answer will greatly harm some innocent people in the procession. And an attempt to save them will require telling an untruth." Here, truth jeopardizes harmlessness! You have to choose.

Obviously, we will continue to fail in the abstentions if our compliance remains only physical (superficial). Yoga would have been another religion if this behavior was ordained for a blind compliance. Instead, at every juncture your thought-watching should create awareness about the pangs and drifts that pull you away from compliance of *yama-niyama*. Then a realization should follow about how that shortfall affected your purification process. A genuine realization leaves you re-dedicated to the total compliance by trying even harder. But most significantly you remain self-motivated in that effort. This eliminates all useless concepts of sin and punishment or god-fearing or god-flattering blind faith.

Later advancement in *dhāraṇā* and *dhyāna* alone will enable you to understand and to comply at the emotional and spiritual (deeper) levels as well. *Yama* and *niyama* cannot be lived automatically and mechanically. Any apparent contradictions at a lower level will also be resolved through awareness of the big picture from a refined thinking process.

But such a complete overhaul of the thinking process comes in stages. It takes a while before we can do the proverbial "out-of-the-box" thinking. The "big picture" thinking takes even longer, as it often seems unfashionable and materially useless. "Spiritual" thinking is almost absurd to the conventional wisdom. Moreover, the world's warring religions have monopolized and hijacked spiritual thinking for ages. Non-violence has to start with tolerance toward contrary ideas and beliefs.

The abstentions ask for compliance at all three levels. Harmlessness, truth, and abstention from theft are actuated on the physical level; abstention from indulgence ("having no lust") is actuated at the astral level, and abstention from avarice is actuated at the causal level.

The greatest challenge in today's material world is "abstention from indulgence" especially when it is more commonly interpreted as "sexual indulgence." It is true that the animal traits in humans, aggravated by modern-day materialism, have placed sex on such a high pedestal that instead of being regarded only as a means of reproduction, it has become an end in itself. Many modern-day psychologists have also placed sex at center-stage in all their diagnoses, as if sex were the fulcrum of human life.

Sage Pātañjali is not recommending vows of celibacy or running away from one's duties. An expanded concept of indulgence is "indulgence of a mind gravitating toward the gratification of the senses." This renders the aspect of sex as "just one avenue" and of only *kārmik* significance. In other words, a couple may discharge its *kārmik* duty of bearing children but keep it just that, a duty. In abstaining from indulgence, Sage Pātañjali is asking us to be desire-less toward every kind of gratification.

Yamas *Are a Universal Mandate*

Each *Yama* is a universal duty, irrespective of race[23], place, time or circumstances (Sūtra 2.7/II.31). The *Yoga-Sūtra* is direct and a "no-nonsense" guidebook. It addresses the whole of humanity and belongs to it by transcending any religion or anthems of morality. Sage Pātañjali says that compliance with the abstentions has to be absolutely total—nothing short of complete—with no exceptions whatsoever, for any shortfall leaves the purification process incomplete.

In today's world, you are conditioned to believe in what is fashionable. One's intellect can find thousand ways of defending anything. Patriotism defends wars, religious interpretations rationalize killings, freedom of speech protects absurdity, retribution justifies aggression, and love proxies for lust. However, in *Yama* abstentions, there is no room for any excuse, however smart, compelling, and politically expedient it may sound.

Excuses make very stealthy inroads. By nature, a human mind can only understand the world in black or white, compulsively ignoring many nuances and thus creating a fragmented reality. A material mind must define and distinguish material objects in order to possess and control them. Isn't it true that you constantly foster a fond identity for yourself through thought or action by distinguishing yourself from others along those lines? Well, groups, communities, nations, and races, do the same. Skin color, language, nationality, likes, and dislikes are all defining, but also

---

[23] *Many authors have preferred a literal translation of the Sanskṛt word* "jāti" *as the caste. If the* sutra *is talking about* yama *being a "universal" mandate, it is unlikely that the intended meaning is caste, a pervert interpretation that plagued centuries in India. Reference is obviously to "the way you are born" and a more appropriate generalized term like "race" needs to be used.*

dividing features. Place and time create historical contexts for all human experiences; but some of them resurrect as "history" to become a cause célèbre. Together, they build insurmountable walls of traditions, norms, customs, beliefs, and cultures that provide passionate justification for exceptions to the abstentions and even lend them legitimacy. Thus, a country might have artificial boundaries but its people create "real" boundaries of unquestionable patriotic history, and sing ballads of victory that marginalize death and misery once inflicted on the defeated. And lastly, emergencies and exigencies are always the compelling "super-valid" excuses, but excuses nonetheless! Sage Pātañjali maintains that any seemingly valid excuse still renders the compliance defective and incomplete. With such a strict compliance of Yama, Yoga begins with a very demanding obligation.

Compliance of Yama

Exceptions and excuses are products of the thinking process. Is fiery aspiration alone enough to overcome such rebellious coups of thoughts that are contrary to Yoga? No; but through practice, **when thoughts contrary to Yoga are present there should be cultivation of their opposite thoughts** (Sūtra 2.8/II.33).

Thoughts always wander, proliferate and gather emotional accretions while they drift. Sometimes the assault of contrary thoughts is so sudden and powerful that an unprepared seeker gets swept away. In anticipation of such an assault, you need to practice *drift watching* and develop a quick-response mechanism.

In order to watch a thought-drift, you have to first become aware of such drifting. Thoughts keep us immersed with their emotional webs. In becoming aware of a drift, you stand aside of the flow of thoughts. The first tangible benefit is that it breaks the runaway thought-chain. Then you have to pick up the most recent thought and retrace the thread backward, along the entire trail up to the point where the thought-drift occurred. Another immediate effect of this practice is that the proliferation of further thoughts is arrested. It allows space for you to reflect on the nature of the thoughts and to review how the drift-chain flourished. You can also detect certain patterns in the drifts and recognize persistent weaknesses, because specific objects or events would be seen to trigger such drifts more often and more easily for you.

To counter the contrary thoughts, Sage Pātañjali recommends cultivation of positive thoughts, which is then a relatively easy step. Such opposite, positive thoughts become our first responders in aborting a thought-chain in its wild marathon, and help us accomplish this task more quickly at each attempt.

Another important effect of this practice is that, in feeling a need for positive thoughts and in a gradual training of the thought process to generate them, your will is energized. The structure of predispositions stands reorganized. Eventually, it takes much less effort to create positive thoughts.

Rhythmic breathing also helps tremendously. Thoughts contrary to Yoga would create mind modifications and an increased emotional turbulence. This would throw the breathing out of rhythm. With slight effort, rhythmic breathing can be restored and mind modifications restrained.

Thoughts contrary to Yoga are:

- Harmfulness
- Falsehood
- Theft
- Indulgence
- Avarice

It is immaterial whether the contrary thoughts are thoughts in action committed personally, caused to be committed, or even approved of; whether they arise from avarice, anger, or ignorance; or whether they are mild, moderate, or intense. These thoughts will always result in ignorance and pain and such realization is how the opposite thoughts should be cultivated (Sūtra 2.9/II.34).

You may notice that the five *yamas* form pairs of opposites with the contrary thoughts, and may wonder why Sage Pātañjali does this repetition of content, which is so uncharacteristic of him. But, in fact, he sends a much wider and deeper message here.

First, he wants to caution us that following the abstentions (*yama*) is not going to be easy. You may resolutely abide by the abstentions and yet see the contrary thoughts continuing to raid. A determined behavioral change on the physical plane will have to be complemented by the cultivation of positive thoughts. But should positive thoughts be created for each and every contrary thought? If the aim is to reduce mind modifications, creating another wave of thoughts, for whatever pious reason, is not really going to help.

Secondly, one should not just watch out for the contrary thoughts; one should also look for their accomplices, which make a veiled appearance in the form of excuses, justifications, explanations, and concessions. To unguarded mind, the contrary actions—direct, indirect, or tacit—may appear to be of varying degrees of severity. The root cause of the action, for example, avarice, anger, or ignorance, may also provide a perfect justification for the contrary thoughts. And the outcome, varying from mild to moderate to intense, may make the actions less or more culpable. The point is that a thought that is contrary to Yoga still remains the cause, and as such, inevitably brings pain and ignorance.

What is the opposite positive thought? Sage Pātañjali appears to be making a potent but subtle point here that *growing awareness* of all of the above dynamics *is in itself* that positive thought, and, therefore, such a "thought" does not add to the mind modifications. The process itself is the solution. You could yourself think of innumerable examples of how contrary thoughts are formed, what weaknesses trigger them, and how we offer justifications that are always sound enough to condone the error. But awareness can be created consciously only through practice. Thus, instead of reacting to the contrary thoughts as they occur, you can learn to have a swift realization of the impending pain that will act "opposite" to the thoughts contrary to Yoga and help *yama* to rein them in.

Results of Practicing Yama

Enriched awareness ushers you into a new world. The success in *yama* will enhance your new experience and protect you from its pitfalls. The new connectedness that you feel has to translate into a bond with humanity, with nature, the flora and fauna, and any enmity or hate will be a major deterrent in that bonding. But while reaching across to establish this connection, your words and acts should carry enough weight. No personal unfulfilled desire should handicap your extended hand in any measure. In all actions you should free yourself from generating new *karma* by fully realizing how the *karma* seeds impregnate repeated births.

Total compliance of *yama* prepares you for undertaking the primary means of Yoga, as:

- All enmity ceases (with harmlessness)
- Words and acts are effective (with truth)
- Any desire is fulfilled (with abstention from theft)
- Creative energy is acquired (with abstention of indulgence)
- Law of rebirth is understood (with abstention from avarice).

ALL ENMITY CEASES

All enmity ceases for one who has perfected harmlessness (Sūtra 2.10/II.35). To maintain harmlessness is not easy, especially when provoked. Harmlessness is a virtue in the strong, but only a pretense of the weak. Mahatma Gandhi said, "I don't like the non-violence of the coward. Non-violence of the brave alone is non-violence." If harmlessness is to be practiced in totality (as Sage Pātañjali expects of everything said in *Yoga-Sūtra*), it would mean not causing an iota of injury to anything or anyone in thought, word, or deed. Harmlessness has to seep in through every pore in every cell of the complex body/mind system and be at the core of your structure of predispositions.

Today, there is no dearth of public figures parroting harmlessness but invariably harboring contrary thoughts or intentions. The champions of passionate patriotism or religious fundamentalism want us to overlook the collateral damage, an ugly offspring of their actions. In Yoga, there is no room for empty talk. In the end, you either do or do not harm; mere preaching is inconsequential and justification is futile. Some people and nations are still obsessed with an instinctive fear of "enemies" that they need to fight against and vanquish.

But how does enmity end in others? The *yogīk* concept of perception needs to be consistently applied here. You see enmity or hatred in others because, in your own self, the seeds of enmity and hatred are still present. These seeds create vibrations that mirror vibrations in the perceived object. Thus, when others (even animals who are traditionally "enemies") do not see nor sense an iota of harm in a *yogī*, no fear or reaction arises in their minds. Thus, all enmity ceases. Unless this happens, there is a long way to go on the *yogīk* path. Initially grasped only intellectually, this concept is eventually realized as the insight, "We see only what we are ourselves" (Sūtra 5.2.1/III.30).

WORDS AND ACTS ARE EFFECTIVE

Words and acts are effective when truth is perfected (Sūtra 2.11/II.36). All truth is relative, and that creates pairs of opposites until you discover the ultimate truth that has no opposites. On the *yogīk* path, self-realization blossoms by peeling away the layers of degenerating untruth. At any time, the prevailing truth appears to be the ultimate, and you are completely consumed by it. Don't we see all the friction in the world as essentially a clash of two relative truths? The friction also causes varying degrees of harm, and the "relative" untruth creates a shortfall in *yama.*

The final layer of relative untruth is painstakingly and resolutely peeled away when as a seeker you understand the purpose of inner evolution, the difference between the form and the formless, and the laws of *karma.* The very process of perception is understood as the breeder of that untruth, with the more significant realization that it is a product of appearances, woven together through colored thoughts and driven by ego's self-serving desires. On the *yogīk* path then, you move away from the objects-dominated source of fragile truth (physical plane), you witness the transient nature of the verbalized thoughts and realize the limitations of spoken words in capturing the truth (astral plane), and finally you experience the power of sound, the vibrations, from which all that is created has emerged (causal plane). Again, this is not an intellectual inference, but the experienced truth that presents the sound as the creator of right words and actions, or even of silence and inaction. Aimless actions, automated reactions, hollow words, and haunting desires melt away in the wake of this realization. *Then*, whatever such an accomplished *yogī* says, happens. Creation follows sound. Most importantly, at that stage of inner evolution, you (then a *yogī*) would remain unattached to the words as well as the actions.

Ordinarily, such creative powers of Yoga always fascinate people, but the cause of this fascination is a flawed perception. These powers appear magical to those who remain anchored in the physical. Such people fail to understand, first, that the possessor of such powers has already traveled a long enough distance on the *yogīk* path that his or her purpose of life has changed completely. The powers are bestowed under the keen watch of the teacher, with strict caveats for their use, either as an investment in further Yoga pursuit or for promoting some common good. Secondly, that the kārmic laws still apply. Should the powers be used for any material gains that breed desire, this will attract an appropriate consequence. In that case, a *yogī* becomes a seeker again and regresses rapidly, finding it harder and longer to catch up on the *yogīk* path.

ANY DESIRE IS FULFILLED

Any desire is fulfilled when abstention from theft is perfected (Sūtra 2.12/II.37). In *yama*, you are not just supposed to refrain from stealing things tangible and physical; the same restraint has to be shown on the astral and causal planes. Perfection means that:

> *[T]he seeker takes nothing; no emotional benefits, such as love and favor; dislike or hatred are not claimed by him and absorbed when they do not belong to him; intellectual benefits, the claiming of a reputation not warranted, the assumption of someone else's duty, favor or popularity are equally repudiated by him and he adheres with strictness to only that which is his.*—Alice Bailey, 198.

Many translators see "any desire is fulfilled" as "all wealth comes to him." Or "all jewels come to him." Those who think of material riches are sadly holed up in the material world and remain spiritually challenged. However, when you perfect abstention from theft in the sense of denying yourself what is not actually your own (a herculean task in today's world) you have already come a long way. As a result, there is a complete transformation of concepts of what is of value and what is desired, if anything, at all. And *that change* is what you get.[24]

CREATIVE ENERGY IS ACQUIRED

Creative energy and indomitable courage are acquired by abstention from indulgence (Sūtra 2.13/II.38). Of all the abstentions, the one from (sexual) indulgence is the hardest to understand and follow. Sexual impulse is seemingly so intrinsic that suppression of it seems like going against one's very nature. First, let us realize that Sage Pātañjali is not advocating suppression of anything, anytime. However, human sexual impulse that demands gratification is not hardwired to the organs of action as it is in the animals. In humans it begins with a subtle sexual desire and gets personalized, articulated, and amplified through a culture-specific thinking process. That is why in the context of all the contrary thoughts and less-than-desired instincts, Sage Pātañjali always proposes a solution for how to work on the cause not on the effect. When one understands the true nature of thinking, one can isolate and extinguish desires requiring no effort or suppression.

A seeker has however to remember that any need for suppression means that one is not ready yet. Initially, one should only try to avoid the unnecessary amplification of an instinct compelling unusual obsession that one would regret later. Understanding slowly emerges that sex has limited purpose connected with nature's scheme of things. On the spiritual path, a discovery of innate happiness also devalues sex as a source of happiness. Procreation as a means of allowing souls to be born again is understood. Nowhere is hermitage prescribed as the only way to abstain from sexual indulgence. In fact, a normal householder's conscious and

[24] *Interestingly, all cravings create* granthī *at* Maṇipūra chakra. *When this* chakra *is refined, a seeker understands the futility of worldly pleasures and develops an inner sense of joy. That is the real wealth. This sūtra literally translates as "[A]ll jewels or wealth comes to him."* Maṇipūra *literally means "City of Jewels," and once the lower animal nature is obliterated, life truly becomes rich.*

relaxed choice of abstaining and not indulging is more severely tested against the backdrop of more challenging circumstances, and hence fortified.

However, there is a much larger dimension to this concept. Yet unknown to the mainstream science is how energy is created on the astral and causal planes. The food metabolism as a source of energy is known, but the *prāṇa* cycle is less understood. One of the most vital discoveries of Yoga masters is that besides *prāṇa*, the life-force, three other energies exist in a human system—the essence of consciousness, awareness, and the will. A human being is created in such a way that from the moment of birth (from the first breath), two celestial functions get activated:

- **Fusion** at the *Mūlādhāra chakra* to energize the essence of consciousness (creative energy) by combining two or more atomic nuclei into one.
- **Fission** at the *Swādhisthāna chakra* to energize the will (indomitable courage) by splitting the atomic nuclei into two or more parts.

Along with the structural changes and the resultant internal purification, these energies start accumulating in micro units over a fairly long period of time. One of the accomplishments on the *yogīk* path is to be able to recharge the higher centers in the body-mind system through these accumulated energies that rise with *prāṇa* through the main subtle channel called *suṣumna* (along the spinal cord). When they rise and activate other *chakras* it results in the energy of *awareness*. (At the pinnacle of Yoga, the awareness dissolves into consciousness, when the two energies merge). Any indulgence saps the energies and prolongs this process of recharging.

Today's scientific community seems largely unaware of these finer sources of energy built right into the human system. These human energies, coupled with the natural self-diagnostic and immune systems, are capable of preventing almost all diseases and suffering. But where we stand today, a lucrative consumption culture glorifies cures and downplays prevention. There is an all-out effort to stimulate every latent human desire begging for satiation. This is a modern form of slavery stealthily unleashed upon us. It ultimately creates our hypnotized mind-state leading to wasteful consumption and a collective dissipation of human creative energy.

The finer energies are creative. As your identification with the physical self grows during adolescence, the generation of physical energy through food takes prominence over these creative energies, whose fountainheads start rusting and eventually cease to function. They are reactivated only with a conscious access to the subtle bodies and the purifying exercises. Hence, the thoughts and actions created by these energies are initially tilted in favor of the physical, but begin shifting in favor of the spiritual as they become refined. Then, creativity becomes more powerful, and as a seeker you possess seemingly magical powers in your words and deeds.

LAW OF REBIRTH IS UNDERSTOOD

Law of rebirth is understood when abstention from avarice is perfected (Sūtra 2.14/II.39). Avarice needs to be understood as distinct from its narrow meaning of greed and grabbing. Abstention from avarice should be taken to mean absence of all desires and longings. Only abstention from avarice will ensure true contentment.

> *We forge our own chains in the furnace of desire, and of a various longing for things, for experience and for form life. When contentment is cultivated and present, gradually these chains drop off and no others are forged.*
>
> —Alice Bailey, 200.

Abstention should not be achieved by suppressing desires but through an awareness of how desires work. Desire propagates a long chain of attachments that lead only to pain. The law of *karma* tells us that since desire must reach fruition sooner or later, naturally the unfulfilled desires in this life entail another life. This holds a key to the secret of rebirth for the seeker. Desire is the root cause of multiple life-terms requiring rebirth. Abstention from avarice is rewarded with a direct knowledge of your own past lives. This is how the seeker learns about rebirth firsthand.

In realizing how avarice brings unnecessary baggage, you would learn the true meaning of the pursuit of excellence for the sake of excellence, and not by betting your contentment on the achievement of an end.

Niyama

If *yama* are external and behavioral, *niyama* are intrinsic and to be imbibed. Perfection in *niyamas* is a moving target. Some practitioners tend to believe that *niyama* is a preliminary practice and its role diminishes once higher Yoga states like *dhyāna and samādhī* are reached. This belief is partly based on narrow interpretations. "Spiritual reading" for example is often taken as a task of reading spiritual scriptures rather than as a rigorous practice of developing spiritual intelligence.

The nature of *niyama* is so intrinsic that any compliance is possible only by transforming yourself. Physical habits, emotional stances and colored concepts, all need to change. And this process takes forever. Failing to understand this is the other factor in undermining *niyama*.

Hence, *niyama* cannot be simply willed and self-initiated. Achieving full compliance is a difficult prerequisite even for an advanced Yoga practice. At times, such a totality of compliance is more bestowed upon than achieved. It really becomes a *collateral effect* of all Yoga practices and comes as its crowning prize.

***Niyama*, the five observances, are** (Sūtra 2.15/II.32):

- *Śauca*, practice internal and external purification
- *Santosa*, live in contentment
- *Tapah*, have fiery aspiration toward Yoga
- *Svadhyāya*, do spiritual reading
- *Īśvara praṇidhāna*, devote to *Īśvara*.

---

1. PRACTICE INTERNAL AND EXTERNAL PURIFICATION

Here again, the intended purification is of all three external bodies—physical, astral, and causal—and their corresponding internal thinking instruments—brain, *mānas*, and *buddhi*. These bodies respectively intake food, *prāṇa*, and thoughts, and they must be regulated for purification.

Incidentally, Yoga is often associated with vegetarianism (meaning "not eating meat" and its variations). However, no such thought seems to be propagated in *Yoga-Sūtra*. The emphasis is on purification. If your food intake is of a kind, consumed at a time, and in such a quantity that it creates undesirable residues in your body, the body needs extra purification. Residue is a function of each individual's metabolism. By expanding this concept, the intake of anything that entails killing of another life would certainly leave behind subtle traces of pain. Instead of taxing the purification process, you may choose not to eat meat in the first place. But that is *your* choice; the sūtra does not narrowly define any such thing. (*Prāṇa* intake is separately dealt with in *prāṇayāma*).

Intake of *thoughts* is a new concept to most of us. A corollary of the *yogīk* framework of gross-subtle matter is that thoughts exist, albeit subtly. Your thoughts are entangled with the very nature of your reality, and are pretty much an open channel to the rest of the world. Your thoughts affect those around you. Your own thoughts about yourself and those of others affect who you are. Thoughts are much more powerful than we may think, they are tangible matter.

In Yoga, it is believed that sense impulses are processed in the frontal lobe of the brain to produce thoughts as vibrations, and coded thoughts are flushed out via the *ājnā chakra* (the point between the eyebrows). Likewise, we attract others' thoughts as sense impulses, as our intake. Other people thus influence us, not just by their overt behavior but also by their covert thinking. This harm is akin to passive smoking, and that is why you are always better off in the company of noble people and well-wishers. Though we cannot prevent intake of others' thoughts, we can certainly build our own protection (a kind of firewall) from them, in the form of an improved structure of predispositions. Doing this would ensure that others' thoughts are not blindly acted upon by us.

A helpful hint may be needed here. We know thoughts only in their blown-up, verbalized version. The thoughts flushed by us or input from others are in a coded form. We will see more of this later.

2. LIVE IN CONTENTMENT

Living in contentment comes from a robust and positive understanding of *karma* cycles. When *karma* is viewed as fatalistic, it creates a sense of acquiescence leading to inertia. Space, the primary causal element, is pregnant with the humongous *karma* algorithm that generates events from the seeds sown in the unfathomable past in anticipation of a learning to occur; a learning that perceives forms and knows the formless. So, a "big picture" perspective of *karma* brings contentment with the circumstances and leads to redemption of *karma*, bringing about a true behavioral change. Redemption is an active engagement with life's situations by dealing with the possibilities they offer instead of facing them with listless inertia. Such an attitude also makes you unattached to the fruits of labor with the realization that an effect is not under your control, and that the effect-producing *karma* cycles may bring in results in their own form and in their own time scale—instantly or after a long while.

3. HAVE FIERY ASPIRATION TOWARD YOGA

Your mind will have no room for any idle thoughts when it is consumed by a fiery aspiration toward the *yogīk* path; a path that is not smooth or strewn with a sweet trail of spiritual accolades. Initially in fact, there are more failures than successes. When cell-level changes occur, they also bring forth a rebellion from the unwilling cells. Only fiery aspiration enables one to stay on the path in the face of repeated failures.

Of course, there is a caveat. Fiery aspiration should not put you in a spiritual overdrive. The pace at which you will be able to progress on the *yogīk* path is not a function of your passion or zeal, but solely depends on your spiritual legacy of earlier lives and your ability to internalize the change now. There are no short-cuts in Yoga and bravado does not work. "Fiery aspiration" mentioned in *Yoga-Sūtra* is more like a flame (like a pilot in a furnace) that you keep alive to kindle your determination every time there is a failure, to continue with your spiritual journey uninterrupted.

4. DO SPIRITUAL READING

A crowning glory of Yoga practice is spiritual reading. Many translations describe this as a meager discipline of "reading of scriptures." There is no other loss in translation as unfortunate as this. How far would just "reading" the scriptures take you if there were no intrinsic change? Recitation may keep the scriptural teachings alive in memory and the sound may create intended vibrations. But the teachings need to be constantly mulled over, assimilated so that they become change agents. There is a greater risk of recital taking prominence over the study.

Then, it is not *what* is read that is important, but *how* it is read. It is a million times better to "read" nature, which holds the real secrets, than to read the scriptures mechanically. Spiritual reading in this case refers to your enhanced perceptive ability to read nature's nebulous patterns that are normally invisible to the naked eye. To be able to *see* the words in the scriptures come alive, in the world around you and within, makes "reading" spiritual. Such reading is deeply penetrating, not limited to the eyes, lips or the brain. Against its probe, time and space are helpless in defining and limiting the objects as they otherwise do, while creating apparently misleading forms. When awareness is elevated to a subtle plane, you witness a pulsating connectivity among all objects—animate and inanimate alike. That is a seeker's truly life-changing experience, and it heralds a dawn of spiritual reading ability.

5. DEVOTE TO *ĪŚVARA*

All the above happens with the consent of and guidance from inner *Īśvara*, who becomes your ultimate teacher. If the very word *Īśvara* makes you visualize an image of God or some almighty super-human deity, in whatever form, this becomes a stumbling block. Any amount of intellectual debate about the existence of God is a waste of time. The debates use words to encase ideas originating from the confines of a limited and colored view of the world. For looking inward, it does not matter if that divine principle is God in any "form." To unshackle these confines, you have to perceive without help from the mind; it is in the moment of such perception that you get a glimpse of *Īśvara*. When that happens, it also obliterates the need to prove anything to anyone. Adoration for your inner teacher springs from the heart. Devotion is not an effort anymore.

As often said here, in devoting to *Īśvara* we are not talking about either a seemingly intense but externalized display of devotion or an improvised emotion, making you kowtow before anything or anybody. In *Īśvara* you immerse, and devotion springs spontaneously, resulting in a loving surrender. Translations like "focusing on god" imply a form and introduce duality in the act. A loving surrender results in a formless and non-dual state.

Results of Practicing Niyama

In fact, practice of *niyama* launches you truly into the spiritual domain. But, one of the early fallouts in this practice is dislike of, even hatred for, your own physical body, which seems to be drawing you away from the newfound spiritual happiness and back into material pleasures. It takes time to realize that *karma* redemption is possible only *because of* the physical body. We learn that the purification is both external and internal, and that all the bodies, gross or subtle, are its candidates. Eventually, *niyamas* deliver purified and harmonized bodies as a foundation for the soul connection. Thus, because of *niyama*:

- Form is seen as a vehicle of divine purpose.
- Bliss is achieved.
- Purification makes all three bodies perfect.

FORM IS SEEN AS A VEHICLE OF DIVINE PURPOSE

Form is seen as a vehicle of divine purpose after internal and external purification (Sūtra 2.16/II.40). It is consistent with the *Yoga-Sūtra* to say that internal purification will lead to a new awareness of the physical body—not as a form but as a useful vehicle for the subtler bodies. Then you will start experimenting with the Yoga hypothesis: "Gross is a manifestation of its subtle counterpart." Eventually, when your own physical body is seen as the external manifestation of the astral body, you should also be able to see in others not a physical form but its cause, the underlying astral body. This would unveil a glimpse of the spiritual Self as the primary initiating principle present in every object.

When you can see an object (but not its form), that creates a desire-less state about appearances. Sage Pātañjali specifically asks the seeker to be desire-less toward own or others' bodies because those are the hardest of the forms to grow unaware of. Bodies are the essential vehicles for subtle-to-gross manifestation. This concept is very important, because the inner evolution in Yoga is the exact reverse, a gross-to-subtle realization. Later, in *āsana*, we will learn about the body and mind postures that reinforce this premise.

Purification is not just external and internal to the physical body, but to the subtler bodies as well, since they are also matter, though composed of higher vibratory frequencies. With growing awareness of the spiritual Self, the subtler bodies start expressing themselves. To make the gross and the subtle coexist, and to allow easy interpenetration at the cellular, molecular, and electronic levels, the purification involves individual fine-tuning of the bodies as well as elimination of the mutual incongruence.

Great advancement has been made in the world of medicine and health, in the areas of physical purification, both internal and external. Psychic purity is the next frontier. Our culture's rapidly growing awareness of spirituality is still mired in the long-standing divorce between science and religion. Moreover, a crucial role of the thinking processes and the *prāṇa* metabolism remains largely unrecognized. It is about time that the psychic dimension of the world is brought onto the mainstream scientific radar, and the psychic laws are studied in their own right as the subtle causes of the physiological laws.[25]

---

[25] *This prophetic thought appears on the website of an anonymous fulltime international team of physicists and mathematicians (facts not confirmed by the author of this book). "Our mission is to finalize an historic discovery of how gravity, electromagnetism, the nuclear forces, space and consciousness are part of the same unified field ... a realm of information, where consciousness literally interacts with geometry at the quantum scale to create everything that we define as reality (Source: http://www.newrealitytransmission.com)"*

The bodies, when purified, work in tandem. The internal purification helps in the external (surprisingly the reverse may not always be true!) and allows the gross to be controlled by the subtle. **Through purification also comes a conquest of the organs, a quiet spirit, concentration, and the ability to recognize the soul** (Sūtra 2.17/II.41). Thus forming a hierarchy of gross controlled by its subtle counterpart: on the physical plane, the sense organs are controlled by *mānas*; on the astral plane, the emotions are controlled by a quiet (gently still) *buddhi*; on the causal plane, the intellectual faculties are *sāttvik*, reflecting the soul in a controlled concentration, so that collectively the three vehicles deliver to the seeker the ability to see the soul. *This ability* is the harbinger of a vision of the soul.

Apart from your beliefs, religious or otherwise, sometimes you are so grounded in the material world that seeking the invisible soul seems vague, if not absurd. Having reached a desired level of purification, the bodies, working together, gradually establish communication with *Īśvara*. Then, the whole thing does not remain so absurd. Eventually, the vision arrives as an admittance card from *Īśvara* that allows you to pursue higher studies in Yoga.

Īśvara is full of love. Its vision unfolds gradually in a manner compatible with the seeker's predispositions. In the early part of the spiritual journey, one venerates the teachers, enlightened individuals and various forms of god. *Īśvara* assumes many such symbolic images for a while before emerging in its full-blown manifestation.

BLISS IS ACHIEVED

Bliss is achieved as a result of contentment (Sūtra 2.18/II.42). The beauty of bliss is such that until experienced, one is blissfully unaware of it and can carry on with life in pursuit of worldly happiness! Among all the changes that take place on the *yogīk* path, even the definitions of happiness change. This is why the five mind-states are described as "painful and not painful" (Sūtra 1.5) to highlight that no mind-state is a real bliss (or rather that bliss is not a mind-state.) Bliss is mentioned only now, for the first time, when the seeker is on the threshold of having a vision; for only now will this be understood.

If you truly understand and appreciate *karma*, then you will be eager to redeem your *karma* by fully living it out. The seeker learns to embrace *karma* redemption dispassionately and to avoid a reflex discrimination of *karma* as a pair of opposites, "good" or "bad." Contentment is, therefore, not a spineless "feel good" relaxation or inaction. Contentment is not blissful inertia; to be content is an active state! You are fully engaged with life, with the three bodies working in unison, instinctively dealing with the forms and yet seeing the form-less. And finally, there is a vision of *Īśvara*. At *that* level, you are in a state of "bliss."

All human endeavors are in pursuit of happiness. But when you expect happiness to arrive from "somewhere," it never does. Happiness is a state that connects you within and exposes the occasional disconnect between being happy and the so-called happiness-producing objects, people, and events. Contentment arriving from nowhere demonstrates this contrast. The happiness-producing objects also produce pain sooner or later. This reality is usually accepted only intellectually, but the moments of happiness anesthetize your ability to think about them. You have to make an extra effort to dissect your happiness. The very definition of happiness then starts changing as the new reality awakens. By forgoing the transient happiness, you seek the permanent one. It is realized then that contentment stops the proliferation of material desires and prevents any need for their transient satiation. Thus, contentment brings bliss.

But there is a long gestation period between contentment and bliss. Bliss is a no-mind state that occurs on the fourth plane, beyond the three planes of the Universe—physical, astral and causal. A glimpse of bliss is experienced in *pratyāhāra*, and it stays and expands itself with further advances in Yoga.

PURIFICATION MAKES ALL THREE BODIES PERFECT

Purification through fiery aspiration makes all three bodies perfect (Sūtra 2.19/II.43). We may lose the substance of this sūtra if we limit the body to mean only the physical, and the senses to mean only the sense organs. As maintained throughout *Yoga-Sūtra*, bodies are physical, astral, and causal, and sense organs precede the sensing that is collectively processed by the brain, *mānas*, and *buddhi*.

The "fire" also needs to be seen on three levels. Fire as metabolism sustains bodies. Fire as destroyer eliminates impurities. Fire as energy rises up the vital centers (*chakras*) in the body to bring about a union with *Īśvara*. Witnessing the presence of *Īśvara* ignites a spark that kindles desire for union.

The often unintended fallout of the ascendant energy is the enhancement of bodily powers; for example, the ability to sense without use of the external sense organs. The brain, *mānas*, and *buddhi* are able to perceive without the involvement of the individual mind. As the intelligence and the powers of the Universal Mind become accessible to the higher awareness, the second-hand knowledge of the colored individual mind would vanish in the process of purification. But most significantly, if a union with *Īśvara* is aspired for and the aspiration is fiery enough, by then you would have lost any attachment to these powers.

Āsana

Sage Pātañjali says that **the posture assumed must be steady and comfortable** (Sūtra 2.20/II.46).

This is the only sūtra that mentions posture. Such a brief reference does not diminish Haṭha Yoga and its whole body of knowledge that includes the discipline of *āsana* (postures). It is a marvelous discipline in itself and of tremendous benefit to health. But on the path of *Yoga-Sūtra*, *āsana* seems prescribed not for the technique, but for its enduring achievement—"steady and easy" postures. Such postures elevate awareness, which is then released and set free from entanglement with a grosser or a sluggish body.

Though a steady posture of the physical body is essential, the physical is the least significant of the postures. Living in today's complex world, you would also need a steadfast astral or emotional body that is not oscillating, and an even firmer and steadier causal body that is unwavering. Sage Pātañjali is referring to this threefold posture, which has to be steady and easy. Such a posture enables a meditative attitude that lasts long.

It is really an unfortunate misrepresentation of the enormous promise of Yoga when people are left to believe that Yoga for physical fitness (meaning "bodily postures alone") is all that Yoga is. Some Yoga teachers correctly emphasize an unhurried, smooth-flowing approach, and encourage their students to let mind collaborate with the body in the culmination of a correct physical posture, reached through a proven rigorous technique. But as long as athletic prowess remains the focal point, and the full spiritual potential of Yoga is not presented to the seekers, a great opportunity is lost. If the purpose of Yoga remains good health of a physical body, which can repeatedly return to the pursuit of material pleasures, you would never question the purpose of life and would not even know how close you were to the doorstep of spiritual bliss.

One wonders why a dedicated Yoga teacher would refrain from discussing the spiritual aspect of Yoga simply for fear of losing students. In the West, religions have kept spirituality a hostage for centuries by forcing its separation from science. True spiritual consciousness is as natural as environmental consciousness. That spirituality is an integral part of *āsana* practice should be a strength and not its awkward secret.

And then, some Yoga proponents present sad examples. Their innovations and improvisations lead to exotic body origami that is sold to the gullible in glamorous marketing packages. Some even get carried away by their own commercial success. They encourage seekers to believe that these hundreds of body postures have their authority in *Yoga-Sūtra*. A lot of merchandise is marketed under the guise of recommended and essential adjuncts to Yoga. The cumulative effect of such a short-sighted approach is that a seeker is further ensnared in the very aspect of life that the Yoga of *Yoga-Sūtra* is trying to uplift.

Posture Sustains Persistent Slight Effort

A physical posture, though important, is not the main point of asana practice, and certainly not the only one. The three bodies serve each other by working as a team. On the *yogīk* path, the subtle astral body learns to rein in the gross in order to arrest the mind modifications. The causal body learns to rein in desires, eventually in order to stop the modifications. Such control is manifested in a steady physical posture, tranquil emotional posture, and concentrated intellectual posture that facilitates *pratyāhāra*.

The center of gravity of concentration can be located inside only when the bodies remain steady and the externally generated disturbance ceases. Then the three bodies are in perfect sync, and the thinking instruments are disengaged from the sense-induced thoughts. With the overcast perceptual fields clearing, the meditating/thinking instruments can now directly perceive *Īśvara*. This, in turn, reinforces the steadiness and ease of the postures.

Steadiness and ease of posture is to be achieved through persistent slight effort and through concentration upon the Infinite (Sūtra 2.21/II.47). But besides the obvious concentration upon the Infinite, "persistent slight effort" in achieving that posture is a key guideline for Yoga practice. *Persistence* is needed because mind and emotions may lose steadiness at the slightest provocation. The effort also has to be *slight* or the effort itself will keep the subtle bodies consciously engaged and away from *Īśvara*. This brings us back to rhythmic breathing as the only solution that can be *persistent* ("continuous") and requires only a *slight effort* to be embedded in your autonomous body functions.

Advanced practitioners of the discipline of *āsana* know that the test of a perfected *āsana* does not lie in the degree of athletic prowess but in reaching that one moment of equilibrium when the awareness of the physique dissolves and disappears from the mind's radar. In that moment, you are aware only of your breathing. While many *āsanas* are designed to regulate bodily functions in order to promote health, a few simple *āsanas* direct us to hold a meditative posture uninterrupted for an extended period. *Sukhāsana, siddhāsana, padmāsana* and *swastikāsana* are recommended by some authors. These are characteristically different (and less glamorous) from other *āsanas* meant for physical fitness. Ironically, when one learns *Yoga-Sutra* and understands how the health of the physical body depends on the health of the astral body, one would also appreciate the *āsanas* not for their athletic challenges but for the opportunities they present to access the astral level.

Sage Pātañjali recommends such *āsanas* because they allow you to lose consciousness of the physical body in order to facilitate rhythmic breathing with persistent slight effort, and to experience astral and causal bodies at the same time.

Posture of Astral and Causal Bodies

Before reaching *pratyāhāra*, when this (steady postures also of the astral and causal bodies) **is achieved, the pairs of opposites no longer impact** (Sūtra 2.22/II.48). The astral body is affected by perception. Duality is inherent in human perception. With ego as the guiding force, you instantly create a distinction between yourself and the rest of the world. Everything is either within or without, mine or not mine. The emotion-laden thinking process oscillates between these pairs of opposites: me and them, here and there, now and then and so on. At the heart of all this tug-of-war caused by the pairs of opposites is intrinsic "relativity."

How is relativity born? The sense data travels linearly, in waves. Awareness of an object is created by related thoughts that occur in succession, "one *after* the other." This succession creates an awareness of a continuum of "time" and creates a sense of "past and the future." Time becomes relative. A sense of time creates a sense of space. The awareness of objects comes bundled with the context of a location. This moment has this context, and the next one has another. Thus, each moment in time is attached to a specific spatial context. Although time and space mean different things to different people, who each have their individualized perceptions of the objects of the world, still we appear to be weighed down by the common denominators of measured time and shared space. That commonality creates a sense of shared reality, and that very sharing reinforces it as "*the* reality." We are left to believe that our world is one; while in view of the relative reality, there are as many worlds as there are thinking individuals!

The pairs of opposites ensure that the mind continues to oscillate at the slightest provocation, like a tuning fork. Getting tossed between opposites becomes bondage. Even the ego (higher, causal body) and sense perception (lower, physical body) act as a pair of opposites. Each squeezes the astral body between them and makes it oscillate. Similarly, there is a need to conquer desire in order to make the causal body steady.

When the three bodies attain a steady posture *together*, they neither feast on the sense data nor dance to the ego's tune. Soon you learn to disengage from the senses and see the "real" perceiver instead of the ego. The world is not seen then as "me and everything else" but as an "interplay between the Spirit and the matter." Thus, gradually, all pairs of opposites cease to prevail and all desires cease to excite.

Posture leads to breathing. There is a complementary give-and-take between rhythmic breathing and the subtle bodies. The rhythmic breathing calms them and lets them attain the right posture, and a calm subtle body regulates breath and makes it rhythmic.

Prāṇayāma

In humans, uniquely, breathing can be brought under conscious control, or be left alone to function autonomously. A human life begins with the first breath and expires with the last. Emotions affect normal breathing, and thus regulated breathing can stabilize emotions. But in Yoga breathing has importance for additional reasons: first, the air that is breathed is subtle matter, and awareness of it can help develop awareness of the subtle world. Secondly, one can carry *prāṇa* with the inhalation-exhalation process of a breath, and thus jumpstart the respiration of *prāṇa*, which serves as a precursor to *prāṇayama,* the control of *prāṇa.*

Prāṇayama is the most crucial Yoga practice. Rhythmic breathing prepares the ground for aligning the regulated breath with the *prāṇa* energy. *Prāṇayama* techniques synchronize the two and bring *prāṇa* respiration up to speed. Eventually, one learns to control the *prāṇa* energy directly, by leaving breath alone and even suspended. The ability to control *prāṇa* complements the state of *pratyāhāra* (explained in the next section) by eliminating any need to attend to the exterior for replenishment of the energy to sustain the inner subtle selves.

In the final grooming of a Yoga master, all practices merge into advanced *prāṇayāma. Prāṇa* in the individual's body at that stage is as purified as *prāṇa* in the environment (the cosmic life-force).[26]

Yoga-Sūtra is widely used, rightly or wrongly, for authenticating many improvisations of breathing and *prāṇayāma* techniques. Practitioners are sometimes asked to follow awkward breathing patterns and a stressful cessation of breaths. Many techniques do provide the necessary exercise to the underperforming or misused breathing apparatus. Such exercise may be useful to an extent, and bring an initial "feel good" sense, but caution must prevail with prolonged use, since some of the techniques may be harmful, especially when practiced intermittently. To add to the risk, many techniques may be based on the following **wrong assumptions**:

- Air is one and the same thing as *prāṇa.*
- Breathing air in a particular fashion *automatically* controls *prāṇa.*

Sage Pātañjali always recommends comprehensive solutions at the subtle as well as the gross levels. Getting carried away by the physical aspect alone may make you miss the golden essence of the sūtra: **when right posture is attained there follows right control of *prāṇa* and proper inspiration and expiration of breath** (Sūtra 2.23/II.49). Here, the goal is to ***synchronize*** *prāṇa* and the breathing. And the golden essence is that breathing drives *prāṇa* only in the initial stages; eventually and ideally, **prāṇa should**

[26] *There is one cosmic* prāṇa, *manifesting in numerous names (pure consciousness, cosmic energy) and forms (cosmic life-force, Universal Mind) in the universe; the origin of everything. In an individual, the* prāṇa *gets caged in, confined to and constricted by the body and gets cut off from its universal source.* Prāṇayāma *enables reconnection of the individual's* prāṇa *with the cosmic* prāṇa *for rejuvenation, purification and finally, a re-union.*

drive breathing. Breathing is only the physical vehicle for the internal *prāṇa* to draw its replenishment from the external *prāṇa*. It works this way:

1. Ordinarily, our breathing is shallow and erratic and is out of step with the *prāṇa* cycles.
2. Yoga practices first make our breathing rhythmic.
3. Then we align the breathing rhythm with *prāṇa* cycles to bring both of them in sync.
4. Soon we consciously make *prāṇa* drive the breath.
5. Eventually, we control *prāṇa* directly, at times making the breath redundant. (*That* is the cessation of breath!)

Swami Kuvalayananda maintains in his book *Prāṇāyāma* (Lonavala, India: Kaivalyadhāma, 2005, 41) that "*śvāsa* and *praśvāsa* which can never mean anything else than the air flowing in and flowing out, make the meaning absolutely clear [that '*prāṇa* is breath']." However, there is a simple problem in equating the two. "Breathing" is a process, while *prāṇa* is a substance. Breathing of air and breathing of *prāṇa* has to be distinct, though initially they may travel together for a while.

He interprets *prāṇāyāma* to mean a "pause in breath." That doesn't appear to be wholly true either. Patanjali's terse sūtras are never elaborative and always compel us to look beyond the literal. What happens *during the pause* is more important than the mere physical act of pausing itself.

Similarly, regulating *prāṇa* would reach its culmination when a *yogi* would consciously circulate that energy and make the breathing of air redundant. Such a cessation (*keval kumbhaka*) of breath is certainly a million times richer experience than a deliberate act of retention or cessation. To begin with a deliberate practice, which ultimately becomes a way of life with conscious control, is more consistent with everything else prescribed by Sage Pātañjali. Swami Vivekananda is also clear about this.

> *When the posture has been conquered, then the motion of prāṇa is to be broken and controlled, and thus we come to Prāṇayāma, the controlling of the vital forces of the body. prāṇa is not breath, though it is usually so translated. It*

is the sum total of the cosmic energy. It is the energy that is in each body, and its most apparent manifestation is the motion of the lungs. This motion is caused by the prāṇa drawing in the breath and is what we seek to control in Prāṇayāma. We begin by controlling the breath, as the easiest way of controlling the prāṇa.—Vivekananda, 214.

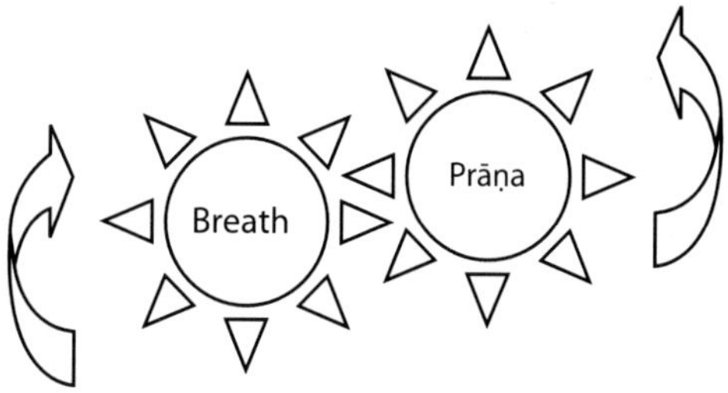

Initially, breath moves prāṇa.

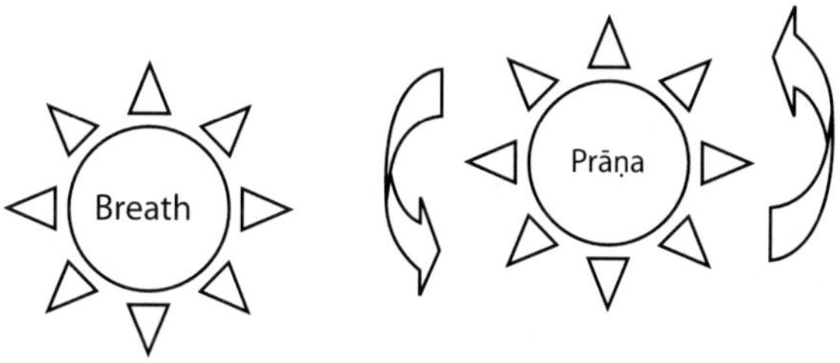

Eventually, however, prāṇa moves breath and like a flywheel keeps rotating even when the breath is suspended.

Figure 2.2: Prāṇa and Breathing

The subtle controls the gross. The astral body, powered by *prāṇa,* controls and invigorates the dense physical body. Hence, physical well-being depends directly on the quality and the deployment of *prāṇa* into the physical body. Ordinarily, *prāṇa* itself cannot be controlled. Hence, initially the control is achieved through breath control when both are in sync. But Sage Pātañjali is giving us a more significant clue, which is reinforced by Alice Bailey:

[T]he key to the just response of the lower (physical body) to the higher (astral body) lies in rhythm and in the ability

> *of [the] physical body to respond or vibrate in rhythmic unison with the etheric* body.*—Alice Bailey, 219. (* "Etheric" means "causal" as used in Bailey's book).

Thus, more than any breath control that requires deliberate effort, the rhythmic (natural) breathing brings about the proper synchronization with *prāṇa* and ensures that quality *prāṇa* is drawn in and sufficiently deployed into the entire body. That is why the rhythmic breathing *itself* is the initial control of *prāṇa*.

There is a give and take again. A steady posture (*āsana*) of all the bodies fosters a "meditative attitude" for the synchronization of breath with *prāṇa*, and properly synchronized rhythmic breathing strengthens the correct posture. The final *prāṇayāma* is a complete stoppage of breath, whether internal or external, while revolutions of *prāṇa* continue. It is like the wheels of *prāṇa* are driven by the wheels of rhythmic breathing. So even when breathing stops, the *prāṇa* continues in its desired momentum. (*Figure 2.2*) This event signifies a total vibrational harmony between the astral and the physical bodies, which makes the physical body (breathing) progressively redundant as the vehicle for *prāṇa* intake.

Thus, in *Yoga-Sūtra* the concept of *āsana* is far wider than mere physical postures and is intertwined with a similarly wider concept of *prāṇayāma*. It also follows that something as profound as this works on the very essence of body/mind functions. To sustain the force of such changes, the body/mind system needs internal purification by means of *yama* and *niyama*, which must go hand in hand with *āsana* and *prāṇayāma*. Any lopsided practice of Yoga is therefore deficient and risky. A simultaneous practice of the first four limbs of Yoga can never be overemphasized. Good Yoga teachers would always take care of this. A good teacher, however, needs to untangle *yama–niyama* from any irrelevant undertones of religious dogmas and explain to the students the complementary nature of the four limbs of Yoga.

Right Technique of Prāṇayāma[27]

Right control of *prāṇa* (the life-force) is external, internal, or motionless; it is subject to place, time, and number and is also protracted or brief (Sūtra 2.24/II.50). This forms the centerpiece of all practices outlined by Sage Pātañjali. It is made cryptic, so that the exact method should not become wrongly exposed and fall into lay hands, which might result in risks to the body/mind. Any half-cooked shortcut to Yoga or any of its exotic adaptations is like playing with fire and may cause bodily and mental harm beyond repair. Let us not forget that *prāṇa* is energy.

All Yoga practices are based on the same threefold structure of a human being. Therefore, any practice has to address the threefold efforts respectively—intense (for physical), moderate (for astral), and mild (for causal).

In this sūtra, some additional specifics are provided. The breath is external, and *prāṇa* is internal. Both can be motionless when *prāṇa* remains temporarily confined around the astral body. This is not the motionlessness of passing out but one of full awareness that ushers in an experience you never had before.

This motionless experience is particularly important as a precursor to *pratyāhāra* and the subsequent states of *dhāraṇā*, *dhyāna*, and *samādhi*. The motionless breath and *prāṇa* open up one's ability to communicate via subtle aspects that do not depend on the sense organs of the physical body. This is an essential stepping stone toward the primary means of Yoga.

The "place," according to the *Yoga-Sūtra* logic now familiar to you, is not a physical location but a place within the body, a *chakra*, where *prāṇa* is located at any given time. "Time" suggests the respective length of the breathing cycles, *prāṇa* rotations, or the motionless states, and "number" suggests the count of repetitions. Of course, these three terms have a deeper meaning as well. For example, *"as the microcosm of the universe, the place in one's*

---

[27] *In this sūtra, Sage Pātanjali alludes to rhythmic breathing, synchronization of breath to* prāṇa, prāṇa *rotations in phase and sub-phase practices, and the details of intermediate steps in other breathing practices. The* prāṇa *rotations are fairly advanced and are available only to eligible disciples.*

body also parallels with a place in the planetary expanse and thus has astrological significance."—Alice Bailey, 224-25.

If we end the *prāṇayāma* discussion here some readers may feel cheated. However, this author sincerely believes that *prāṇayāma* is not something that can be learned by reading. Dear readers are requested to seek a good teacher with whom they can discuss the above aspects to their satisfaction, and only then commence the practice without forgetting that *prāṇayāma* is *one* of the eight limbs of Yoga.

Pratyāhāra

It is important here to recap the underlying thinking process as implied in *Yoga-Sūtra*. There is an important difference between the "thinking instruments" (brain, *mānas*, and *buddhi*) and the "thinking process"; just like a difference between a sense organ (for example, an eye) and the sense (optical signals).

The brain, the physical thinking instrument, is composed of the fore brain (the frontal lobe, the conscious brain) with its registration area (with four layers—intellectual-emotional-sexual-movement), together with the hind brain (occipital lobe) and the mid-brain (temporal lobe) with their memory pools.

Electromagnetic vibrations arrive from the environment—received as sense impulses which travel throughout the nervous system by means of the spinal cord and enter the brain at the thalamus (see *Figure 1.2*). These vibrations are transferred to *mānas* flowing over the memory pools on the way to the frontal lobe, via the parietal lobe. The energy of the incoming sense impulses stirs the structure of predispositions embedded in the memory, and these impulses attract near-identical memory patterns from the memory pools which are filled with past-experienced emotions. Ideal thinking would be a process wherein the mind acts only as a catalyst in helping the brain to see the impulses as they are. Instead, however, the untamed mind interacts with the threesome—the impulses, the near-identical memory patterns, and the associated emotions—in the registration area. This creates vibrant "individualized" thoughts causing mind modifications.

In the registration area, thoughts are formed with a blend of four layers. *Buddhi* brings in the intellectual layer that makes an individual's signature on the thoughts, *mānas* brings in the emotional layer that is judgmental, and the brain brings in a highly physical/ sexual orientation. Together they create mild or intense mind modifications.

For appreciating the value of mind's non-attachment in the state of *pratyāhāra* we have to properly grasp mind's indulgence first. Under the influence of *tamas*, mind conceals that the incoming impulses are mere appearances. Moreover, such a shallow perception is further affected by a conditioned cognition—one that uses only known patterns in the memory. Lastly, the emotional gloss creates attachment to the objects, and the mind lets us believe that such colored and deformed perception gives us our "only reality." Such indulgent mind deserves to be kept aside.

In *pratyāhāra*, even though the flow of sense impulses continues, the mind remains non-attached to the process, so that the calming and control of the senses result when sense organs withdraw from the object likewise (Sūtra 2.25/II.54). Thus, *pratyāhāra* is a process in which you would consciously separate the mind from the thinking process and not allow them to engage and interact. This is achieved by diverting the flow of impulses away from the normal passage at the thalamus so that the thoughts are not formed and one thus remains in a meditative mode. This is neither an accident nor a psychic adventure; it happens at will. That is why it's a breakthrough.

For reaching this milestone the secondary means of Yoga contribute collectively—*yama-niyama* compliance eliminates causes of alternating mind-states, *āsana* steadies and stills the physical body to remove any residual agitations, and *prāṇāyāma's* regulated breathing does the same to the astral body by eliminating the sentimental swings.

But what happens to mind is even more significant. All along, mind has been actively participating in the thinking process to *generate* knowledge even if it is conditioned, individualized and sentimental. Through the Yoga practices, mind evolves into its original self, the Universal Mind, and starts sourcing spiritual knowledge. Thus, in a dramatic turnaround, the brain and its partners stop creating defective knowledge and become users of exact knowledge. Mind can return to its original role of a catalyst and not indulge. This is non-attachment.

In fact, it is difficult to capture the experience of *pratyāhāra* in words. It is detachment without physically detaching yourself from the world; it is the intended "freedom from longing for all objects of desire."

In *pratyāhāra*, there follows a complete subjugation of the sense organs (Sūtra 2.26/II.55). The sense organs are habitually outward-bound. They follow the energy of desire, and extend their subtle tentacles to caress the perceived objects. This engagement gives an object its perceived form or appearance, which creates sense impulses. However, it is important to remember here that your perception is not invited by the perceived object; but the real initiator is the perceiver, your own self, and the motivator in that act of perception is your desire.

It is tough to control the sense organs that owe their natural outbound tendency to a human legacy of millions of years. Instead of reining in the sense organs, it is easier to snap the link between sensing and thinking. Doing this blocks the desire on the causal plane, disabling its instigation to the sense organs. With desire made inoperative, the senses and the sense organs are rendered totally redundant. During spells of ill-health or an emotional disturbance, it is our common experience that otherwise favorite things appear temporarily unworthy of attention. In Yoga, you can bring about such a state consciously in a positive way. But importantly, this withdrawal of the senses is not caused by any temporary affliction, and there is no hatred for the objects, because hatred is only another form of attachment. This inattention results rather from a relaxed indifference.

This is a difficult achievement, and by then a lot of structural changes have already occurred in you. With the sensory input becoming redundant, the sense organs become ineffective in driving the thought mill.

> *[N]ot only must the outer conduct be corrected, not only must the inner purity be arrived at, not only must the right attitude towards all things be cultivated, and the life-currents consequently controlled, but the capacity to subjugate the outgoing tendencies of the five senses must be worked at.*—Alice Bailey, 229.

It also implies that the astral body now becomes your primary body, and gets detached at will from the outbound physical, which now becomes secondary. A sense of this can be only grasped intellectually until you learn to do it consciously after arduous and patient Yoga practice.

Pratyāhāra is considered a breakthrough because, in that state, the freedom from longing for all objects eliminates the outward bound orientation of your perception. Instead of repeatedly *forcing* your attention inward, your perception would come to reside there peacefully, at will. Desires are defused, perception is direct and independent of sensing, the sense organs are retired and mind is no more agitated. Once settled inside, the awareness recognizes *Īśvara* and that gives enough reason to continue to stay there.

Vision of Īśvara

Our usual reflex thinking directly connects the sense organs with the organs of action, resulting in an automated behavior / response. With the sense organs withdrawing from attachment to objects, the organs of activity are relieved of their bondage of compulsive habits and are brought under full conscious control. As a seeker you develop a relaxed indifference toward objects, people, and events that, until then, had held you captive. You are not drawn to them by ordinary reflex thinking anymore, and yet that does not bring any sense of deprivation. You do not become impassive, either. Moments of joy or empathy become purer, because there are no strings attached. The control is willed and not done under duress or with effort. This control brings a new quality to living; a freedom in the true sense of the term.

In the process, your awareness expands and embraces something new within—*Īśvara,* whose glimpse *pratyāhāra* brings for the first time. Awareness of *Īśvara* opens several doors for you. *Īśvara* is poised to become the ultimate teacher on the *yogīk* path. That is vital for the primary means of Yoga (*dhyāna, dhāraṇa* and *samādhi*). A pre-requisite of these advanced end-states is an engagement with the subtle objects in the inner domain, and such engagement contains many delicate lessons. For instance, only the subtle images as the object of meditation can eventually enable meditation without any objects at all. *Iśvara* abides in that apparent "nothingness." But it all happens in several progressive phases. Let's see how.

First, a "Pause"

***Nirodh pariṇāma,* a state of mind transformation**, is the silencing of the senses leading to an **"involuntary pause"** in the following sequence:

- **The brain reacts** to that which is seen **(*saṃskāra*).**
- Then follows a **moment of restraint (*nirodha*).**
- Then ensues a moment wherein the **mind responds to both** these factors.
- **Both factors momentarily hold each other out and the perceiving consciousness has full sway over that moment** (Sūtra 2.27/III.9).

A complete subjugation of the sense organs neither happens suddenly nor is sustained for a long period. At first, the snapping of the link between sensing and thinking happens in a flash, for a fraction of a second. Though this pause leaves a beautiful memory, it remains an involuntary occurrence. During that pause, when thinking is suspended, the consciousness perceives a glimpse of a vision. You need to cultivate the ability to interrupt thinking by a willful pause in order to hold on to that.

Ordinarily what one does is think and act in an automatic reflex. Most of our behavior is learned. Even when it is not, one continues to react to a new situation from a comfort zone of what is already known, until eventually the new becomes familiar. The thinking process is a substantial cause of such a reflex.

In reaching the *pratyāhāra* stage, a seeker gains the ability to develop a conscious response rather than an automatic reflex. A response leads to a willed pause in this way:

1. You are concentrating on some object and are slowly becoming aware of the act of concentrating itself. To that awareness, the *act* of concentration becomes an object. This stimulates the mind into thought-forms and results in mind modifications.
2. But now any modification is immediately followed by a different awareness, a need to control the modifications, and this brings in your will to stop the form creation, and the mind momentarily ceases to modify itself. But this control itself generates mild modifications.
3. The above "modify and control" sequence goes on for a while, but you persist and eventually manage to be aware of both triggers almost simultaneously. *"Recognition of the object and the immediate control of the responsive* citta *(mind) occur like a flash of lightning."*—Alice Bailey, 260.
4. Then it happens—a willed pause. Both sensing and willing are delicately balanced and consciously suspended. Neither the object nor the controlling creates any mind modification. Your awareness suddenly elevates itself because there is no medium for perception. With nothing to obstruct the view, *Īśvara* thus appears on its own plane to offer a vision, though it is gone the next moment.

Only a practitioner knows how an effort to control the mind is counterproductive, because the controlling thoughts create mind modifications and increase the mind turbulence. Early attempts at concentration become frustrating, because even with the eyes closed and the body stilled, either the object of meditation (if one has such an object) or the awareness of your act of meditating itself creates mind modifications.

> *If there is modification which impels the mind to rush out through the senses and the disciple tries to control it, that very control itself will be a modification.*
>
> —Vivekānanda, 221.

The thinking instruments and the thinking process have no agenda of their own. They can lead the individual in circles of bondage or on the swings of freedom with equal ease. However, given the stimuli of today's material world, they are prone to gravitate more toward physical gratification, and hence towards bondage when left to themselves. Yoga practices make the parasympathetic nervous system operative.

Once the thinking instruments and the individual thinking process are so equipped, it is easier to apply the will to excite or inhibit the nerves and thus control the thoughts and actions. This ability further facilitates a willed pause that leaves space for the arising of spiritual perception.

Then, Steadiness of Spiritual Perception

The gradual activation of the parasympathetic nervous system helps in supporting the "spiritual perception" that replaces the ordinary physical one. Day by day, a greater automatic control of the will follows, and both the thinking instrument and the thinking process assume a "steady posture (the *āsana*)."

Through the cultivation of this habit of "pausing" there eventually occurs tranquility and a steadiness of spiritual perception (Sūtra 2.28/III.10). Here, Sage Pātañjali is laying special emphasis on the *cultivation of habit* from what first occurs as a one-of-a-kind involuntary flash. This is a long and often frustrating process. But despite its momentary nature, the initial vision is alluring enough. The vision is life-changing; it brings the intellectual concept of "illumination" into the practical realm. The so-called esoteric becomes a viable way of life. Now, even that momentary flash assures you that you can still the mind, make the brain responsive (and not reflexive), achieve the pause, yearn to revisit the vision again and again, and finally hold it at will for uninterrupted contemplation.

Then, a Constant Power to Contemplate

What happens when the vision is firmly installed? *Samādhi pariṇāma,* a constant state of contemplation, keeps you unfazed in the face of distractions that still continue to barge in. The ability to separate the thinking instrument and the thinking process takes root at long last. **When this becomes a habit and mind's thought-form making tendency is arrested, that eventually results in a constant ability of meditation** (Sūtra 2.29/III.11). The intellectual-emotional-sexual-movement registration areas in the brain do not activate, as they used to even at the slightest sensory provocation, and thus the thought-churning tendency is voided.

However, contrary to a naive belief, this silencing of the thought process does not render you any less capable of living in the ordinary material world. Let us not forget that it is a purely conscious, willed silencing. Secondly, your ordinary perception is not simply replaced by the spiritual perception, but your knowledge is now rooted in the omniscient Universal Mind. You are perfectly capable of discharging your worldly duties. In fact, you would do so without inviting attachment and the resulting pain. In this way you will be better equipped to deal with the circumstances of life, because your contentment does not depend on those circumstances. This is the way a meditative attitude is established, and there remains nothing magical about it.

Again, only a practitioner will realize that although the pause, a steady spiritual perception, and an ability to contemplate are linear progressions, the three are miles apart. They are also signs of the seeker graduating into a *yogī*, a *mahāyogī*, and eventually a *paramayogī* (Yoga master) through these radical changes.

Also, Bodily Perfection

Still living in the ordinary material world, now the seeker-turned-*mahāyogī* would be a different individual, with all three bodies having undergone structural changes. **This also results in mastery over five basic elements and bestows bodily perfection** comprising symmetry of form, beauty of color, strength and the compactness of a diamond (Sūtra 2.30/III.46).

The physical body of a *mahāyogī* would acquire a graceful, symmetrical form. Each of its constituent parts would be geometrically perfect. Ordinary actions would appear nicely choreographed to a quiet rhythm and under absolute control. The astral body, devoid of all colors of emotional modifications, would become beautiful, translucent, and clear. The causal body would vibrate in the strength of a spiritual will, signifying power of the highest order. Thus, the bodies would collectively reflect a physically perfect form, emotional compassion, and subtle power. Such perfect bodies are a product of many years of inner evolution. Together they produce the compact effect of a diamond whose indestructibility coheres like its fourth dimension.

Rewards fall in the seeker's lap in the form of peaceful control over the elements within the physical body, leading to rhythm and balance in *guṇa* and finally, some *siddhī* (powers). But such powers are difficult to maintain. Even a diamond may have flaws, and a flaw can resurface over time, even on the most brilliant diamond. Behind the powers lurks temptation to use them, and the dividing line between the use and the misuse is thin. Any temptation may invite a desire-driven cycle of mind modifications. That's the potential flaw.

Now, Transfer of Awareness

Is such a radical change in you ordained or willed? Sage Pātañjali says, both. Evolution is a continuous and ceaseless process. Everyone knows that everything changes from moment to moment, though the world stands fragmented in conflicting beliefs about what is the purpose of change and what is its cause. The propositions range from a speculation of absolute randomness to an affirmation of an intelligent hand behind it.

The conventional theories of evolution are mono-dimensional, because they are based on a physical and seen world alone, and the causes of evolution are either inferred or hypothesized. *Yoga-Sūtra*'s subtle-to-gross paradigm lends more dimensions and evidence in place of inferences. It also takes the evolutionary process beyond planet Earth and makes it truly Universal, as it should be. It finally connects the "survival of the fittest" principle on the gross plane to the "subtle-to-gross" creation on the subtle planes. This makes "choice" and "creation" as collaborators in the universal framework of involution–evolution and not as mutually exclusive options.

Sage Pātañjali makes a definite statement that **the transfer of awareness from a lower vehicle (body) into a higher (astral and above) is the greatest creative and evolutionary process** (Sūtra 2.31/IV.2). It is creative because it is built upon the individual's choices. It is evolutionary because it is transformational. This is *jātyaṃtara pariṇāma*, a conscious transformation process, brought about by the overwhelming extant intrinsic elements.

Sage Pātañjali thus subscribes to a unique position. He proposes a cyclical occurrence of an epoch with two phases: evolution (from subtle to gross, or the progressive unfolding of fine matter into gross, inert matter) followed by involution (gross to subtle, or progressive realization of gross to fine matter). This creates trillions upon trillions of random possibilities in each phase, but the phases by themselves remain inevitable in either direction. A corollary of the above proposition is that the cause of change is always *awareness* that in evolution continuously degenerates into grosser bodies, or in involution elevates into subtler bodies. Thus, in evolution, all humanity is *ordained* to realize its true (subtle) self at its own pace and in its own way. But a will can be summoned through Yoga for an accelerated inner evolution.

The accelerated inner evolution (involution), achieved by upgrading inner awareness through persistent Yoga practices, brings about an increased vibrational tone that requires a more cultivated and sophisticated form to sustain. Though the changes mainly occur on the astral and causal planes, consistent changes are also needed in the more gross and dense (physical) vehicle. The changes occurring at all levels—electronic, molecular, and cellular—bring about a complete metamorphosis.

> *This metamorphosis follows three stages: With the desires shifting from lower to higher and worldly to esoteric, there is a transfer of consciousness. Since the energy follows thoughts, the transfer brings about an elevated vibrational tone corresponding to the higher objectives. This brings about structural changes through transmutation within the human being that makes the three bodies congruent to the new finer thoughts and desires. All this culminates into*

transformation, as a permanent change.—abridged from Alice Bailey, 382.

A similar inner evolution occurs, though on a different scale and level, in every species, both flora and fauna. Unlike other life species, however, human evolution can be a conscious process for those who choose it and Yoga shows the way.[28]

Then, what is the impediment to this conscious evolutionary process? So far, you were thinking that *guṇa* was the "final frontier," and that with mind's non-attachment to the thinking process, the final link with *guṇa* is snapped. Now you realize that the energy of *guṇa* may be creating a form, but it does not induce perception at its own volition. A perception is our own mind's activity instigated by our desire to perceive, and that remains the main culprit. Desire seeds *karma*.

Desire, the Final Conquest

The activities of a Yogī are free from causing new *karma* cycles; while for others they continue to so cause, on three different planes: physical, astral and causal (Sūtra 2.32/IV.7).

No New Karma *Cycles*

For a *yogi*, who can remain in the state of uninterrupted meditative attitude, and who is desireless while going through the daily chores, the generation of new *karma* cycles ceases. It may be reiterated that in such a state you need not appear any different, renounce the world, or retire into a vegetating inactivity. As a truly free person, free even from creating new *karma*, you can and do devote yourself to worldly activity with a meditative attitude, desiring nothing in return.

[28] *If it is not abundantly clear to the reader already, Yoga practices refer to no patented processes of any particular school of Yoga, or any particular religion, or any particular part of the world. Any sustained effort at soul-unfoldment and self-realization that leads from one milestone to the other as shown on the* Yogīk *Path is a valid Yoga practice, by whatever name it is called.*

The principle of redemption itself is important to meditate on. Though the cause of *karma* exists on the subtle plane, the experiencing occurs on a grosser plane, and hence the redemption from *karma* must also occur there. That is why a human birth is valuable—to be able to redeem the *karma*. In fact, even an ordinary worldly person has abundant opportunities of redemption. But with heightened spiritual awareness, beyond the ordinary, you would learn to glide on the physical plane without the mind's attachment. And *karma* is not fully redeemed until then.

We cause three kinds of *karma*:

- On the *physical plane,* through an activity that is wicked, and depraved. This may occur out of ignorance (for which knowledge is the redemption), or out of indulgence in the dense physical realm (for which spiritual awakening is the redemption). However, where the actions are the product of a deliberate choice, in spite of knowledge or in deference to the contrary inner voice, total destruction of the decayed personality and even of physical existence is the only redemption. (This truth applies to all behavior contrary to *yama* and it can be seen afresh in this light.)
- Blind reactions to the pairs of opposites perceived on the *astral plane*. Here, one does not commit deliberate actions but, by oscillating between the pairs of opposites, reacts to the external situations reflexively. The reactions represent swings between love and hate and the resultant array of emotions. Restoring the equilibrium, balance, and harmony, through purification and contentment is the redemption. (*Niyama* deserve another look in this context.)
- Whether externally manifested or not, the desires continue to inflict pain on the *causal plane* of the seeker who has not yet perfected and sustained the meditative attitude, and this results in a turbulent spiritual journey. Continuous improvement and elevation of awareness is the redemption.

The law of *karma* seeds an inevitability of a gross-to-subtle inner evolution as an effect of innumerable causes. Any object is only a gross manifestation, and the subtle element, its real cause, remains veiled. Until the subtle real cause is known to you and its meaning understood, the law of *karma* ensures that you are repeatedly presented with the same gross manifestation in the guise of events in your life which are enacted differently only in the context of space and time. Thus, *karma* is an occurrence awaiting redemption. Upon your realization of the subtle cause, the particular cycle of occurrence ceases. Please note that looking only at its appearance, we perceive *karma* as happy or painful, but by itself *karma* possesses no such quality.

"Good *karma*" and "bad *karma*" is also a convenient and simplistic misinterpretation. For example, when we put a car in a "drive" mode (the cause) it inevitably rolls on (its effect). If, at the time we are on the road, it is a "good" *karma*, but if we happen to be right on the edge of a cliff, it is "bad."

Forms No More Needed as Karma's *Effect*

The law of *karma* dovetails with the law of reincarnation.

> *In every life, as it comes into physical manifestation, are latent those germs or seeds which must bear fruit, and it is these latent seeds which are the efficient cause of the appearance of the form. These seeds have been sown at some time and must come to fruition. They are the causes which produce those bodies in which the effects are to work themselves out. They are the desires, impulses, and obligations which keep the man upon the great wheel which ever turning carries a man down into physical plane existence, there to bring to fruition as many of those seeds, as under the law, he can handle or deal with in one life.*—Alice Bailey, 393.

The seeds of *karma* are subject-specific and emerge from thinking. Depending on the three basic types of thinking associated with the intellectual, emotional, and sexual registration centers, **three kinds of *karma* seeds are born with forms which are necessary for the fruition of their effects** (Sūtra 2.33/IV.8). Each of these in turn would need a particular type of body-mind system, family-social environment, and other peripheral aspects for its fulfillment. And that may not be present all the time.

Then the unfulfilled, residual seeds create a legacy of potencies for the next life, and the legacy is instrumental in choosing the most fulfilling environment to come to life into. In this sense, you are fully responsible for the conditions of your future birth. Residual potencies—memory with structures of predispositions and functionality—are the cause that determine the type of body-mind system you will be born with. These potencies also shape the entire spectrum of structures within which you will think and act.

However, this inevitability is not as severe as it appears to be. Though the legacy of residual potencies is certain, its redemption, a function of human will and diligent efforts, is the unpredictable variable in the equation. Thus, you also become an architect of your own life when you realize your spirituality and the redemption begins. That is why at the pinnacle of Yoga, when all *karma* is redeemed and the enlightened seeker (now a *mahāyogī*) creates no new *karma* cycles, the need for life on the physical plane ceases, and such an individual may consciously pass through the final death of the last physical body.

Mind-Created Forms Have No Known Beginning

If all desires come from experiencing, where does the desire to live come from, in view of the fact that one has not died yet? This desire, then, must be a residue of the last birth. But in that case, if every desire to live must germinate from the previous experience of death, the backward chain of previous births will extend unendingly. **Desire to live being eternal** (and forms originate in desire) **mind-created forms have no known beginning** (Sūtra 2.34/IV.10). Then, a desire to live cannot be primary, and death may not be putting any real end to life. Death must be then a transition, just marking the expiration of a physical body in order to release its astral counterpart to carry on its life. And why this astral body needs to return to its manifestation into a physical form again and again must be for what is then possible, experiencing. Thus, a desire to experience comes first, and then all the other desires follow.

The concept of cyclical epochs of involution and evolution is like "chicken and egg." If involution follows evolution and vice versa, what is the primary cause; and if the Universe too is an object, how did it originate? The wisdom of the Vedas about the origin of the Universe is hard to conceptualize. The hypothesis is that involution and evolution are coextensive and occur continuously within each entity—whether a single atom or the whole universe—at its respective scale of space and time. "To be born, to live and to die" is the common code. In living, one dies; in death, one is born.

The universal evolution unfolds over a seeming eternity and breeds *avidyā* and *karma*. The word used here is *avidyā* (ignorance) and not "sin." Only in the post-*Vedik* period did the priest class contort *karma* into "sin" and invent "rituals to avoid punishment" for their own selfish material gain. *Avidyā* is the fruit of evolution, and once it sets in, it is difficult to be free from its oppression through *tāmasik* desires and negative thoughts. Forms so generated are the cause of future existence and of a strong desire to live.

Sage Pātañjali points out that the eternal desire to live continues to warrant an endless cycle of births and deaths, with no known beginning. But more than what is said, the sūtra is important for what it left unsaid: "Though the beginning is not known, it is possible to *end* the cycle," a concept so vividly developed in the foregoing sūtra.

Not Karma, *but "Form-Creating Desire" Is the Cause*

Though the end of *karma* cycles would also mean the end of "birth and death" cycles, *karma* is an effect and not the root cause. **As forms are created through desire and held together through the will to live, when the desire (cause) ceases to attract, then the form (effect) ceases to exist likewise** (Sūtra 2.35/IV.11). The subtle desires result in the grosser personality that gives a collective form to the three bodies. A desire manifests itself in the mental vitality or a will to live. The will to live perpetuates another effect—the "outgoing life" that initiates perception and creates forms of other objects. These two pairs of cause and effect emanate from desire, and one form creates another form and one life creates another.

To a seeker, whose feet are still glued to a living and gratifying world, a desire to live is a fundamental premise, absolutely not accessible for review. It is so integral to our personality that a mental state of a "lack of desire to live" appears to be weird. The only way you can relate with this world is through the objects and their forms. That alone makes "sense." From such a point of view it is a quantum leap to even imagine that somewhere on the *yogīk* path there may be an important milestone of "having no desire to live."

However, "no desire to live" should not be construed as a wish to end life. Living life fully with a total indifference toward death is that mind-state. What is emphasized here is the fact that it is the most fundamental desire and the last one to be given up. Thus, when there is no desire to attract and no requirement of compulsive perception, there is no reason for any form to exist. In the process of becoming a Yoga disciple, "living without desire to live" becomes a far distant yet real possibility. This realization does not arrive like a thunderbolt but evolves ever so gently when the vision of *Īśvara* becomes a beacon. Almost from nowhere arrives a conviction that one can die consciously and may not want another life for the physical body.

Vision

A vision visits you as a disciple in many ways. You are able to en-*vision* the *yogīk* path, and that is instructional. A visionary realization that desire is the final conquest is a profound revelation. But the real game-changer is the one-on-one vision of *Īśvara* that remains an out-of-this-world experience.

Vision paves the way for a breakthrough point on the *yogīk* path—*pratyāhāra*. First occurring as an accidental pause in thinking, it soon becomes a conscious willed action that makes the primary means of Yoga possible. From this point onward, when the pupil is ready, the Master appears as *Īśvara*. This inner guru guides the seeker, while the individual mind gradually reduces its engagement with the overpowering brain to let in awareness of your essential spiritual nature.

Now the egoistic self lovingly surrenders the reins to *Īśvara* who can deliver the ultimate truth. The seeker is now an ardent *disciple* of that truth.

Chapter Two: Rearranged Sūtra: (Number in brackets is conventional sequence)

2.1 (I.34) **प्रच्छर्दनविधारणाभ्यां वा प्राणस्य॥**

pracchardana-vidhāraṇābhyāṁ vā prāṇasya

The peace of mind is **also** brought about by the expiration and retention of *prāṇa* . . . (continued in next Sūtra)

2.2 (I.35) **विषयवती वा प्रवृत्तिरुत्पन्ना मनसः स्थितिनिबन्धनी॥**

viṣayavatī vā pravṛttir utpannā manasaḥ sthiti-nibandhanī

. . . or through direct perception of the object, a perception that is higher and beyond sense perception . . . (continued in next Sūtra)

2.3 (I.37) **वीतरागविषयं वा चित्तम्॥**

vīta-rāga-viṣayaṁ vā cittam

. . . or the mind is stabilized and rendered passionless as the lower (sex-dominated) nature is refined, purified and is no longer indulged in.

2.4 (II.28) **योगाङ्गानुष्ठानादशुद्धिक्षये ज्ञानदीप्तिराविवेकख्यातेः॥**

yogāṇgānuṣṭhānād aśuddhi-kṣaye jñāna-dīptir ā viveka-khyātiḥ

When the eightfold Yoga has been steadily practiced and when impurity has been overcome, spiritual enlightenment culminates into full illumination.

2.5 (II.29) **यमनियमासनप्राणायामप्रत्याहारधारणाध्यानसमाधयोऽष्टावङ्गानि॥**

yama-niyamāsana-prāṇāyāma-pratyāhāra-dhāraṇā-dhyāna-samādhayo "ṣṭāv aṇgāni

The eight limbs of Yoga are: the 5 abstentions (*yama*), the 5 rules (*niyama*), the posture (*āsana*), right control of life-force

(*Prāṇayāma*), the abstraction (*pratyāhāra*), concentration (leading to *dhāraṇā*), meditation (leading to *dhyāna*) and contemplation (leading to *samādhi*).

2.6 (II.30) **अहिंसासत्यास्तेयब्रम्हचर्यापरिग्रहा यमाः ॥**

ahiṁsā-satyāsteya-brahmacaryāparigrahā yamāḥ

Harmlessness, truth to all beings, abstention from theft, indulgence and avarice, constitute the *yama*, the 5 abstentions.

2.7 (II.31) **जातिदेशकालसमयावच्छिनाः सार्वभौमा महाव्रतम् ॥**

jāti-deśa-kāla-samayānavacchinnāḥ sārvabhaumā mahā-vratam

Yama, the 5 commandments constitute the universal duty and are irrespective of race, place, time or circumstances.

2.8 (II.33) **वितर्कबाधने प्रतिपक्षभावनम् ॥**

vitarka-bādhane-pratipakṣa-bhāvanaṁ

When thoughts contrary to Yoga are present, there should be cultivation of their opposite thoughts.

2.9 (II.34) **वितर्का हिंसादयः कृतकारितानुमोदिता लोभक्रोधमोहपूर्वका मृदुमध्याधिमात्रा दुःखाज्ञानानन्तफला इति प्रतिपक्षभावनम् ॥**

vitarkā himsādayaḥ kṛta-kāritānumoditā lobha-krodha-moha-pūrvakā mṛdu-madhyādhimātrā duḥkhājñānānanta-phalā iti pratipakṣa- bhāvanaṁ

Thoughts contrary to Yoga like harmfulness etc., whether committed by oneself, caused through others or approved of; whether arising from avarice, anger or ignorance; and whether mild, moderate or intense would always result in pain and ignorance. Such realization is how opposite thoughts should be cultivated.

2.10 (II.35) **अहिंसाप्रतिष्ठायां तत्संनिधौ वैरत्यागः ॥**

ahiṁsā-pratiṣṭhāyāṁ tat-saṁnidhau vaira-tyāgaḥ

All enmity ceases in others in the presence of one who has perfected harmlessness.

2.11 (II.36) सत्यप्रतिष्ठायां क्रियाफलाश्रयत्वम्॥

satya-pratiṣṭhāyāṁ kriyā-phalāśrayatvaṁ

When truth to all beings is perfected, the seeker's words and acts are immediately effective.

2.12 (II.37) अस्तेयप्रतिष्ठायां सर्वरत्नोपस्थानम्॥

asteya-pratiṣṭhāyāṁ sarva-ratnopasthānaṁ

When abstention from theft is perfected, the seeker can have whatever he desires.

2.13 (II.38) ब्रम्हचर्यप्रतिष्ठायां वीर्यलाभः॥

brahmacarya-pratiṣṭhāyāṁ vīrya-lābhaḥ

By abstaining from indulgence creative energy and indomitable courage is acquired.

2.14 (II.39) अपरिग्रहस्थैर्ये जन्मकथन्तासम्बोधः॥

aparigraha-sthairye janma-kathaṁtā-saṁbodhaḥ

When abstention from avarice is perfected, there comes an understanding of the law of rebirth.

2.15 (II.32) शौचसंतोषतपःस्वाध्यायेश्वरप्रणिधानानि नियमाः॥

śauca-saṁtoṣa-tapaḥ-svādhyāyeśvara-praṇidhānāni niyamāḥ

Internal and external purification, contentment, fiery aspiration, spiritual reading and devotion to *Īśvara* constitute the *Niyama*, the 5 rules of life.

2.16 (II.40) शौचात्स्वाङ्गजुगुप्सा परैरसंसर्गः॥

śaucāt svāṅga-jugupsā paraiḥ-asaṁsargaḥ

Internal and external purification produces indifference towards forms, both one's own and all the forms in the three worlds.

2.17 (II.41) सत्वशुध्दिसौमनस्यैकाग्र्येन्द्रियजयात्मदर्शनयोग्यत्वानि च॥

sattvaśuddhi-saumanasyaikāgryendriya-jayātma-darśana-yogyatvāni ca

Through purification also comes a conquest of the organs, quiet spirit, concentration and ability to see the Self.

2.18 (II.42) संतोषादनुत्तमसुखलाभः ॥

saṁtoṣād anuttamaḥ sukha-lābhaḥ

As a result of contentment, bliss is achieved.

2.19 (II.43) कायेन्द्रियसिध्दिरशुध्दिक्षयात्तपसः ॥

kāyendriya-siddhir aśuddhi-kṣayāt tapasaḥ

Through fiery aspiration and through the removal of all impurities, comes perfection of the bodily powers and of the senses.

2.20 (II.46) स्थिरसुखमासनम् ॥

sthira-sukham āsanam

The posture assumed must be steady and comfortable.

2.21 (II.47) प्रयत्नशैथिल्यानन्तसमापत्तिभ्याम् ॥

prayatna-śaithilyānanta-samāpatttibhyāṁ

Steadiness and ease of posture is to be achieved through persistent slight effort and through concentration upon the Infinite.

2.22 (II.48) ततो द्वन्द्वानभिघातः ॥

tato dvandvānabhighātaḥ

When this is achieved, the pairs of opposites no longer impact.

2.23 (II.49) तस्मिन्सति श्वासप्रश्वासयोर्गतिविच्छेदः प्राणायामः ॥

tasmin sati śvāsa-praśvāsayor gati-vicchedaḥ prāṇāyāmaḥ

When right posture is attained there follows right control of *prāṇa* and proper inspiration and expiration of breath.

2.24 (II.50) बाह्याभ्यन्तरस्तम्भवृत्तिर्देशकालसंख्याभिः परिदृष्टो दीर्घसूक्ष्मः ॥

bāhyābhyantara-stambha-vṛttir deśakāla-saṁkhyābhiḥ paridṛṣṭo dīrghasūkṣmaḥ

Right control of *prāṇa* (the life-force) is external, internal or motionless; it is subject to place, time and number and is also protracted or brief.

2.25 (II.54) स्वविषयासम्प्रयोगे चित्तस्य स्वरूपानुकार इवेन्द्रियाणां प्रत्याहारः॥

sva-viṣayāsaṁprayoge cittasya svarūpānukāra ivendriyāṇāṁ pratyāhāraḥ

Abstraction (or *pratyāhāra*) is a withdrawal of mind from the sense experience so that the calming and control of the senses result while sense organs withdraw from the object likewise.

2.26 (II.55) ततः परमा वश्यतेन्द्रियाणाम्॥

tataḥ paramā vaśyatendriyāṇāṁ

As a result, there follows a complete subjugation of the sense organs (in *pratyāhāra*).

2.27 (III.9) व्युत्थाननिरोधसंस्कारयोरभिभवप्रादुर्भावौ निरोधक्षणचित्तान्वयो निरोधपरिणामः॥

vyutthāna-nirodha-saṁskārayor abhibhava-prādurbhāvau nirodha-kṣaṇa-cittān-vayo nirodha-pariṇāmaḥ

The silencing of the senses results in the iterations of sensing and controlling giving way to mind's simultaneous response to both that leads to a moment of voluntary "pause" when the perceiving consciousness has full sway.

2.28 (III.10) तस्य प्रशान्तवाहिता संस्कारात्॥

tasya praśānta-vāhitā saṁskārāt

Through the cultivation of this habit of "pausing" there eventually occurs a steadiness of spiritual perception.

2.29 (III.11) सवार्थितैकाग्रतयोः क्षयोदयौ चित्तस्य समाधिपरिणामः॥

sarvārthataikāgratayoḥ kṣayodayau cittasya samādhi-pariṇāmaḥ

The establishing of this habit (of pause) and the restraining of the mind from its thought-form-making tendency eventually results in a constant power to contemplate (*samādhī*).

2.30 (III.47) रूपलावण्यबलवज्रसंहननत्वानि कायसम्पत्॥

rūpa-lāvaṇya-bala-vajra-saṁhananatvāni kāya-saṁpat

This also results in mastery over five basic elements and bestows bodily perfection comprising symmetry of form, beauty of color, strength and the compactness of a diamond.

2.31 (IV.2) जात्यन्तरपरिणामः प्रकृत्यापूरात्॥

jāty-antara-pariṇāmaḥ prakṛity-āpūrāt

The transfer of consciousness from a lower vehicle into a higher is part of the (Nature's) great creative and evolutionary process.

2.32 (IV.7) कर्माशुक्लाकृष्णं योगिनस्त्रिविधमितरेषाम्॥

karmāśuklākṛṣṇaṁ yoginas tri-vidham itareṣāṁ

The activities of a Yogī are free from causing new *karma* cycles; while for others they continue to so cause, on three different planes: physical, astral and causal.

2.33 (IV.8) ततस्तद्विपाकानुगुणानामेवाभिव्यक्तिर्वासनानाम्॥

tatas tad-vipākānuguṇānām evābhi-vyaktir vāsanānāṁ

From these three kinds of *karma* emerge those forms which are necessary for the fruition of their effects.

2.34 (IV.10) तासामनादित्वमं चाशिषो नित्यत्वात्॥

tāsām anāditvaṁ cāśiṣo nityatvāt

Desire to live being eternal mind-created forms are with no known beginning.

2.35 (IV.11) हेतुफलाश्रयालम्बनैः संगृहीतत्वादेषामभावे तदभावः

hetu-phalāśrayālambanaiḥ saṁgṛhitatvād eṣām abhāve tad-abhāvaḥ

As forms are created through desire, the resultant personality and held together through the causal vitality (the will to live) and resultant outgoing life—when the desire (cause) ceases to attract, then the form (effect) ceases to exist likewise.

Chapter Three: Yogī and Insight

3rd Milestone

An assuring vision of *Īśvara* would launch you on a long journey into spiritual consciousness. At that point the goal is known and the path is seen. But still it is an alien territory. Will the newly acquired clearer perception and sharper reasoning be enough to face the new challenges?

By now, chasing indiscriminate happiness has greatly subsided as its sources appear transient. A new sensitivity has developed since the objects, people and events present themselves as effects and not as the causes. The law of *karma* further reveals that the mind-induced hindrances cause the lures of *guṇa* to hide. In this condition of discipleship, you make desire your target, since it is seen to excite the *guṇa* in the first place. From a disciple on the way to becoming a *yogī*, you transform this new sensitivity into insight or mature emotional intelligence. (Ordinarily, the term "disciple" refers to allegiance owed to an external guru. Here, having already envisioned a glimpse of the ultimate truth, the allegiance is to your "search for truth." The external guru is only an aid and not a prerequisite anymore.)

Your inner evolution as a disciple brings you in touch with the subtleness within, and that awareness develops new insight into the whole world that exists outside of you. The interplay of mind and spirit becomes evident in all objects. Your mind relates with a mind without, and all minds appear as one, giving you some idea of the virtual Universal Mind.

Till this point in your life, you have lived with a reflex discrimination between yourself and the rest of the world. Such a separation is prompted by a deep rooted physical awareness and an overarching ego. The new awareness of subtlety dissolves the artificial walls of separateness and brings home a new harmony. All objects, from the tiniest to the largest, present themselves as a single family to you. Thus starts your experimentation with the third Yoga hypothesis, *Macrocosm, the universe and microcosm, the human being, are alike.* You are moving towards realizing why your mind is also one amongst the many objects of matter.

New awareness of a meta-mind brings you closer to the spiritual Self within. Before you know it, your reading of situations and understanding of objects also turns spiritual. The reflex segregation between the self and all the rest makes way for a new commonality in all the objects, since each has the spirit and the mind-matter. The Yoga methods and practices continue with inner purification, and bring you to a point where you are not only aware of your astral self, but also remain primarily identified with it—and it becomes your *new* self. You are no more a slave to unremitting physical urges and unruly emotional swings. From devoted discipleship, you would become a *yogī* who knows how to harness emotional intelligence on the *yogīk* path.

In this phase: transition of a śiṣya into a yogi

Yoga hypothesis	Macrocosm, the universe and its microcosm, the human being, are alike.
Know through experience	An interplay of Mind and Spirit; singularity of mind and plurality of matter
Involuntary control	Discriminative thinking
Achieve Voluntary control	Spiritual reading
Become	A devoted disciple
Be	A *yogī*

New words used in this chapter

mūlaprakṛtī	Five basic elements in the composition of all matter
ākāśa	Space
madhyama-nāda	Range of sound vibrations belonging to the astral plane, 25 percent as powerful as *paśyanti*
paśyanti-nāda	Range of sound vibrations belonging to the causal plane, 25 percent as powerful as *para*
para-nāda	Range of sound vibrations belonging to plane beyond the three planes of physical, astral and causal
Mantrās	Incantation; such text that is designed to create certain vibrations
Siddhī	Perfection; psychic power
samāpattiḥ	Complete absorption; total merging at equilibrium
kriyā-yogaḥ	Yoga of action; practice addressed to controlling *prāṇa* through body-mind actions
kaivalyaṃ	Non-dual state; the ultimate state in Yoga
prajñā	Intuition; revelation

Existence and Creation

Though practice is the key, a journey into spiritual consciousness requires a more elaborate framework of reference for the physical-emotional-intellectual world, in order to make the practice insightful. Now you know, *experientially* as a disciple, that there is a lot more to this universe than what is seen. There is a more subtle world beyond or besides the physical world that interpenetrates the physical and makes it alive. The physical world is an effect, and the subtle world is its cause.

If the cause precedes the effect, then the subtle world must also owe its origin to something subtler. What does such precedence lead to? Does a hierarchy exist?

What you know

Let us begin with what you know about yourself.

Your physical world has three components:

- Body, containing various organs with bones, flesh, glands, blood, gasses, etc.
- Awareness (of self and the world), created in the brain through the senses and sustained by the nervous system that make the organs functional
- Energy generated by the metabolic mechanisms working on food, oxygen and *prāṇa* which sustains both of the above—the body and the awareness.

It is reasonable to conclude that a subtle body also has subtle counterparts for each of these physical components. However, the world of subtle bodies is not "out there" somewhere. We must revisit our limited concepts of "within" and "without" as suggested earlier. The subtle and the gross form a single continuum. Hence, the subtle world interpenetrates the physical world, and the subtle components remain integral to the physical components. The two worlds coexist virtually.

What you are about to know

You, as a "disciple of truth," are now given another hypothesis to test: Macrocosm, the universe and its microcosm, the human being, are alike. You are yourself an object that lives amidst a vast array of other objects, from atoms and particles to giant planets and the universe. The hypothesis challenges you to discover that each of these objects, from the tiniest to the largest, varies only in scale but not in composition.[29] The gross, subtle, and subtler components are present in each of them.

We have seen the gross-subtle continuum like an ever-extending stick. If the grossest physical bodies are at our end of this spectrum, the subtlest must be at the other end. If the gross emerges from the subtle, where does the subtlest emerge from? You can find a key to this question by carefully looking at the three physical components again. The **body**, as a configuration of bones and flesh, is an "inert" mechanism without life. Life is motion manifesting in **awareness** that is provided and sustained by **energy**. However, the last two are not physical, but subtle phenomena themselves. While a body and awareness are "created," energy is by itself. Hence, beyond the subtlest, only energy would prevail. Energy is essentially the Consciousness.

The life span of the bodies is finite, and the life span of the physical world is shorter than its cause, the subtle world. Though immeasurable by humans, even the subtlest at the other end of the spectrum must have a finite span. All the bodies, whether gross or subtle, are manifestations and collectively form our universe, let us call it "Existence." But in turn, the objects owe their existence to the womb of life that must be beyond or before Existence, where the gross-subtle world remains in conception, let us call it a state of "Creation."

The *Vedas* give us the following elaborate framework.

---

[29] *"We didn't get here by accident. Fractal geometry, a mathematical understanding of the universe, is revealing the truth of the spiritual maxim 'as above, so below.' Fractal geometry demonstrates the scientific nature of that belief system, showing that images repeat themselves throughout life."—Bruce Lipton and Steve Bhaerman,* Spontaneous Evolution: Our Positive Future and a Way to Get There from Here (*Hay House*, 2010).

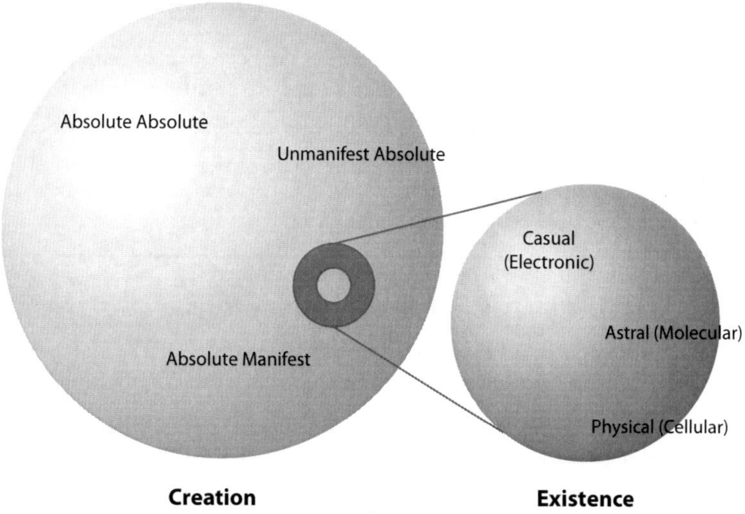

Figure 3.1: Creation and Existence

Descriptions and even illustrations like the above are generally somewhat "flat" because beyond a point our brain ceases to understand even the concept of subtlety. Our brain itself is an organ, and in spite of its subtle counterparts like *mānas* and *buddhi*, our thinking keeps the awareness lead-footed and limited. So, we can be aware of milk but cannot fathom the yet uncreated cream that lies within it, right in front of us.

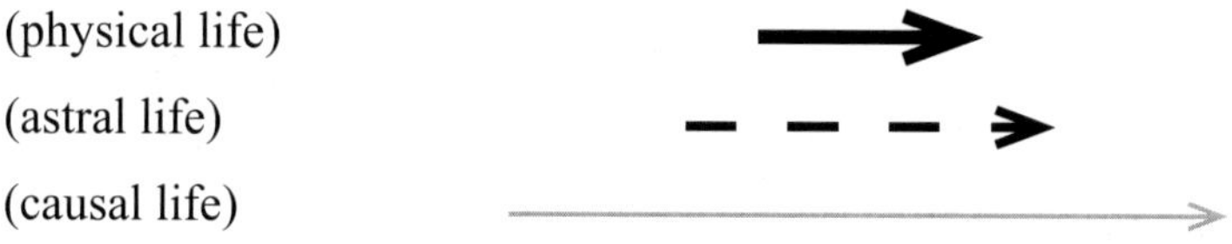

Figure 3.2: Life-span

The astral body survives the physical, and the causal body survives the astral. What happens at the end of the life span of the subtlest causal body? With no physical, astral, or causal body around, there is only awareness and energy left in the state of Creation. Awareness is finite and characterized as mind-matter;

energy is infinite, as the Spirit, and that still presents a duality. Ultimately, when even awareness ceases, everything collapses into a Dimensionless Point that simply is, an infinite ocean of energy. This is the state of non-duality, abiding in itself, a subtle truth.

Accelerated *Yogīk* Path

In evolution, the whole of humanity is *ordained* to realize its true (subtle) self at its own pace and in its own way. The real sequence of *Yoga-Sūtra,* revealed here, shows a clear path for a seeker who can become a disciple, then a *yogī*, then a *mahāyogī*, and finally a *ParamaYogī* (Yoga-master). But is this the only path? Sage Patanjali makes us aware that it is not, and that "will" can be summoned through Yoga for an accelerated inner evolution. Such "will," a function of the spiritual legacy of past lives, enables you to hasten the evolutionary progress. **Attainment of spiritual consciousness is rapid for one who seeks it wholeheartedly with an intense urge** (Sūtra 3.1/I.21).

Acquiring a skill of *pratyāhāra* is a major achievement for a seeker who, at the doorstep of advanced Yoga, commences a real ascent on the *yogīc* path. The journey beyond this point is in the subtle inner domain and strictly under *Īśvara's* watch. But, how soon and/or easily one reaches this point differs from seeker to seeker.

Attainment of spiritual consciousness is a piecemeal process. For a while, spiritual consciousness plays hide and seek, thanks to the obstacles. The Yoga practices do nothing directly to remove the obstacles but instead bring about a gradual internal change that eliminates the cause of the obstacles and their ability to obstruct. Working on the causes and not the effects makes Yoga an irreversible transformation process, but that also makes it a very long one, possibly extending over many lifetimes. However, Sage Pātañjali provides some solace and shows ways in which the progress on the *yogī*k path can be accelerated by those who are eligible.

Karma accumulates and gets carried over from one life to the next; and so does the spiritual legacy. Another bit of good news is that action in spiritual practice needs no redemption, and that proficiency only accumulates in every lifetime that you walk the spiritual path. We see many individuals turning "spiritual" suddenly—and at times, inexplicably—after living a conventional (even indulgent) materialistic life. In fact, abilities like judicious thinking, one-pointedness, compassion, goal-orientation, or inner quest are visible traits in many achievers who are genuinely "spiritually" oriented without wearing that label. Sometimes their material achievements make them restless and thus they recognize their spirituality within. (Here "spiritual" means altruistic or a calling beyond the ordinary; not religious, which in this context is a misnomer.) Once on a spiritual path, these dedicated individuals can redirect the same shining traits they used for material accomplishment, toward a new, higher purpose and progress rapidly.

Those who embark on a spiritual path at an early age tend to experience fewer obstacles since they need to do less unlearning. For them, the spiritual path is embraced as a natural course of things and not as a cure for the ills of material life. With an energetic commitment they revive the spiritual legacy of their earlier lives expeditiously.

Spiritual legacy

In the distant past, people were more easily disposed toward the spiritual path of *bhaktī*, devotion. Many among us still inherit that legacy. A path of devotion followed in past lives yields quicker spiritual attainment for many seekers early in this life, and provides abundant energy for the spiritual quest. To build on their legacy of devotion, many will pursue the path of spiritual attainment through self-realization (the subject-matter of *Yoga-Sūtra)* in their current or subsequent lives. The process of realization needs devotion to turn into a loving surrender to the inner teacher, but buttresses it with an iron will and strong, unswerving endurance.

Spiritual devotion in earlier lives is more likely to manifest at a younger age for those who want to be on a path to self-realization. The *yogīk* path may appear to be one path, but there are as many tracks as there are seekers. Your will and tenacity determines the rapidity of the progress, and the physical, astral, and causal are its three dimensions. **How rapid depends on whether the practice is intense, moderate or gentle** … (Sūtra 3.2/I.22). The extremely **strong-willed** may make an **intense** journey, but such seekers are likely to be handicapped by slower assimilation of their new "self," which can lead to a risk of constant conflicts. The **less strong-willed** may make **gentle** progress and may need to compensate for that with more tenacity and devotion in order to deal with repeated failures.

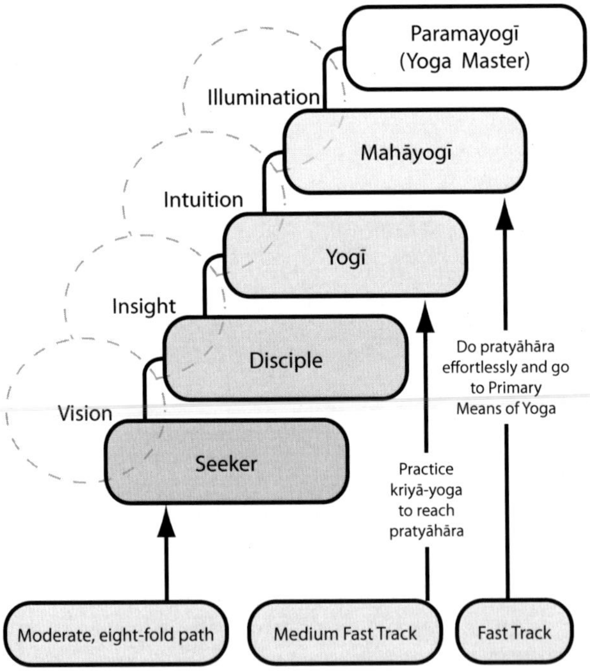

Figure 3.2: Spiritual Legacy

The **moderately willed** would balance the will and tenacity, and would also have a **moderate** share of risks and failures. This even-paced moderate track appears to be well suited to the householder's mode of life.

What we bring to the present life as a spiritual legacy of our previous lives makes us one of the three types of aspirants—with high, medium, or low spiritual legacy. *Yoga-Sūtra* prescribes three different kinds of *sādhanā* (paths) to these three classes of aspirants. Prescription for the high legacy aspirant is **fast track** practice of meditation on *Īśvara* and non-attachment to restrain the modification of the mind-stuff to enter into *samādhī*. For the medium legacy aspirant, a **medium fast track**, called *Kriyā Yoga*—humility, absence of desire, spiritual reading, and devotion to *Īśvara*—are prescribed. For the low legacy aspirant, the **moderate** eightfold *sādhanā* is prescribed (as described in Chapter Two—*yama*, *niyama*, *āsana*, *prāṇayāma*, *pratyāhāra*, *dhāraṇā*, *dhyāna*, and *samādhī*).

Yet another way

The other half of Sūtra 3.2/I.22 is, **but** (in attainment of true spiritual consciousness) **there is "yet another way."** In *Yoga-Sūtra* this "another way" is only indicated and not explicitly shown. It appears to indicate that the legacy of thousands of years of "devotion" is a good foundation for obtaining direct blessings from *Īśvara*. However, implied in such devotion is totality. This devotion is not just externally exhibited in chanting this or worshipping that; and is not a function of how often one performs rituals perfunctorily; rather, this degree of devotion springs from every cell of the body, and it is quite a challenge to let it do so unhindered. You can't just put it there.

This apparently easy but extremely tricky path is feasible only to a worthy few. An absolute devotion to *Īśvara* can lead you to the same seemingly normal state of *saṃyama* that can be reached after the otherwise strenuous practice of *dhāraṇā*, *dhyāna*, and *samādhī*. This individual is able to live on two different levels of awareness simultaneously—appearing to live the normal householder's life and also continuing to be in the super-contemplative state, not just as a practice but as a continuous state of pure awareness, as exemplified by the Indian Saint Meerābāi.

Fast Track

One who has accrued considerable inner evolution on the *yogīk* path earns a natural ability of *pratyāhāra*, thus qualifying directly for the Primary Means of Yoga without following the Secondary Means. The earlier stages can be quickly passed so that a seeker can directly turn into a *mahāyogī*. *Pratyāhāra* signifies a profound change in perception.

The act of perceiving, as we have seen, occurs at various levels:

1. **Form (Physical)**: At the most mundane level, it is an act of seeing and form-sensing through the sense-organs, processed by the brain.
2. **Word (Astral)**: In the process of cognition the sense data travels with *mānas* on the astral plane, the sensing gets verbalized and drives the emotion-laden thoughts.
3. **Idea (Causal):** At the highest level of recognition, its cause, concept, or essential idea is sensed intellectually, by *buddhi*.

Thus, the process touches all three levels—form (physical), word (astral), and idea (causal).[30]

Judicious Reasoning and Beyond

Falling into a groove and adopting a habit comes naturally to us. A "routine" is our comfort zone guarded by the structure of predispositions. Our bodies prefer familiar environments because they are less threatening than the ones we don't know. Thus, the target object referred by the form, word and the idea being the same, we tend to use the three interchangeably. For example, within the domain of physical attraction, the word "love" and the basic instinct are all taken as one and the same. How many challenges such a mix-up creates for us?

---

[30] *When we see a mango, for example, it is perceived on the physical plane in terms of its vibrant color, alluring smell, large size, and rounded shape. It is cognized on the astral plane as the "king" mango that "tastes as wonderful as it always did during the "feasts" with the loved ones. And intellectually it triggers a sense of luxurious satiation of a craving.*

In any new environment, thoughts are complex; knowledge is imprecise, incomplete, and slow to evolve; the underlying emotions are turbulent; and the resulting mind chatter is unending. In the midst of a hazy mess of crisscrossing thoughts, one has to struggle to reach a stable thought that makes sense. This very process of making sense of a challenging situation builds a new algorithm in our brain and stores it in the memory. This new faculty is called "judicious reasoning" and the structure of predispositions is adapted accordingly to accommodate it. But on the fast track, one can quickly go beyond it.

When among the form, word, and idea, each is distinctly perceived it is judicious reasoning, but when the three appear blended together it is a perfect perception (Sūtra 3.3/I.42). While judicious reasoning remains a deliberate mind-driven activity, a perfect perception is intuitive and highly contemplative wherein the "divisive" mind stays non-attached. Mind does not engage with the brain to create thoughts knitted around the forms and words; but acts as the pure catalyst that it really is. This blending affords a perceiver direct awareness of an object's essential meaning. That instant journey from sensing an object to penetrating its core makes the form dissolve and expression wither away. You see right through an object!

Until you arrive at this stage (as a *mahāyogī*, described in Chapter Four) you cannot avail of the gift of intuition. Hence, till then, the next best alternative is judicious reasoning—though you keep struggling with the choice of words used, weighing the multiple implied meanings, and figuring out how best to deal with them. Judicious reasoning can also be translated as "discrimination" and intuition as "discernment." Judicious reasoning is the most that objective thinking can be. On the contrary, intuitive perception is not borne out of any thinking process in the domain of individual mind, but is rooted in the Universal Mind.

Through such refined reasoning you learn how, under *guṇa*'s influence, the thinking process cognizes independent aspects of an object and braids them into a collective sense. On the *yogīk* path, you would eventually learn how to perceive on the transcendental fourth plane, a great transition that occurs only when the limitations of judicious reasoning are fully understood.

Judicious reasoning is still supported by the scaffolding of things already known and is still influenced by the associated emotions. When judicious reasoning matures into intuitive spiritual perception, the individual mind no longer engages with the brain for cognition, and the dominance of memory and emotion-soaked thinking is set aside. You recognize the form, the word, and its idea instantly, just by looking at an object. All at once; all as one. That is intuition.

On the fast track, you arrive up to this point in quicker steps. Earlier, the divergent and collectively chaotic sense impulses triggered thoughts, which flew in all directions. But now, the newly refined and less rigid structure of predispositions would allow much larger chunks of incoming impulses to flow unhindered. Hence, such "unqualified" impulses would fail to collect any near-identical memory patterns, therefore triggering no thoughts. Thus, often free from compulsive reflex thinking, and no more "kicked in" by each impulse passing through, the thoughts shrink in volume and slow down. Besides, the thought formation needs less back-and-forth loops through the memory pools, so the process of thought formation picks up pace. Now, disparate thoughts do not clutter the thinking instruments. Thus, the thoughts are fewer, more coherent and processed instantly. This transition results in a quiescent state of mind. A quiet mind is less indulgent, which provides a gap in thoughts ready to behold a vision of *Īśvara*.

Reasoning of any kind requires active brain-*mānas-buddhi* to get some help in cognition by digging into the memory; but that ends up coloring the perception. On the fast track, intuition disables a compulsive access to memory, the only bondage, by bypassing it[31] and quickly acquiring the ability of spiritual perception.

---

[31] *Thought is a process of amalgamating incoming impulses with near-identical past memory patterns soaked in past emotional experiences and creating a fresh, but nearly similar, new thought frame. These frames are then "excreted" in coded patterns from the point ājnā*—located in the brain's frontal lobe—*to become another person's incoming impulses, with one true copy going to our memory pool. If one were to study this process of near-similar thought frames moving at a speed of 120 frames per second, it would be like viewing a movie. This whole process is destroyed during a direct perception—there is no other*

Spiritual Perception

A *mahāyogī* may not even need judicious reasoning as a stepping stone to spiritual perception. In other words, it is not always necessary to first sense the form, to comprehend the associated word, and then to grasp the idea. You need not sense these three as distinct components of the object and then "judiciously" blend them in the process of cognizing it. That elaborate process is an effort. It is possible to set aside judicious reasoning and still understand the object intuitively. **Intuition (perception without judicious reasoning) gushes forth when memory no longer colors and the awareness entangled in the word and the form is transcended making only the idea to present in a Meta context** (Sūtra 3.4/I.43). Intuition brings everything into an instant perception. Though the sources change, it still remains a cognitive activity. In contrast, a vision of *Īśvara* is a direct perception, without any mind-assisted cognition. Such a true contemplative perception is the next progressive ability.

Knowing by the appearance and concoction of suitable words (sound patterns) comes essentially from the memory pools. There is a certain give and take between memory and thinking, since during cognition thoughts draw near-identical known patterns from memory. The marginally different "new patterns" are, in turn, lodged back into the memory for future use. This is conventional incremental learning.

How is the memory progressively bypassed? It uses an accelerated biological evolution of the brain itself. The disciple's journey on the fast track *yogīk* path is evidenced by certain cell-level changes in the body-mind system. The most significant change is the rerouting of sense impulses traveling through the brain. Now, the side

---

way to be free from this bondage. Now, one is able to close the circuit between the base of the spine, taluka and ajna, and rotate prāṇa *within the circuit for the cleaning process—this is what Sage Pātanjali refers to as the "internal purification." When "devotion to* Īśvara*" is added to this, one can see, know, and be guided by the spiritual Self within. All obstructions and obstacles are thus destroyed.*

Later, in intuition, doors are closed (at taluka*) even to the incoming impulses. In this way we can totally isolate ourselves from the world (temporarily) without running away from it. The intuitive state can be used for higher spiritual practices, and one returns to a lower state for household obligations. But this, then, is a conscious choice, not a compulsion as before.*

passages of the brain are cleared and used by the sense impulses to travel to the frontal lobe, bypassing the top of the brain route where memory pools are lined up (see progression from insight to intuition in *Figure 4.1*). Thus, the memory-driven inferential and dogmatic thinking process that leads to judicious reasoning is set aside and transcended. The forms no longer create the appearance of distinct objects, and their verbal labels no longer inhibit or excite.

The same contemplation, with or without judicious reasoning, can also be applied to things subtle (for eventually reaching the state of *samādhī*) (Sūtra 3.5/I.44). The gross emerges as articulation or manifestation of the subtle. Hence, the subtle remains present in the gross form of each object as its cause. As the gross can be perceived with or without judicious reasoning, the subtle can also be so perceived. (The gross matter and the subtle elements have the relationship shown in *Figure 5.1*).

Intuition strips the words off any associated emotive overlays and receives them only as sound. The relation between *ākāśa* and sound is the most significant. We have seen (in Chapter Zero) how Spirit becomes matter when perceived. Matter in its subtlest form is the Universal Mind and its first manifestation as matter is *ākāśa*. *Ākāśa* is the primary matter from which air, fire, water, and earth elements are successively born, thus creating through their infinite permutations and combinations the whole material world.

One can contemplate the whole world subtly by knowing the sound (vibrations) alone.

> *Every form is the result of thought and of sound. Every form veils or conceals an idea or concept. Every form, therefore, is but the symbol or attempted representation of an idea...*—Alice Bailey, 124.

To be able to look at an object and its form and to perceive the causal idea and the specific impulse lying latent in it is spiritual reading. Thus, those with high spiritual legacy can quickly regain the ability of non-attachment and spiritual reading, and then directly proceed to *dhāraṇā*, *dhyāna*, *samādhī*, and *saṃyama*.

Medium Fast Track (*Kriyā Yoga*)

Those with medium spiritual legacy can follow the Yoga of techniques to elevate awareness (*Kriyā Yoga*). Instead of following the long and winding practices of the Secondary Means of Yoga, such privileged aspirants are already *yogīs* and can concentrate only on the three most demanding *niyama*: fiery aspiration, devotion to *Īśvara*, and spiritual reading to reach *pratyāhāra*. Spiritual reading as a way of life holds together and reinforces the fiery aspiration and the devotion. *Niyama* is a tricky endeavor. It is, on one hand, an essential practice for a seeker. Yet many times, success in *niyama* remains elusive, even when *yama* are adhered to and proficiency is achieved in *āsana* and *prāṇayāma*. For the fortunate ones, if you recall, fulfillment of *niyama* is more bestowed upon than earned, and becomes a culmination of Yoga that ends in the states of *dhārana*, *dhyāna*, and *samādhī*. In this culmination, *niyama* is thus the end of the road as much as the journey.

The three basic Yoga avenues (taking *Jnana Yoga* and *Rāja Yoga* together) are:[32]

- ***Karma Yoga*** (comprising *Hatha Yoga*, the Yoga of physical postures, and *Laya Yoga*, the Yoga of the body's force fields) guides a disciple on the physical plane.
- ***Bhakti Yoga*** guides the disciple on the astral plane and shows how to bring into submission one's emotions and feelings to devote them toward the sole longing for *Īśvara*.
- ***Raja Yoga*** that Sage Pātañjali is teaching us in *Yoga- Sūtra* is on the causal plane. It is the science of mind and shows how to make the will purposeful and any desire non-existent in order to bring one's being on all three planes in

---

[32] *Here is an interesting analogy with* chakra*:*

1. "*Karma Yoga* resulted in the awakening of the three *chakra* below the diaphragm (*mūlādhāra*, *swādhisthāna*, and *maṇipūra*).
2. Bhakti Yoga resulted in their transmutation and transference into heart (*anāhata*) and throat (*viśuddha*) *chakra* above the diaphragm, and
3. Rāja Yoga synthesizes all the forces in the body in the head (*ajna*, *bindu*, and *sahasrāra*) *chakra*, and from there distributes and controls them.

Rāja Yoga, which Sage Pātanjali primarily deals with, includes the effects of all the others."—Alice Bailey, 122.

harmony so as to dissolve its awareness, establishing the way for *Īśvara* to manifest.

Kriyā Yoga takes an aspirant on a medium-fast *yogīk* path that hastens the inner evolution and brings about a quicker culmination of *Rāja Yoga*. ***Kriyā Yoga*, yoga of action, leading to union with the soul, is threefold** (Sūtra 3.6/II.1):

- **Fiery aspiration**: The subjugation of the physical self is possible only when each physical cell embarks on a mission of change. *Yoga-Sūtra* uses the word *tapaḥ.* Some interpreters have also used expressions such as "penance" or "austerities." However, one cannot simply will oneself into penance because the moment the effort ceases, the physical cells are prone to regress. Austerities should be effortless and become one's natural way of life; that is possible only when Yoga's purifying exercises are carried out unceasingly. Thus, fiery aspiration should be invested in *yogīk* practices and not just in external measures, so that every atom of one's body is afire with zeal and resolve. In a way, this is sublimation of the physical plane.
- **Devotion to *Īśvara***: When the outbound senses are turned inward and the thinking process is made more composed and even-paced, a window of opportunity opens. A gap in thoughts allows perception to occur without judicious reasoning or discrimination. Such direct perception establishes communication with *Īśvara*. All the distractions then wither away and there is only one longing—to be aware of *Īśvara*. On the astral plane, this results in every thought being focused on this alone. In a way, this is sublimation of the astral plane.
- **Spiritual Reading**: Spiritual reading, too, becomes a way of life. Earlier, it was mentioned that ceaseless practice of internal and external purification exercises are rewarded in the form of effortless practice of *niyama* and its culmination in a gift of spiritual reading. The ability to read everything spiritually brings about a critical shift. The self-view and the world-view converge into a single spiritual consciousness, and "I" dissolves into soul awareness.

> Omnipresence of *Īśvara* becomes a new reality. In a way, this is sublimation of the causal plane.

> *The organs are the horses, the mind is the reins, the intellect is the charioteer, the soul is the rider, and the body is the chariot.*—Vivékananda, 168.

The chariot noted by Vivekananda will reach its destination only if the organs are controlled by the mind, if the mind's reins are well held by the intellect, and if the intellect is fully devoted to the soul. The aim of three-fold *Kriyā Yoga* is to bring about the soul vision and to eliminate obstructions, hindrances, and distractions. When all *niyama* are fully established, you are truly no longer the same person. The vision is like a divine touch (*sparś*), and once you have *Īśvara* as your guide, you would willingly and lovingly surrender. That self-dissolution is quite distinct from any dogmatic devotion that is just a skin-deep behavioral expression. But the journey still goes on, and the *yogī* is not there yet. *Īśvara* is still only a visualized image, not an experience.

The obstructions to the physical control and the behavioral changes are still being eliminated. Hindrances on the astral plane obscuring the vision are still being removed. There are distractions on the causal plane that still create difficulties in holding on to the soul vision. **The aim of three-fold *Kriyā Yoga* is to bring about the soul vision and also to eliminate these afflictions (obstructions/ hindrances/ distractions)** by burning their seeds and rendering them infertile (Sūtra 3.7/II.2).

The seeds of afflictions, either carried over from past lives or created from the present life, need conscious redemption. By now, the *yogī* has also undergone structural changes, and the accompanying rhythmic breathing practices help in pre-empting the creation of any new seeds.

Thus, as we saw at the end of Chapter Two, eliminating the form-creating desires is the goal. It can be achieved through an accelerated medium-fast track that quickly turns the seeker-disciple into an accomplished *yogī.* An alternative laborious journey of the secondary means of Yoga, the "moderate" pathway, is explained next.

Moderate "Eightfold" Pathway

The elaborate eightfold pathway takes you to *pratyāhāra*. It takes longer, but Yoga is not about any kind of competition anyway. In Yoga, the duration and the quantum of efforts bring no proportionate results or rewards.

We know that people often turn to spiritual things inexplicably in the midst of their ordinary lives. We also know that a certain type of "part-time" spirituality is alluring for a while, as you can return to your "normal" life and let the material and spiritual lives conveniently coexist. Initially, there is neither real understanding of the spiritual path nor any fiery commitment to it. However, actively turning toward the search of truth is hardly an accident, and once you are back on the spiritual track, its purpose is better served by investing real energy in the spiritual journey.

Exceptionally few are *born* spiritual. But those who take up the spiritual path—whether sooner or later in life—are really catching up with their spiritual legacy, unbroken by death. And until that point, they are simply living out the associated *karma*. If the legacy is not enough to put you on a fast or medium-fast track, you belong to a vast majority, and should follow the moderate, *aṣṭānga* (eight-limbed) path. Sage Pātañjali assures you that even this moderate path leads to enlightenment.

Still, why does it take longer? Those with a strong spiritual legacy find it almost natural to withdraw their attention from the luring objects at will, a state of *pratyāhāra*. *Yogīs* on the fast track are born with that ability, and those on the medium-fast track acquire it quickly. Those without that ability, like most of us, have to learn this major transition. Most of the Sūtra commentators have addressed all the eight limbs rather inaccurately . . . presenting them on a single dimension. They have almost forgotten to tell us about the inter-relationships among the Secondary Means, and a crucial transition called *pratyāhāra*. This passing over, from the external domain of objects to the subtle inner domain, facilitates a quantum leap from the Secondary Means of the eight-limbed pathway to its Primary Means.

Transition to a World Within

Terms like "turning inward" and "looking within" have lost their real significance through vernacular overuse. The perception process is so inevitably outward bound that any turning inward is an adventure, and staying anchored in your internal domain is an Everest expedition. But, to move towards the pinnacle of Yoga you have to take that leap without which, breaking away from the compulsive thought process, and learning at the feet of *Īśvara* would never be possible.

You cannot be focused inside merely by closing your eyes. The inner domain is not accessible to the sense organs. The preliminary exercises and the Secondary Means of Yoga equip your senses to get connected to the *chakras* of the astral body, which act like mini-brains and do the sensing without the sense organs.

Initially, in place of the objects, this inner attention will allow you to get engaged solely with the images, and then slowly move away from the stored images altogether to engage with the intuitive symbols, coded signals and finally nothingness. *Samādhī* belongs to this domain, but unless you transition to it from the external domain the eightfold pathway does not work.

What comes naturally to those who embark on the fast or medium-fast tracks has to be earned on the moderate path through concerted hard work of the Secondary Means of Yoga. Then you can remain anchored within, even with eyes wide open. But, before making this critical transition, we must understand the subtle inner domain.

Objects, Interplay of Mind and Spirit

Objects are multi-layered; but our mind does not allow us to look at them that way. What would happen to a disciple once all the mind afflictions were eliminated? A disciple would become free from the compulsions of object-oriented living. But this freedom is not to be confused with any abandonment of material life. You will continue to live your life, yet it is not the same world, because you would not be the same person anymore.

All along, Sage Pātañjali has talked about understanding the thinking process and its relationship with the thinking instruments. A disciple learns to unhook the thinking process from the mind, at will, and not to get swayed by a torrent of sense impulses. Setting the mind aside as a catalyst must be practiced in order to be able to perceive directly.

> *He stands then apart from the great illusion; the bodies which have hitherto held him no longer do so; the great current of ideas and thoughts and desires which have their origin through the "modifications of the thinking principle" of men imprisoned in the three worlds no longer sway or affect him; and the myriad thought forms which are the results of these currents in the causal, astral, and physical worlds no longer shut him away from the realities or from the true subjective world of causes and of force emanations.*—Alice Bailey, 165.

Simply put, it is realized that the "seen" world is our own fabrication born out of our mind modifications. This is not synonymous with a more folksy but an obviously wrong statement that the "world is all imaginary." *Yoga-Sūtra* does not seem to make such a naïve assertion and nowhere is the word *māyā* (illusory) used. On the contrary, it is affirmed that this world exists in reality; that the past and the present exist in reality, that to forsake them, to run away from them, to dismiss them all as *māyā* is fruitless and a sign of ignorance. But it is also important to recognize that some mind is always at work in the conception, creation, transformation, and destruction of each object. And that your reality at any given point in time is always an inferred approximation of *the* unchanging reality that is framed in a relativistic mode. Ironically, such a perception of the unchanging reality keeps constantly changing.

Objects do exist, but we see them as what we are conditioned to see, and that is not real. The *yogīk* path shows how to stand in the inner consciousness of the spirit rather than stay in such a personalized view of the world of objects. Thus, even though the objective world does not cease to exist, it ceases to affect or lure us. In broad daylight, the objective world dissolves for such a disciple—first momentarily, and later at will; and then in its place stands a glimpse of the celestial world that one intuitively knows is the real home. This is an important moment on the *yogīk* path.

For one who has achieved Yoga (the union) the objective world ceases to be though it continues to exist for those who are not yet free, thus creating as many virtual worlds as there are beings (Sūtra 3.8/II.22). The perennial question is: Does the objective world exist independent of all the beings? First, any answer is almost impossible for us to fathom because our testimony to existence is our perception of the world, and that is limited by the sensory experiences and the thinking instruments. And, for those who transcend the senses and the thinking instruments, it does not matter anymore. But it is important to realize that the laws of the three worlds do not change; *a yogī only transcends them*. What makes this possible is an elevation of the awareness to a new level.

On the *yogīk* path, you must have a whole-hearted participation in the world and be able to make *niyama* a way of life. A disciple who acquires the ability to do spiritual reading stands in the midst of the worldly objects, yet they don't exist. They exist for those who can't read spiritually, and simultaneously they don't exist for the disciple. The objects continue to challenge and strengthen the disciple's ability and application of spiritual reading.

At this stage, a disciple acquires a beautiful ability to be fully aware of the world around and yet be isolated from it. In such an isolated participation, the dynamic life ceases to swirl around. It becomes possible to consciously connect with the world on subtle levels. This reveals the past and future of the ever-changing gross. That picture is more stable, more durable, and more real.

Mind and Spirit, the Primary Pair of Opposites

Once we move away from the world of objects as they appear and dive into the world of mind and Spirit, the concepts from here on are really understood more by experiencing than by reading about them even if put into such revealing words.

The mind-matter (the perceptible range from the subtlest Universal Mind to the grossest inanimate substance) and the Spirit (the all-permeating principle beyond ordinary perception) is the primary pair of opposites. **The understanding of the nature of the perceived as well as the Perceiver is produced by virtue of the association of the soul with the mind** (Sūtra 3.9/II.23). In the process of perceiving and experiencing any object, the mind-matter and the spirit come together for its composite appearance.

To say that "mind-matter and spirit come together" is a profound statement, because mind is perceivable but the spirit is not. A human experience is a skit scripted by the Spirit that lends energy to the perceived object in the form of live *guṇa*, and into the perceiving object in the form of awareness. But the mind for its part creates an illusion that the object is, what it is perceived as. Then, the *guṇa* is mistaken as the truth, and the instruments of perception—the pseudo perceivers on the causal, astral, or physical planes—are mistaken as the real perceivers, thus ushering the coup of the "I" identity.

This "I" is inconspicuously present in all human experiencing. You don't need to go far for a demo. Listen to your next conversation, or overhear any conversation between others, and count the "I"s. You will find out how flooded you are by these big I-megaphones. (And then listen to your own internal dialogue!)

On the physical plane, an experience is in the form of awareness of a physical state; on the astral plane, in the form of feelings and thoughts, and on the causal plane, in the form of desires and concepts. However, the underlying commonality is the inseparable "I" that also starts falsely owning the objects, feelings, and thoughts that are only the impressions of the process of experiencing.

> *Vivéka, (discrimination) slips through the cracks of thoughts. Like music, vivéka can be thought of or read about but is real only when known directly. It is critically important, therefore, not to try to establish vivéka mentally. The self-sense (asmitā) is always almost subtly present, avoiding detection as it lays claim to experience, and it is compelled to "own" everything, even non-mental insights.*—Chip Hartranft, 29.

So, the "I"-centric experiencing concretizes a divided view of the world, the "self vs. not-self" that appears to contain mind-matter alone. The interplay of mind-matter and the Spirit produce innumerable pairs of opposites. Realization that matter and Spirit are poles apart is the first step of divorce from the "self vs not-self" discrimination. Slowly, a discerning process of "Self and not-Self" dawns in its place. Matter is not just in the form of objects, but even perceiving sense organs, senses, and the mind are all matter, while the Spirit is the soul, the real Perceiver. This is followed by the second important realization that all the deceptive experiencing occurs only because of the alleged union between the two brought about by the very process of perception. Then, in *pratyāhāra* a disciple takes a giant step of separation—to let pure awareness prevail, thus letting matter be matter and the Spirit be Spirit. It is needless to emphasize, though, that this occurs progressively and ever so gradually. Just the "theoretical learning" of the philosophies does not take one far, and any deliberate mental acrobatics to rein in mind modifications are counter-productive. It takes years of dedicated Yoga methods and practices, and patient drift-watching, to discern your thought processes. We are ordinarily so immersed in thoughts that "thinking" about thoughts appears to be a waste of already scarce "free" time. Discerning is also to be aided by awareness-enhancing practices, and by the ability to hold a meditative attitude resulting from the structural overhaul of the body-mind.

And lastly, a vision of *Īśvara* is still playing hide and seek at this stage. You also must yearn for the moments of pure awareness, because without its help you may know *about* the interplay between mind and the Spirit but may not know *why*.

Avidyā, *Cause of the Interplay*

The cause of this alleged association between mind-matter and the Spirit is *avidyā* (ignorance) that must be overcome (Sūtra 3.10/II.24). Why does this omniscient Spirit (soul) get entangled with the ignorance of matter in the first place? In the soul's desire to experience, it ends up using the outgoing senses as vehicles, which brings about its identification with the phenomenal world. Then how could pure awareness prevail? By reversing the process; by letting pure awareness slip-in, in place of the ignorance that withers away in stages. Hence, as the awareness of the spiritual Self grows, the experiencing of the material world is punctuated by a certain reluctance, and instead there is a greater desire to know your own spiritual nature. Eventually, the expanding consciousness brings home awareness that matter and the Spirit, the mother of all pairs of opposites, are two distinct entities. The seeds of ignorance are thus removed slowly, and the need for any outbound-experiencing itself is preempted. Even when you experience, it is no more drawn reflexively toward the pairs of opposites to taint the thinking with a tension between the opposites that makes it sway.

What do we mean by "pairs of opposites"? The relative reality plays this trick on us. Everything becomes subject to time and space keeping our comprehension of reality diffused over a range of possibilities. A *guṇa*-based perception makes it worse by creating ever-changing impressions. And the center-stage "I" makes a reflex discriminative judgment about everything, creating false distinctions of self and not-self. By stretching the contextual dimensions of time and space long enough, any phenomenon can be rendered as "only relatively true," thus creating pairs of opposites forever. At the heart of this "relativity" is duality that stops only at the Spirit which is absolute and cannot be perceived by itself, making time and space redundant.

A progressive dissolution of ignorance becomes manifest in the evolution of "I," the personality. The wrong identification ceases with the dissolution of the false personality that otherwise colors the individual mind. Eventually, the individual mind becomes as pure as the Universal Mind that brings direct perception in place of thinking and knowing. It is realized that the real Perceiver cannot experience its own self and can only *be* that. Pure awareness that resides within, simply is, and cannot be sensed. Thus, pure awareness occurs only when *avidyā* (ignorance) ends.

Complete End to Avidyā*, a Great Liberation*

When ignorance is brought to an end through a *complete* non-association with the things perceived, this is a great liberation (Sūtra 3.11/II.25). The perceived objects external to the self do not trigger an experience alone. A human mind can be self-indulgent and engage in auto-generated loops of thoughts within its own confines, thanks to the self-triggering memory pools. Memory seeds explode and puff up on their own, releasing more seeds in the process. Hence, it is also important in the end that the memory itself is bypassed.

Sage Pātañjali says that *avidyā* is "brought to" and not "comes to" an end. This refers to the seeker's conscious efforts to bring mind modifications under control, to establish the discerning ability and to be in the state of pure awareness. Only in conscious discernment does a seeker use discrimination "without being discriminative," and continue to be in a physical world without experiencing or having any need to do so. Discernment between mind and the Spirit has to be interiorized as a way of connecting with the world, even while dwelling in the inner domain.

Discernment between Mind and Spirit

A sensory response and a thought process of an "uninterrupted" discernment first seeds itself as a concept in the mind of a disciple. Then it arrives on the astral plane as active, discriminative discernment. The disciple starts analyzing the thoughts as they occur. However, it takes a long time for the stubborn reflex discrimination to melt away before you can effectively discern on the emotional and the physical levels as well. And it takes even longer for **discerning instinctively and overcoming the stage of bondage of *avidyā* through uninterrupted discrimination** (Sūtra 3.12/II.26).[33]

We need to understand the words—"discrimination" and "discernment." It is our inborn tendency to classify and differentiate in

[33] Sūtras *II.22 to II.26 may sound repetitious. When deeply meditated upon, one finds that they are not; in fact, nothing else in* Yoga-Sūtra *is this way. Each* sūtra *has a definite and profound lesson.*

order to comprehend. This gets first articulated in our instinctive differentiation between self and not-self. On the spiritual path as our understanding of the spiritual "Self" grows, initially Self (the soul) is still a part of our not-self. This is a very important point to note. When you invest more in the physical aspects of a practice, in your worship of the gurus and in adulation of the books, but do not witness any transformation within yourself, you need to check if all your "spirituality" is still anchored outside. That is when you need to practice and start proper discernment to spontaneously recognize a differentiation between matter (to which "self" belongs) and "Self," the Spirit.

Throughout this process as you remain vulnerable to the assault of habitual reactive thinking, and must therefore return to the initial discriminating state time and again. This is a losing battle until the collective practices on the *yogīk* path bring about a change at the cellular level. Then, any ground gained in this way is permanent, and the disciple inches toward the state of uninterrupted discernment. But at no stage on the path can one afford to be lax, because the tendency of the self to associate with the objects is built into the process of perception.

As *avidyā* is superseded by *vidyā*, the inspired quest for truth slowly yields "perception without judicious thinking" and finally, "spiritual reading." Only then is the uninterrupted discernment possible.

> *The aspirant then definitely assumes the attitude of higher polarity (the spirit manifesting as the soul, or the inner ruler) and seeks in the affairs of every day to discriminate between the form and the life, between the soul and the body; between the sum total of lower manifestation (physical, astral, and mental man) and the real self, the cause of the lower manifestation.*—Alice Bailey, 171.

Thus, uninterrupted discernment (as Self-consciousness) is really the absence of discrimination (as self-consciousness), as the distinction between mind and the Spirit becomes a part of life, making any discriminative thinking redundant. This also brings you closer to your Self, requiring no effort to pull you away from the outbound attention.

Culmination

On the *yogīk* path, no achievement at any stage occurs by destroying anything. Destruction goes against the very essence of Yoga. Instead, all afflictions are conquered by knowing and then going past or beyond them. So, the end of discriminating knowledge comes when the nature of the Spirit and its distinction from the mind-matter is fully known, and hence discrimination is made inconsequential. One does not stop at merely discerning between the mind-matter and the Spirit in the perceived objects. The same discernment is present in you, as the perceiving object, and, thus within you there is a natural separation occurring between mind-matter and Spirit even as you experience objects; and this natural separation thereby denies any excitement to *guṇa.* A union (Yoga) happens only after such isolation of the Spirit in you and others, and that is the real point of culmination.

Discipleship: Under *Īśvara*'s Tutelage

With your new-found ability to settle firmly in the inner domain at will, *pratyāhāra* brings forth a vision, in more than one way, for your transformation into a *yogī.* It brings about contact with the soul, *Īśvara*, which itself is a significant happening. It offers a glimpse of the state of *samādhī.* And then, as a disciple, your Yoga practices and most importantly **spiritual reading results in contact with the soul** (Sūtra 3.14/II.44). A contact with *Īśvara*, initiated with a vision, signifies an acceptance of a disciple for further Yoga studies, and the role of the external teacher comes to an end.

Acquiring the ability of spiritual reading is an immensely substantial achievement. Now you continue to live in the midst of myriad objects with their forms, and yet see them not. You perceive only their veiled substance. A fluid universal synthesis and a common thread of divinity are discovered in all the objects. When the objective forms cease to exist, that also brings an end to any identification with them. Born instead, is identification with the indwelling divinity itself. This is a complete transformation.

Īśvara, *the Goal*

> *Dedicating oneself to the idea of pure awareness has little to do with the emotion of devotion. Rather, it is the orientation one takes as every thought, word, or deed comes to serve the goal of knowing pure awareness.*—Chip Hartranft, 36.

The apparent acceptance of a disciple by *Īśvara* is the beginning of a journey and not an end. A lot of hard work is still in balance, except that it is made lighter by your conscious and loving dedication of everything to *Īśvara*. A vision of *Īśvara* also brings unprecedented happiness to which your body-mind system latches on. When distracted, a longing for the vision brings your devotion back on the track. **Through devotion to *Īśvara* the goal of meditation is reached** (Sūtra 3.15/II.45).

One of the important initial instructions from *Īśvara* is how to say "AUM" properly (explained in detail in Chapter Five). The resonance of AUM gently lifts awareness from gross to subtler bodies, until eventually only the pure awareness prevails as pure consciousness. The *yama*, *niyama*, *āsana*, and *prāṇayāma* continue jointly to cause internal and external purification. This brings harmony to all the bodies, so that together they provide a vehicle for a meditative state. Though the thinking is stilled, the bodies are active, and every thought, word and deed is devoted to *Īśvara*. The world is still full of objects, but there is an instant awareness of their true divine reality, and that knowledge is available for all the bodies to act upon. Now the soul perceives directly in the true sense of the term.

Scholars have debated the idea of "devotion" in *Yoga-Sūtra* because it is an apparent departure from the *Sāṃkhya* philosophy. In fact, the concept of *Īśvara* itself is a departure. Without going into the intricacies of the debate, it can be said that a true practitioner needs devotion to survive the "battle of two selves"—the physical and the spiritual. At this stage, devotion is purely an aid. Any such debates may be good for the scholars, but are wasteful intellectual battles for a disciple that can never substitute for the rigors of the practice and self-realization. Awareness of *Īśvara* arises like a flower blooming—ever so gently and unannounced. Then, no second-hand proof and no winning argument is needed to prove it.

One-Pointed Perception

Though the mind's indulgence in the thinking process stops, it can still stray and needs control, making the new steady postures of the three bodies difficult to hold on to. But, when all the impurities are gone and weaknesses are removed, right postures become a natural phenomenon and need no control. Breathing becomes rhythmic and steady, the thinking instrument is calm, and the thinking process is stilled at will. The individual mind now remains a catalytic agent letting pure perception prevail. The frequency of thought formation drops below a critical level, from where each thought can be watched. One-pointedness becomes a natural state.

One-pointedness becomes your new ability that is at first directed to the perceived objects of material life. A one-pointed perception of an object is possible when a stilled mind allows closely similar (and not wavering) thoughts to form in an easy procession. But as you begin to dedicate all actions to *Īśvara,* and start perceiving not an object but its substance, the one-pointedness shifts from the object's explicit form to its implicit cause. Individual mind slowly becomes inoperative as an indulgent agent. Eventually it could become a catalyst again.

By now you can also use "one-pointedness" incisively, to know a person, an event, or an object in terms of the following:

- cause(s) leading to this particular present form
- how its structure of predisposition prevented any other
- its present form in the context of the ladder of evolution.

One-pointed is a state where mind control and the controlling factor are equally balanced (Sūtra 3.16/III.12). In one-pointedness, only as much mind control is required as to equally balance the effect of the memory pool from which the emotion-soaked patterns emerge. Any excess control is counterproductive; anything less is inadequate. A conscious effort to stop sensory input is likewise unnatural. Practice makes it possible to disengage the thought-making process from the sensory input and let useless impulses flow in and out by themselves (see *Figure 4.1*). Then the brain's oscillations stop, and the mind modifications are rested, leaving the mind in a calm state and awareness steady. Only then can a vision of *Īśvara* present itself without any hindrance.

Elevated Awareness

A shift in awareness from the object's form to its cause is threefold. First to appear on your radar is, of course, the form. In fact, a form is a result of sensory engagement with the object. Form is ever-changing, though the elements that compose it remain the same. To the disciple it reveals its past, because only through successive transformations of the elements has the object come to bear its present form.

Now you understand the object's biography—an historical journey of the object that has brought it to its present form. It flashes like a series of snapshots, showing a meaningful progression. Simultaneously, through one-pointed perception, arises awareness of that meaning. Each snapshot has its attendant time-space context, and from one snapshot to the other there is an inherent cause-and-effect relationship. It is known how and why the object got transformed. The fluidity of this knowledge consists not only of the life manifest in it but also the veiled consciousness of the object itself. This consciousness lies hidden as a potential of future forms. Then it is a short step fast-forward to know the object's possible future state(s). **Thus, through one-pointed perception the aspects of every object—the form, what it symbolizes and the attendant time-conditions—are known and realized** (Sūtra 3.17/III.13).

In this entire process, you touch the essential oneness of all objects, animate or inanimate. The distinguishing external aspects melt into the generic essence of the objects. In this sense, consciousness "exists" in the "timeless" present state and the forms "exist" only as a function of the past and the future. This present state is never-changing. A crude parallel in pottery is of vases, plates, and pots, a spectrum of forms at different points in time depending on different prevailing conditions, while the essential lump of clay remains present in them at all times, whatever the external form may be.

At this stage in your self-realization process, the disciple of truth understands why newer dimensions of the world keep unfolding. The key, it is realized, is the elevated awareness of the self. Awareness of subtler levels within the self leads to an evolution of the mind. In one-pointed perception, the individual mind becomes as clean and all-knowing as the Universal Mind because it is no longer involved with any thinking instrument. Thus, nothing is hidden from view, and one gaze at the object yields all its aspects and its present state on the evolutionary ladder; whatever be the object—a person, a star, or the universe itself. It is significant to note that this is not just an inquisitive knowing or intellectual reckoning (something that involves "thinking") but an intuitive knowing before which everything lays itself bare and transparent.

There are some significant effects of this intuitive knowledge sourced from Universal Mind. You learn firsthand that the gross-subtle hierarchy is scale-invariant. Macrocosm and its microcosm have only external differences, while the essential structure of gross-to-subtle elements is the same. In this way, the third Yoga hypothesis is validated.

Growing knowledge of a transparent world also brings home the real meaning of *māyā*. The apparent and transient forms appear unreal, and their core consciousness as real. Only then, at such a juncture, the world could be called *māyā* or illusionary. Those who are not "there" yet, may find it paradoxical and senseless, and may continue to offer a tongue-in-cheek giggle to this apparently exotic idea.

Spiritual Reading, a Structural Shift

All that we have discussed above brings us to a pivotal question: If the core is one and the goal is one, why are the characteristics of the objects (apparent and inherent) so divergent? And the apparent answer is that each object contains in its "present" the imprints of the past transformations and promise of the future ones. If one were to see this entire spectrum of each object at once, the world would have many more dimensions than three. All matter is a manifestation of the three *guṇa* in myriad permutations and combinations. Depending on the subjective time scale of perception, **these perceived characteristics are acquired (past), simultaneously manifesting (present), or latent (future)** (Sūtra 3.18/ III.14). All matter emerges from the omnipresent, infinite, vibrant *ākāśa*. *Ākāśa* unfolds or *involves* into forms, and forms fold back or *evolve* into *ākāśa*.

Any specific stage of evolution portends infinite potentialities that the law of *karma,* cause and effect, tapers down into finite possibilities. A disciple can read all this and thus does not remain engrossed in the forms any more. Realization of the third hypothesis provides a spiritual vision of the universe full of apparently divergent but essentially similar objects, rendering them scale-invariant and with only pure consciousness at their core, in spite of the simultaneously manifesting outer states. Divergence is a product of an individual mind; *pure consciousness is without mind.*

Thus, in becoming a *yogī,* the ability to read the latent dimensions takes the disciple beyond the manifested, to know:

- When would the object's structure of disposition change?
- What form(s) will it acquire in the future?
- When would the object reach its culmination of purpose or liberation from bondage?

Though the eye of a disciple is physically no different, the perception has now completely transformed. It is like acquiring a "third eye" in this sense. What was once opaque to the physical eye is now transparent; everything can be perceived—the **acquired** form comprising the basic elements, the **manifesting** *guṇa* in whatever state of balance, and the **latent** nature *mūla-prakṛtī* pregnant with future forms. This is spiritual reading.

Powers: Omnipresence, Omniscience, and Omnipotence

Acceptance by *Īśvara* follows a disciplined process progressing through one-pointedness, and the ability to read the subtle aspects with heightened awareness as if reading a transparent object, and culminates in spiritual reading. Now, the discriminative understanding is to be taken to another level with *Īśvara*'s blessings.

Though we often talk about it, we have a very vague idea of "soul." It is often described as the divine fragment entrapped in the body-mind. Though it is essentially infinite Spirit, soul has temporarily acquired a finite form. Quite a challenging concept this, until you realize the deeper meaning first hand at the feet of *Īśvara*. **One who can discriminate between the Soul and Spirit achieves supremacy over all conditions and becomes omniscient** (Sūtra 3.19/III.49).

The ability of spiritual reading offers to you an opportunity to see a soul in each object and to realize the unity of your own soul with that of all others. This is the first vision of **omnipresence**. Spiritual reading also dissolves the limitations and conditioning of the individual mind, which regains its original state of the Universal Mind that knows all that is to be known, without any adaptation. The otherwise opaque world is now clear and transparent to you. But more importantly, the ordinary reflex divide between self and not-self disappears to make way for discerning insight of "Self and not-Self." This is the next stage of **omniscience**. This eventually leads to understanding the secrets of the universe. The subtle controls the gross, and when you know the subtlest, anything and everything can be controlled. This is **omnipotence**, yielding all the powers that could be.

The Secondary Means of Yoga bring about so much internal and external purification that the body-mind system, now a three-tiered unified vehicle, is capable of pure awareness. All three bodies acting as one vehicle for reaching the goal of pure awareness are ready to release the soul from its entrapment and to let it be the Spirit that it is. The highest awareness resulting from discernment between the soul and the Spirit implies dissolution of the physical body-mind system which is now ready for a conscious death, whenever it occurs. (It is readiness, not an invitation to death!)

The abode of the Spirit is Creation and not Existence where the soul has taken a temporary shelter. Unless one has traveled enough on the *yogīk* path, these words are mere words and incapable of delivering any sense. But having traveled this far, the disciple is now gifted with at least a conceptual knowledge of Creation that could be absorbed only in the inner domain.

Intuitive Knowledge

All *perceived* life is **scale-variant**. Each object has its own cycle of manifesting and dissolving that results in shorter or longer life spans. Each object is committed to a process of evolution bound by time-and-space dimensions on the physical plane. This process brings an object into manifestation from subtler elements, and consigns it back to those elements after the life cycle is complete. All physical elements (air, fire, water, and earth, in that order) emerge from *ākāśa* and finally dissolve into it (in the reverse order).

When perception ceases and *pure awareness* prevails, the universe becomes **scale-invariant**. You realize that the past and the future are only sequential states resulting from a human thinking process. Since the sensory input is serial in nature, as we have seen earlier, the resultant cognition is sequential, and that creates a sense of time. When you know anything intuitively, that knowledge is instantaneous. Without time-embroiled perception, there is only the "present."

Time has a spatial context that gives birth to a sense of space. In the absence of time, space is an ever-present context. With time and space becoming transparent, you (now an apprentice *yogī)* can perceive directly as well as know everything, instantly. This intuitive knowledge is omnipresent and omniscient. Hence, Sage Pātañjali says, **this intuitive knowledge is a great deliverer and is omnipresent and omniscient, includes the past, the present and the future in the Eternal Now** (Sūtra 3.20/III.55). You know your own past lives and understand all the pending *karma* firsthand. With blessings and guidance from *Īśvara*, you are ungrudgingly keen on redeeming the remaining *karma* in the firm knowledge that you can traverse to the "other" shore only when you carry no baggage.

All along, it has been said that the bodies are the soul's vehicle for experiencing. Now, with the bodies purified, the soul finds all the atoms, molecules, and cells of the bodies vibrating at a frequency completely harmonized and attuned. The soul that was once blocked by "I"-centric physical experiencing can now project itself unhindered on all the three purified planes of existence.

In fact, because there is no experiencing needed any more, the soul can also project itself on its own spiritual plane. **When all the bodies and the soul have reached the condition of equal purity then true one-ness is achieved and the soul is liberated** (Sūtra 3.21/III.56).

As an orientation into the world of Creation, *Īśvara* begins further training for an aspirant *yogī*. Sound being the original creator, a disciple is introduced through a series of practices (starting with saying "AUM" correctly) for learning higher sounds—*madhyama-nāda*, *paśyanti-nāda*, and *para-nāda*.[34] This is tough training, because these sounds belong to high states of Existence and Creation.

A Caveat to Powers

Milestones on the *yogīk* path do not come without traps. On the path, when the physical identity starts fading, the void is often filled by a "holier than thou" attitude. That is still a mind-game. Worldly name and fame are often replaced by spiritual accolades and recognition. A disciple fantasizes a spiritual aura, and his or her new uncluttered thought process creates a false sense of "knowing all." There are many examples of failed preachers with a disguised corrupt mind that present a revealing commentary on how rigorous the real path is.

Until you have the spiritual vision, and until you are firmly rooted in the purification processes, the goal on the *yogīk* path remains blurred or elusive. You remain only vaguely aware of the soul. The flashes of saintly appearances and divine revelations in the initial days are mostly delusional or imagery. The association with the physical body is still intimate and returns to haunt every now and then. What you seek is what you get. Nothing really changes until you evolve on the *yogīk* path and your awareness rises from lower to higher selves.

---

[34] *Para-nāda* (which does not belong to Existence) is the highest range of vibrations that can potentially disintegrate the three worlds, and hence a *mahāyogī* is trained in *para-nāda* only by *Īśvara*. Sensing of higher vibrations enables understanding of the astral and the causal worlds.

The powers of the lower (animal) self are carried across many lives via incarnations. These are physical in nature and keep the self tied to sensory gratification. Only when you realize that unfulfilled *karma* is the cause of reincarnation do you start seriously questioning the futility of repeated experience cycles brought by *karma*. And only when there is a sincere desire to redeem yourself you can move to the higher planes.

Sage Pātañjali also deals squarely with another legitimate question a disciple may have. To the untrained eyes **there appears to be a similarity between higher and lower powers gained by incarnation and also by or use of incense or drugs, *mantrās* (incantations), prayers, through plain compulsive rituals or meditation** (Sūtra 3.22/IV-1). Do drugs, various types of incense, and religious rituals really produce influence on the astral plane? Surely they do. The astral plane, though subtle, is still matter. The biological effects that drugs and incense produce as external change-agents are also produced internally through penance and other rituals.

The prayers and *mantrās* work on the causal plane with the power of words or sound. This is a limited creative power. Compulsive or an intense desire works on the intellectual plane. However, though one uses subtle bodies, any awareness so generated is transient and is not at will. As soon as the agents cease to exist, the awareness gravitates to the grosser planes. Besides, any abilities, skills, and powers that are developed using these means may become self-locking. Such means to higher awareness soon become ends in themselves.

This is the reason why meditation is set apart from the rest. The gross to subtle planes are inclusive in nature. That means that any act on the higher plane subsumes the lower one. Meditative processes begin as conscious exercises, but in the true meditative state you are not conscious of the process. This eliminates the risk of getting locked up in it.

Meditation acts on the highest plane. On this plane, the intense desire is channeled to the spiritual Self. In this way, any entrapment of the lower powers is recognized and is left behind. However, this is still knowledge and not experience. When the intense desire turns itself into spiritual will, you go beyond the domain of knowledge.

This sūtra speaks about *siddhī*. In the strict sense of the term, *siddhī* means a state where the components are in balance. Any "sense" of power is only its fallout. On the lower planes, the psychic powers can keep the disciple trapped, because the corresponding consciousness in balance is of a low order. In meditative *siddhī*, because the consciousness is now spiritual, the entrapment of powers is less compelling, though the powers are significant. At this stage, the real battle for a disciple is with the temptation to project a spiritually superior self-image. This continues to happen until there is a complete surrender to *Īśvara*.

Sage Pātañjali also wants us to remember that not only the above change-agents, but also the **Yoga practices and methods by themselves, do not bring about elevation of consciousness, but only serve to eliminate obstacles** (Sūtra 3.23/IV-3). Having described the obstacles and afflictions, and having initiated the seeker in practices and methods for removing them, Sage Pātañjali now finds it necessary to clarify this important aspect.

The practices may till the soil and methods may remove the weeds, but the crop is still a product of the latent seeds. The practices do not grant emancipation nor lead to illumination; they remove the obstacles that prevent it from happening. If it is not in one's structure, all the practices and prayers of the world will not create transcendence.

> *A farmer does not actually create a crop such as apples; rather they are the product of apple trees, each one the latest in a long line of predecessors. The ancestry of each apple tree stretches back to antiquity, every generation depending for its existence on a fruitful convergence of seed, sunshine, water and nutrient soil. [The] [f]armer, as the current agent of the convergence, is a proximate cause of the apple's existence, having obtained the seeds, planted them in rows of soil, irrigated and fertilized them, and finally harvested the fruit. One would even call the*

> *product "the farmer's apples." But it is primarily the seeds that determine the apple's essential attributes—color, texture, taste, shape, content, life span, and potential to reproduce—even though each of these may be affected by proximate causes.*—Chip Hartranft, 62-63.

Methods and practices together serve to remove the *granthī* blocking the energy flows and bring about the inner biological development to withstand the higher vibrations of illumination. Such removal of doubt should help you in developing a correct perspective. There is no need to be casual and lax about the practices and methods, nor to be idolizing them or treating them as ends in themselves.

We have seen that your spiritual progress has continuity across lives. You resume spiritually where you left it off in the previous life. The practices and methods only hasten up the resumption of the spiritual journey in your present life. When the spiritual journey begins, it first manifests on the astral and causal planes. The ordinary swings of emotions subside, and a deeper understanding of emotions leads to a control over them as the awareness elevates.

Insight, the Emotional Intelligence

The Yoga practices bring about bodily purification so that awareness gets transformed and released from bodily bondage. Expanded and elevated awareness radically changes the composition of thoughts. The dominance of physicality (sexual component) recedes, and refined emotions and sharpened intelligence start taking over. Memory's hold goes away, the structure of predispositions is altered, mind modifications slow down, and the seeds of *karma* get burned out. There is a distinct realization that soul alone is the goal; prayers, penance, and philosophy are all peripheral; practice (*Yoga abhyāsa*) is the only path; reflex thinking is slavery to the emotions, and discerning thinking is emotionally intelligent. This is the new insight.

This insight drives further transformation, by knowing:

- How personality is acquired

- How memory sustains personality
- How the structure of predispositions can be dissolved
- How all structures are fabricated in *guṇa*
- What brings *guṇa* back into balance and harmony
- Why there is one mind but many forms
- Why we see what we are ourselves
- Why *Īśvara* is the *real Perceiver*

How Personality Is Acquired

If your spiritual destiny is a legacy of your previous lives, you may question why in the present life you have to start all over again, with a painful material existence for any length of time, before catching up with that legacy. The reason is simple. *Karma* is neither good nor bad. All the seeds that remain dormant must germinate in a new life. But life itself is a result of the dominant seeds of the desire to live.

Sage Pātañjali describes, as the "effect-producing causes," several perpetrators of *karma* like,

1. the incoming impulses
2. past memory patterns soaked in emotions
3. the *guṇa* latent in them
4. the desires and motives that constantly orient materially
5. the conscious brain with its oscillations
6. the individual mind that remains involved with the brain processes after losing its ability to throw light, and finally,
7. the big "I"-centered awareness, the main culprit.

The "I am" consciousness is responsible for the creation of the organs through which the sense of individuality is enjoyed (Sūtra 3.24/IV-4). The physical body and the mind are designed to be the vehicles for experiencing the sentient world. They cause the creation of sensory organs for that purpose, and warp awareness into an outward orientation in order to enjoy a sense of individual personality. The sensory data that is brought back may be divergent and disparate but it is impregnated by a unifying ego-sense making it "my own experience." Thus the initial design goes awry, and this forms a self-fulfilling vicious cycle of *avidyā*. As long as the outbound sensuous desires continue to reign, the sense gratification and perception of objects continues. The cycle is broken only by your sincere realization that no real joy lies in sense perception and its outgoing tendency. *Avidyā* is then slowly replaced by *this* knowledge and the spiritual Self starts expressing itself.

Bookish knowledge and the myths surrounding the powers and *siddhīs* sometimes create anticipation. That ironically strengthens the "I"-consciousness because it provides one extra reason—being "holier than thou"—to distinguish yourself from the rest. The vision of *Īśvara* is the first major milestone that exposes the confinement inherent in "I"-consciousness. Even then, surrendering "I"-consciousness requires great courage, because the whole self-view and the world-view are tightly woven around it. The self/not-self divide is so ingrained in our thinking that it is hard to imagine that others, especially the poor, the sick, and the needy, have the same glorious divine fragment that we have discovered in ourselves. This uncommon sense of commonality shakes the foundation of personal existence. Only a true devotion to *Īśvara* makes the surrender of individuality possible.

How Memory Sustains Personality

Our personality is built bit by bit from our thoughts. The structure of predispositions is partly inherited from previous lives, but largely fabricated by reflex thoughts in this life. To form a thought, as we know, one needs:

- An incoming impulse (the cause and the energy)
- A series of patterns in the memory nearly identical to the impulse (that piggyback).

The brain's memory is coded as patterns, but that is not the only memory we have. Memory is subtle; functional memory exists in each atom, molecule, and cell. Hence it is almost indestructible. **There is an uninterrupted sequence between karma and its manifesting cause as there is identity of relation between memory and cause, even when separated by stage of evolution, time and place** (Sūtra 3.25/IV-9). Thus a cause of *karma* can dutifully surface across many lives, millennia, or geographies.

This is why exercises and practices in Yoga are aimed at a cell-level purification and change. A change in personality is its cumulative effect. Yoga practice also alters the thinking process by reorganizing the contents of the brain's memory pools. First, when the brain's side passages open up for the incoming sense impulses to travel to the frontal lobe, the new route allows you to bypass memory pools on the older route from back and top of the brain. Secondly, your simplified filters of predispositions reduce the dependence on memory in thought formation. Thus your memory is used less and less in the generation of colored and emotionally-charged knowledge, and more and more as a receiver and repository of higher spiritual knowledge.

But perhaps the most revealing message here is that *only those impulses enter your thought process that are identical to the memory patterns you hold and refuse to throw or burn away.* This means that impulses substantially different from the existing memory patterns fail to create thoughts—or at best, they would create a damaging bias by heavily skewing towards the memory patterns. This is what sustains a "personality." This is why different individuals end up thinking differently in apparently similar circumstances. And this explains the phenomenon of "selective listening."

The second important message is that this dominance of memory patterns creates "habitual" thinking orchestrated by the structure of predispositions. Knowing this, you need to remain alert—such habitual thinking should be a red flag, and you must not allow such thinkingto remain, and revel in its comfort zones. At any time on the *yogīk* path, the residual memory seeds can germinate into thoughts that are contrary to Yoga as long as this structure of predispositions exists.

How Structure of Predispositions Can Be Dissolved

The past and the future exist in the present. The form assumed in the (time concept of) **the present is a result of the developed characteristics and holds latent seeds of future qualities** (Sūtra 3.26/IV.12). As conceptualized in Eternal Now, the perceived manifestation occurs only in the present, and thus the past exists in the present as its cause, and the future resides in the present as its potential effect. Any given state of an object or a phenomenon is always an effect of a cause that existed in its immediately preceding condition. All worldly objects and phenomena present a succession of such states as effects and causes. Because a structure of predispositions drives perception, and that perception necessitates the perceived object taking a form, this process links the past, present, and the future in a sequence. To understand this sequence is crucial to Yoga.

This logic can be further extended across lives. Our present body is fabricated on the basis of our final structure of predispositions at our previous death; our future body will be fabricated based on the structure that we will build and leave behind at the time of ensuing death. This recognition contains both a warning and a promise. The warning is that *that which exists subtly cannot be destroyed and must be lived through (and thus redeemed)*; the promise is that *that which does not exist subtly will never be manifested* (and thus preempted) and *that* is in one's control.

The compulsive cycle of past, present, and future is broken and destroyed when you internalize this realization. Then, one can turn inward and be fully determined to change the structure of predispositions (*saṁskāra*). Not creating any new seeds of *saṁskāra* is the only solution for avoiding the future effects. Our reflex thinking generates the seeds. Thought-watching as a part of Yoga practice reveals to a disciple which external and internal triggers launch habitual reflex thinking. A conscious effort of stopping the runaway thought-trains and reviewing them in reverse, and in slow motion, gives an ability to erase the reflex triggers.

Why the thinking process is often a reflex has a lot to do with memory that is soaked in the past emotions. Emotions act as the triggers and also as a magnet. A disciple's transition to becoming a *yogī* is signified by an increased awareness of how emotions work. In fact, very often you would be mistaking sentiments, which are ego-centric, with genuine emotions, which are generic. Getting swayed by sentiments masquerading as emotions or trying to suppress reflex thinking are both wasteful efforts. What leads to real insight is the ability to recognize the power of true emotions as the subtle cause of the physical phenomena. Not just your own, but all phenomena are driven by the underlying structures of predisposition. That realization also allows a disciple to have a subtle emotional view of other people (or even animals and inanimate objects) with whom it then becomes easier to empathize. That is emotional intelligence.

How All Structures Are Fabricated in Guṇa

The characteristics (of the perceived universe), whether latent or potent, are fabricated out of the three *guṇa* (Sūtra 3.27/IV-13). This includes all objects, animate and inanimate, and all life, including human beings. The fabrication depends on each individual structure of predispositions. What events are to follow and what type of existence you must have are also naturally dependent upon your structure of predispositions.

All the objects in the universe are in a continually migrating state on their own individual time scale. When we perceive them it is at a given point in time within our own time scale, which gives them the appearance of being (relatively) animate or inanimate in our individual reality.

The denseness of objects is also relative. Each object is a finite configuration of atoms and sub-particles that are bound together because of certain forces in nature (*mūlaprakṛtī*). These forces excite the *guṇa* and give each particle a migration path, and all particles together create a composite image of simultaneous migrations that appear dense. Collectively slower migration paths create the appearance of a more dense, and hence inert, object. How dense also depends upon the time scale of the perceiver and the level of awareness.

The three forces of *guṇa* (*tamas*, likened in the scientific jargon with the strong force; *rajas*, with the weak force and gravity; *sattva*, with the electromagnetic force) have an energy vibration frequency that lends a form to an object through myriad permutations and combinations. A human being also has his or her own cumulative *guṇa* combination and structures.

As long as you do not recognize *guṇa* as the causal force, and instead react to an appearance of an object that is created by the incoming vibrations, you will not realize the irony of "subjective" objectivity that thinking breeds, and would remain in the hypnotic spell of the *guṇa*. In Yoga terminology, in most of the objects the *guṇa* are not only in imbalance but are in a perpetually dynamic and excited state.

With help from *Īśvara*, a disciple can experientially understand *guṇa* as a stand-alone energy, independent of the form. Also understood is the *nature* of *guṇa*, why they appear to behave as they do, and what causes their imbalance in all the worldly objects. This alone helps, and further motivates in getting rid of the structure of predispositions. The *guṇa* are thereby left alone, to remain unexcited and in perfect balance and harmony within an object, even when perceived.

What Brings Guṇa *Back into Balance and Harmony*

When P. G. Wodehouse writes that his hero looked "with unseeing eyes," he is referring to a state in which the mind is not involved in the sensory process of "seeing," though the eyes are. A form or appearance of an object does not exist by itself; it is a product of sensory perception. The form exists because you see that it does. **The one-pointed unification of mind, the thinking instrument, with the object causes the forms to manifest** (Sūtra 3.28/ IV-14). When the "I am" consciousness is completely immersed in the physical world, the mind's engagement with a given object through sensory perception is one-pointed and a form is perceived. The perceived forms constantly change. They are intrinsically transient at their respective rates of dissolution. However, perception gives them a relative "real" existence at a point in time. For example, because of an extremely slow rate of dissolution, the perceived form of an inert object like a building may not change over time; but that of a flying bird will change every second.

This is also why those who acquire conceptual knowledge of spirituality but whose "I" consciousness does not change, fail to escape the captivity of forms. This is why idol worship and compulsive rituals dominate the early spiritual path. Idols and rituals have some utility in their own place provided you do not get hopelessly locked in. The role of a true external guru is to ensure that you don't.

A major transformation occurs when "I am" gives way to "Thou art only." When you lose obsession with your own form, and have no agenda for the structure of predisposition, the perceived objects lose their forms. *Guṇa* are perceived as *guṇa* and are left unexcited, thus remaining more in balance and in mutual harmony. That is why forms dissolve. Then the abilities of one-pointedness and the mind's non-attachment can be directed in the inner spiritual domain. After that, it is a journey with an insight into the formless.

Why There Is One Mind but Many Forms

Before dealing with the formless, we need answers to some profound questions about forms. Does an object exist independent of its perception? Would this be a real world if objects disappear when nobody perceives them? ("If a tree falls in a forest and there is no one there, does it make a sound?")

These questions appear to be profound only when one instinctively takes a human being as the center of the universe. Fortunately, that is not the case! All matter, from particles to the universe, animate to inanimate, has life. All life impulses use the respective objects as vehicles to flow through. Every form in manifestation is a result of a perceiver's thought. You need only to look at your own thinking process to know how mind works. The process does not change. It is scale-invariant in a vast spectrum from a microcosm (say, a particle) to the macrocosm (the universe). From the energized *guṇa* to the Universal Mind, there is one unifying entity, the mind. Its impulses give the forms of the objects a sense of real existence. **The many modifications of the one mind produce the diverse forms which depend for existence upon those many mind impulses** (Sūtra 3.29/IV-16). Thus, *"all these forms ... are dependent upon some life, endowed with the capacity to think, and through thought impulses to modify and influence sentient substance, and build it into forms."*—Alice Bailey, 408.

What makes it so difficult for us to even conceptually accept one mind in many forms? The pressure of the automatic working of the *guṇa* holds human brains and the senses hostage. The deluge of sense impulses is as overwhelming as a tsunami. And this dominance of the senses is only compounded by habitual reflex thinking.

Besides, time, a product of an individual mind, creates sense-based awareness "from moment to moment," and each moment registers a "location" for each object. That makes time and space purely relative and gives each mind its own measuring periodicity. Thus, if there *are* time and space scales beyond the range of human minds, they are difficult to fathom, which is one of the reasons why the astral and causal worlds remain "un-scientific" to many scientists.

Your mind's own pre-conditioned scales, structure of predisposition, and thought reflexes give it an appearance of uniqueness. Ironically, when the same mind is used to perceive mind in another person or an object, that mind appears to be unique too. Then it becomes impossible to recognize all the individual minds as only different editions of Universal Mind.

Sometimes, conceptual knowledge stored in the scriptures appears to be lost, hidden away, or institutionalized and tampered with. As a result, it remains inaccessible without the intermediaries. The importance of *Yoga-Sūtra* is that they show us the way to work without intermediaries and to seek and obtain direct guidance from *Īśvara*, so that your individual mind can become the Universal Mind that it essentially is. After all, the forms are born only when cognized by the individual mind.

Why We See What We Are Ourselves

These forms are cognized or not cognized according to the qualities latent in the level of awareness (of the perceiver) (Sūtra 3.30/IV-17). **We see what we are ourselves.** When you see a form, it is not because the form presents itself to the sensory perception of its own volition. Your structure of predispositions invites it to become that form. It dictates what vibrational frequency you would resonate with and draw to yourself. The *guṇa* latent in an object simply manifest accordingly.

Thus, you do not see a soul in another object only because you are not yet aware of your own soul. The brilliant point made here is that the *guṇa* could be rendered powerless if the level of perceiving awareness does not engage and unify with them. But for this to happen, the passive habit-ridden awareness must transform itself into more subtle awareness. The refined energy of higher awareness that becomes pure consciousness can only transcend sensory perception. And as a consequence of that consciousness, the form dematerializes from cognition. With no sensing, no *guṇa*, and no form, only insight prevails and the veil is lifted to reveal that "I" was only a pseudo-perceiver; the real one was *Īśvara.*

Why Īśvara *Is the Real Perceiver*

Through spiritual reading the disciple learns to discern and separate the soul from matter. The "form," the "word," and the "idea" all belong to matter. This way, you start to understand the underlying truth that is your mission as a disciple. The soul is recognized as the vestured *Īśvara*, that is seeking liberation from bondage of the bodies used for experiencing. This liberation is not achieved by breaking out from the bodies but by dissolving them within. The intention is not to abandon bodies but to purify them and tune them as one ensemble that can be erased from the "awareness radar" at will.

But the path is not straight, and there are no easy solutions. Just because the truth is understood conceptually does not mean that there is a shortcut to Yoga. The seeds of *karma* continue to be sown as long as the structure of predispositions is active. Unless all *karma* is redeemed, there is no liberation, even if living extends over many lives. *Karma* is a self-created bondage, and only you can unburden yourself from it. A disciple also realizes that the practices that are of tremendous help on the *yogīk* path, and indispensable in the initial stages, by themselves do not bring any liberation. An unflinching devotion to *Īśvara* is not a mere sentimental expression; it becomes a demonstrated unwavering way of life.

A few words again about *Īśvara*: *Īśvara* is not "God" in any conventional sense of the term. This life is no grant or favor from anyone, nor death any punishment. You become aware of "something" that stands aside, independent of all thoughts, when you watch your own thoughts. That something can still watch it even when the "I"-sense shifts from physical to astral and to causal. And that means it is independent of the astral and causal selves, as well. *Īśvara* is "that something," the real perceiver that is experiencing life through the causal, astral, and physical vestures. We say, "The sun is hiding behind the clouds." The reality is that the sun is where it always is; clouds have moved in between the sun and us to blind us. Likewise, *Īśvara* is always there; it is our "I" awareness that is flirting with the bodies and fooling us by hiding *Īśvara* from our awareness.

The vision of *Īśvara* changes all that. As the inner impurities are slowly removed, a paradigm shift occurs in a disciple's perception. The habitual self-view and the world-view start dissolving to make way for a new understanding that the self and the not-self, both, are matter, and that is distinct from the Spirit. The world of matter appears as nothing but mind's interplay with the Spirit, and its real role is now understood.

As the astral body becomes the primary body, emotions no longer drive the thinking process. Thinking becomes more fluid and perception more penetrating, as the physical pre-eminence in the thinking process evolves into an emotional intelligence. With this insight firmly rooted, you, the disciple, are now a *yogī* and ready for a real grooming with *Īśvara* as your Teacher.

Chapter Three: Rearranged Sūtras: (Numbers in the brackets are from the original sequence)

3.1 (I.21) **तीव्रसंवेगानामासन्नः ॥**

tivra-saṁvegānām āsannaḥ

Attainment of spiritual consciousness is rapid for one who seeks it wholeheartedly with an intense urge.

3.2 (I.22) **मृदुमध्याधिमात्रत्वात्ततोऽपि विशेषः ॥**

mṛdu-madhyādhimātratvāt tato"pi viśeṣaḥ

How rapid depends on whether the practice is intense, moderate or gentle. But (in attainment of true spiritual consciousness) there is yet another way.

3.3 (I.42) **तत्र शब्दार्थज्ञानविकल्पैः संकीर्णा सवितर्का समापत्तिः ॥**

tatra śabdārtha-jñāna-vikalpaiḥ saṁkīrṇā savitarkā samāpattiḥ

When among the appearance of an object, its associated description, and the idea (or meaning) behind it, each is in turn distinctly perceived it is called "judicious reasoning"; when the three appear blended it is the perfect perception of the "Perceiver."

3.4 (I.43) **स्मृतिपरिशुध्दौ स्वरूपशून्येवार्थमात्रनिर्भासा निर्वितर्का ॥**

smṛti-pariśuddhau svarūpa-śūnyevārtha-mātra-nirbhāsā nirvitarkā

Intuition (perception without judicious reasoning) results when the memory no longer colors and both, awareness entangled in the verbal description and the appearance are transcended and only the idea behind the object is present.

3.5 (I.44) **एतयैव सविचारा निर्विचारा च सूक्ष्मविषया व्याख्याता ॥**

etayaiva savicārā nirvicārā ca sūkṣma-viṣayā vyākhyātā

The same contemplation, with or without judicious reasoning can also be applied to things subtle.

3.6 (II.1) तपःस्वाध्यायेश्वरप्रणिधानानि क्रियायोगः॥

tapaḥ-svādhyāyeśvara-praṇidhānāni kriyā-yogaḥ

The Yoga of action (Kriya Yoga), leading to union with the soul, is threefold: fiery aspiration, devotion to *Īśvara* and spiritual reading.

3.7 (II.2) समाधिभावनार्थः क्लेशतनूकरणार्थश्च॥

samādhi-bhāvanārthaḥ kleśa-tanūkara-ṇārthaś ca

The aim of threefold Kriya Yoga is to bring about the soul vision and to eliminate obstructions/hindrances/distractions.

3.8 (II.22) कृतार्थं प्रति नष्टमप्यनष्टं तदन्यसाधारणत्वात्॥

kṛtārthaṁ prati naṣṭaṁ apy anaṣṭaṁ tad-anya-sādhāraṇatvāt

For one who has achieved Yoga (the union) the objective world ceases to be though it continues to so exist for those who are not free

3.9 (II.23) स्वस्वामिशक्तयोः स्वरूपोपलब्धिहेतुः संयोगः॥

sva-svāmi-śaktyoḥ svarūpopalabdhi-hetuḥ saṁyogaḥ

The understanding of the nature of the perceived as well as the Perceiver is produced by virtue of the association of the soul with the mind.

3.10 (II.24) तस्य हेतुरविद्या॥

tasya hetuḥ avidyā

The cause of this association is *avidyā* (ignorance) that needs to be overcome.

3.11 (II.25) तदभावात्संयोगाभावो हानं तद्दृशेः कैवल्यम्॥

ad-abhāvāt saṁyogābhāvo hānaṁ tad dṛśeḥ kaivalyaṁ

When ignorance is brought to an end through non-association with the things perceived, this is the great liberation.

3.12 (II.26) विवेकख्यातिरविप्लवा हानोपायः॥

viveka-khyātiḥ aviplavā hānopāyaḥ

The stage of bondage is overcome through uninterrupted discernment.

3.13 (II.27) तस्य सप्तधा प्रान्तभूमौप्रज्ञा॥

tasya saptadhā prānta-bhūmiḥ prajñā

At the culmination, attained progressively, the seeker gains sevenfold knowledge or illumination.

3.14 (II.44) स्वाध्यायादिष्टदेवतासम्प्रयोगः॥

svādhyāyād iṣṭa-devatā-saṁprayogaḥ

Thus, spiritual reading results in contact with the soul.

3.15 (II.45) समाधिसिद्धिरीश्चप्रणिधानात्॥

samādhi-siddhir Iśvara-praṇidhānāt

Through devotion to *Īśvara* the goal of meditation is reached.

3.16 (III.12) ततः पुनः शान्तोदितौ तुल्यप्रत्ययौ चित्तस्यैकाग्रतापरिणामः॥

tataḥ punaḥ śāntoditau tulya-pratyayau cittasyaikāgratā-pariṇāmaḥ

When mind control and the controlling factor are equally balanced, then comes the condition of one-pointedness.

3.17 (III.13) एतेन भूतेन्द्रियेषु धर्मलक्षणावस्थापरिणामा व्याख्याताः॥

etena bhūtendriyeṣu dharma-lakṣaṇā-vasthā-pariṇāmā vyākhyātāḥ

Through one-pointed perception the aspects of every object—the form, what it symbolizes and the attendant time-conditions—are known and realized.

3.18 (III.14) शान्तोदिताव्यपदेश्यधर्मानुपाती धर्मी॥

śāntoditāvyapadeśya dharmānupātī dharmī

The perceived characteristics of every object are acquired, manifesting or latent.

3.19 (III.49) सत्वपुरूषान्यताख्यातिमात्रस्य सर्वभावाधिष्ठातृत्वं सर्वज्ञातृत्वञ्च॥

sattva-puruṣānyatā-khyāti-mātrasya sarva-bhāvādhiṣṭhātṛtvaṁ sarvajñātṛtvaṁ ca

One who can discriminate between the Soul and Spirit achieves supremacy over all conditions and becomes omniscient.

3.20 (III.55) तारकं सर्वविषयं सर्वथाविषयमक्रमञ्चेति विवेकज्ञानम्॥

tārakaṁ sarva-viṣayaṁ sarvathā-viṣayaṁ akramaṁ ceti vivekajaṁ-jñānaṁ

This intuitive knowledge, which is the great Deliverer, is omnipresent and omniscient and includes the past, the present and the future in the Eternal Now.

3.21 (III.56) सत्वपुरुषयोः शुध्दिसाम्ये कैवल्यम् इति॥

sattva-puruṣayoḥ śuddhi-sāmye kaivalyam iti

When all the bodies (physical, astral and causal) and the soul have reached the condition of equal purity, then true one-ness is achieved and liberation results.

3.22 (IV.1) जन्मौषधिमंत्रतपः समाधिजाः सिध्दयः॥

janmauṣadhi-mantra-tapaḥ-samādhi-jāḥ siddhayaḥ

The higher and lower powers are gained by incarnation, or incense/drugs, or prayers/incantations, or obsession or meditation.

3.23 (IV.3) निमित्तमप्रयोजकम् प्रकृतीनां वरणभेदस्तु ततः क्षेत्रिकवत्॥

nimittam aprayojakaṁ prakṛitīnāṁ varaṇa-bhedas tu tataḥ kṣetrikavat

The practices and methods are not the true cause of the elevation of consciousness, but they serve to eliminate obstacles.

3.24 (IV.4) निर्माणचित्तान्यस्मितामात्रात्॥

nirmāṇa-cittāny asmitā-mātrāt

The "I am" consciousness is responsible for the creation of the organs through which the sense of individuality is enjoyed.

3.25 (IV.9) जातिदेशकालव्यवहितानामप्यानन्तर्यं स्मृतिसंस्कारयोरेकरूपत्वात्॥

jāti-deśa-kāla-vyavahitānām apy ānantaryaṁ smṛti-saṁskārayor ekarūpatvāt

There is an uninterrupted sequence between *karma* and its manifesting cause as there is identity of relation between memory and the cause, even when separated by stage of evolution, time and place.

3.26 (IV.12) अतीतानागतं स्वरूपतोऽस्त्यध्वभेदाद्धर्माणाम्॥

atītānāgataṁ svarūpato "sty adhva-bhedād dharmāṇāṁ

The past and the future exist in the present. The form assumed in the (time concept of) present is the result of developed characteristics and holds latent seeds of future qualities.

3.27 (IV.13) ते व्यक्तसूक्ष्मा गुणात्मानः॥

te vyakta-sūkṣmā guṇātmānaḥ

The characteristics, whether latent or potent, partake of the nature of the three *guṇas*.

3.28 (IV.14) परिणामैकत्वाद्वस्तुतत्वम्॥

pariṇāmaikatvād vastu-tattvaṁ

The one-pointed unification of mind, the thinking instrument, with the object causes the form to manifest.

3.29 (IV.16) न चैकचित्ततन्त्रं वस्तु तदप्रमाणकं तदा किं स्यात्॥

na caika-citta-tantraṁ vastu tad-apramāṇakaṁ tadā kiṁ syāt

The many modifications of the one mind produce the diverse forms which depend for existence upon those many mind impulses.

3.30 (IV.17) तदुपरागापेक्षित्वाच्चित्तस्य वस्तु ज्ञाताज्ञातम्॥

tad uparāgāpekṣitvāc cittasya vastu jñātājñātaṁ

These forms are cognized or not cognized according to the qualities latent in the level of awareness.

Chapter Four: *Mahāyogī* and Intuition

4th Milestone

Contact with the soul is truly life-changing. A whole new world opens up within, and the real Yoga journey begins. The external world of objects becomes exciting too when you are able to see them deconstructed at a micro level of five basic elements. It appears as if the world has acquired five new dimensions and that is quite empowering. Your once emotional roller-coaster now becomes a smooth-sailing cruise, when you harness the newfound emotional intelligence. Intuition replaces the flawed thinking process to transform a *yogī* into a *mahāyogī*.

Even when engaged with a world full of objects, now you stay connected with the spiritual Self within. The ordinary perception becomes spiritual, and you know intuitively that, in all the experiencing, *Īśvara* has always been the real Perceiver. The multilayered identity of any object is recognized at a glance and its past and future instantly known. You are blessed with a few powers that under your guru's strict watch will be used only for advancing on the *yogīk* path.

The Yoga practices bring about bodily perfection that prepares you to sustain higher frequencies of the subtle world, and communication is now established with *Īśvara*. You are ready to resolve some of the most intriguing challenges. A fine distinction among soul, *Īśvara*, and *Purūṣa* is now understood, and you advance to the fourth Yoga hypothesis, "Īśvara *is a perceivable version of* Purūṣa *and souls only appear to be many.*"

The *yogīk* path is now even more challenging because the obstacles are very subtle, and though the means appear to be around the corner, they remain elusive. The teaching too is very intricate. It requires a total and loving surrender to *Īśvara* and a sustained fiery aspiration. Under its stern tutelage, you learn the skills of concentration, meditation and contemplation. These skills may be directed to external objects first, but are later honed in a truly subjective mode within. Gradually, the emotional intelligence is superseded by the spiritual intelligence.

On this advanced *yogīk* path you stand completely transformed, your purpose of life stands completely altered, and the once overpowering ego stands completely dissolved. There are many psychic and spiritual powers that fall in your lap, which would ordinarily make you feel superior, but that kind of vanity does not lure you anymore. The walk on the *yogīk* path is grueling but nearness to *Īśvara* is an unprecedented bliss that makes oneness with *Īśvara* your only goal. You have attained a higher state of awareness and are now truly a *mahāyogī*.

In this phase: a transition from Yogī to a Mahāyogī

Yoga hypothesis	*Īśvara* is a perceivable, *guṇa*-based version of *Purūṣa*
Know through experience	*Īśvara* as the Real Perceiver
Involuntary control	Concentration, meditation and contemplation in the objective domain
Achieve Voluntary control	*Dhāraṇā, dhyāna,* and *samādhī* in the subjective domain
Become	An initiated *yogi*
Be	A *mahāyogī*

New words used in this chapter

Purūṣa	Pure consciousness; beyond *guṇa*; imperceptible
saṃprajñātaḥ	Samadhi with illumination
praṇidhānād	Devotion; loving surrender
sabījaḥ samādhiḥ	*Samādhi* with seed
nirbījaḥ samādhiḥ	*Samādhi* without seed
ṛtambharā	Full of experience; cosmic harmony
vaikharī-nāda	Range of sound vibrations belonging to the physical plane, 25 percent as powerful as *madhyama-nāda*

The Soul Connection

You are still standing at the doorstep of *Īśvara*. The fourth plane, the abode of the soul or the Self, is beyond all three—physical (form), astral (word), and causal (idea). There is a certain hierarchy in this. For example, when you are aware of *guṇa* and captivated by them, you see a form, but when you could recognize and isolate *guṇa* at a higher level, the form is not perceived. It is the same process in going beyond. When you learn to pierce through the verbal expression, the spiritual essence is perceived, and *guṇa* cease to matter. Finally, when there is identification with the soul, nothing else matters or exists.

Fourfold Nature of Objects

A refined emotional intelligence brings **full awareness of an object by concentrating on its fourfold nature—a form** (appearance), **through observation**; **the *guṇa*** (word), **through discrimination** (engagement); **a purpose** (essence), **through insight; and the soul, through immersion** (Sūtra 4.1/I.17). Such ability prepares ground for the higher practices of *pratyāhāra*, *dhāraṇā*, *dhyāna*, and *samādhī*.

The erstwhile disciple in you is now an accomplished *yogī.* You can concentrate and be *one-pointed* at will. New insight fortifies your ability to read spiritually, which brings awareness free from biases and conditioning. An object can now be seen at once on all the three planes—in its appearance, identity, and meaning.

A pulsating life is evident as the common core of all the distinct objects making them "one big family," so to speak. A new connectivity emerges as awareness becomes evident in both the perceiver and the perceived. It is then understood why this subtlety is lost in ordinary perception. Such perception of an object is only its appearance. It does not go beyond a superficial engagement of one's structure of predispositions. Such superficial engagement involves only slight awareness and thus sees only a hint of life, if any at all, present in a gross perceived object.[35]

The ability to read everything spiritually is a gift earned by a *yogī,* as an aid for further studies and experiments. It is an instrument of inquiry—for observation, discrimination, insight, and immersion. At this stage, this inquiry is invested in the process of self-realization. Now you are eager for a life-changing learning experience. It is a serious inquiry and not a hollow one born merely out of idle inquisitiveness.

You have by now mastered the rhythmic breathing as well. The subtle relation of the process of perception, predispositions, emotions, thoughts, the mind modifications, with *prāṇa,* and in turn with breath and its rhythm, is now recognized. *Īśvara* would eventually teach you how to synchronize your breath with the awareness present in the perceived object so that there is an instant identification and knowledge. But this is possible only when you are fully established as a *yogī* and are on the way to becoming a *mahāyogī.* To become aware of the object's fourfold nature, you

---

[35] *My Guru, S N Tavariaji, says that anything that is created on our planet or in the Universe, not just human beings but all other life—the animal, vegetable, and mineral kingdoms—contains and functions with some measure of awareness. If the Universal Mind is 100 degrees of awareness, inanimate objects have roughly 5 degrees of awareness, normal human beings about 25 degrees, and great personalities around 50 degrees. Sometimes one is born with high awareness or one cultivates it through life. It is secondary whether such an individual labels it as "spiritual" awareness or not. However, to take one beyond 80 degrees of awareness, some form of practiced spiritual advancement is needed.*

would have already experienced a state of *samādhī*. Contrary to popular understanding, in *samādhī* and *dhyāna* one may or may not be sitting cross-legged and immobile with eyes closed. In becoming a *mahāyogī*, all external activities are quieted since the memory is bypassed. As a result, the thinking instruments are silent, memory-soaked emotions are sterile, and all the internal noise is muted.

Perception Does Not Need External Stimuli

A deeper concentration is achieved when the one-pointed thought no longer depends on external stimuli and is responsive only to the (subjective) latent impressions (Sūtra 4.2/I.18). Emotional intelligence gives us insight into "personality" and its driver, the "I" awareness; now, in a *yogī's* next lesson, you would understand awareness itself.

In the fourfold perception of an object (corresponding to the four states) ending with immersion, its form melts away, unable to provide a predominantly external stimulus for thoughts. Ordinarily, the external impressions reach the mind via the senses. However, when a *yogī* is able to control the sense-perception, the external stimuli are less successful in hijacking the thinking process. As a result, the thinking instruments become quiet and still, and there are fewer (and at times, no) mind modifications.

But the latent impressions that lay hidden like landmines in the memory pool still remain potent and feed themselves to the thinking process, thus replacing the externally stimulated mind activity with the internally stimulated one. We are familiar with this "mind chatter." The subjective impressions, when stripped of unnecessary emotions, are in the form of subtle shapes, patterns, images, and concepts that become more and more accessible on the advanced Yoga journey. When directed at such subtle impressions, one-pointed concentration serves as a generic ability in *dhāraṇā*, *dhyāna*, or *samādhī*.

With the physical brain stilled, the other subtle intelligence centers (*chakra*) are activated as subtle "mini-brains" capable of communicating on the higher causal plane and occasionally with the

Universal Mind. This brings about many changes in the cellular, molecular, and atomic/electronic bodies. *Yama* and *niyama* no longer require conscious efforts and become a way of life. *Āsana*, the postures, of all the bodies are stable and easy, and the *prāṇa* regulation ensures harmony and balance among the bodies.

But the most significant change that occurs is twofold: you learn to bypass memory pools infested with latent impressions. And, even these stored impressions become more and more *sāttvik,* less agitating and more revealing to let you understand the new soul connection. Gradually, you can concentrate unhindered.[36] But this concentration is still anchored in the grosser bodies and a *yogī* can only remotely perceive the soul's abode.

At the Door of the Soul's Realm

However, even the stilled bodies take a *yogī* only to the door of the soul's realm, because one still remains bound to the phenomenal world (Sūtra 4.3/I.19).[37]

Life exists simultaneously on the physical, astral, and causal planes. If we are aware of a form, or a word, or an idea, it only means our perception is keeping us locked in the respective plane. But, subtle perception enables communication with the subtle life in general, thus opening up labyrinthine possibilities of developing psychic powers and the risk of stagnating spiritually. *Yogī*, you are now at a tricky juncture!

Why are you still at the door? There is a huge distance to travel between knowing "about" the soul and the final union with the soul. Ability to concentrate, free from both the external stimuli and the latent internal impressions, introduces the ardent *yogī* to a

---

[36] *The daily life of a* yogī *stands transformed. Now, the* Yoga *practices attain the highest priority. Twenty-four/seven rhythmic breathing is the natural breathing. Refining and corrective practices keep guard all the time. The* yogī *can hold the fifth step of the upgrading of awareness practice for a minimum of ten minutes. He is practicing advanced* prāṇāyāma *exercises.*

[37] *Sutra I.19 refers to* vidéha *and* prakṛtīlaya. *These refer to upward and downward arcs of life patterns on the molecular plane, respectively.* Vidéha *are those who intensely meditate on the grosser and resolve into the subtler so that the latent impressions migrate to the subtler bodies at death.* Prakṛtīlaya *are on the opposite, the evolutionary, arc. Today they are redundant for the* Yoga *path, because we are ascending on an involutionary quest.*

new world. The concept of soul is now grasped, because only now you perceive without sensing. New vistas open up as awareness shifts from the physical to the astral plane.

Now is the time to know "how to strengthen a link with the soul," so that the soul experience gets conveyed to the brain and you can "understand" the process of enlightenment.

Process of Enlightenment

As a *yogī* you would stand out with a new charm in the presence of family and peer groups, even in odd situations. Thanks to the psychic powers, it would be easier now to decipher complex situations, to read other people's minds, and to know answers to life's challenges. Your personality would radiate an endearing equipoise when influencing people and situations. A majority of aspirants are likely to become seduced in the lure of these early psychic powers, because results are palpable in their immediate physical surroundings.

This is that "tricky juncture" mentioned earlier. It would be tough to not fall for these seductions, and only an exceptional few will bear a genuine disinterest in such powers, treat them as an inevitable effect, and maintain apparently deceptive "nondescript" demeanor. These wise practitioners also know that any powers on the *yogīk* path are to be harnessed strictly for further spiritual progress alone. Such *yogīs* are ready for the next big step—a shift in awareness from the astral to the causal plane.

Direct Perception

At this point in the journey, chakras, the subtle mini-brains, can communicate with the causal plane as well as cohere as one and share communication. This would bring you closer to the soul and into the realm of divine powers in place of psychic. Recognition of the soul would bring you closer to understanding the Spirit. But this process unfolds in stages. Sage Pātañjali says that **the discernment** (between pure Spirit and the world of mind-matter) **occurs through belief, followed by energy, memory, and meditation, and culminates in right (direct) perception** (Sūtra 4.4/I.20).

First, there is a belief or a **concept** that the soul does exist independent of the world of mind-matter. This belief is only an anchor. The word *shraddhā* is misconstrued by many interpreters as "faith," albeit a blind one. This connotation is contrary to the theme of *Yoga-Sūtra*. Here, the right word is "concept," which is much more analogous to a "hypothesis" that eventually emerges as a proven principle of one's experienced knowledge. However, without a hypothesis there is no starting point for any quest.

Another viewpoint is that Yoga is a holistic discipline and requires validation of a series of hypotheses to finally realize the whole truth. On the *yogīk* path, you cannot follow the footsteps of science and try to infer a whole principle by putting together piecemeal findings or simply wait for a "Eureka" moment.

But a quest is like an expedition where a concept alone is not enough; **energy** is needed next in the pursuit of that hypothesis. When awareness shifts from the physical to the astral plane, the *prāṇa* sheath is activated and the degenerated *vayūs* in the bodies start getting purified. Yoga exercises and practices foster proper breathing. Breathing and *prāṇa* have a close correlation. Hence, the next step is to harness more pure and potent *prāṇa* to energize the subtler body-brain systems.

Now, the object-dominated, chaotic **memory** is exiled and is replaced by a memory of spiritual reading. This way, self-chosen and self-created impressions of the soul-realization process are transferred to memory. In the process, the structure of predispositions stands completely remodeled.

With this, the purpose of life itself changes. It is the soul-realization that you now **meditate** upon. In fact, this is how the soul-realization is conveyed to the physical brain and gets woven into the fabric of your daily life. This is the meditative attitude that finally leads to a **direct perception** and creates enormous, powerful, and creative energy (of a fourth or even third grade of higher *prāṇa*). Now, *Īśvara* will not meet a *yogī* in sporadic, involuntary flashes; Its presence can be willed. This also enables you to start understanding *Īśvara* as divinity. That becomes an experienced truth and validates the initial concept.

Knowing Īśvara*, the Concept*

Īśvara, *Purūṣa* and the soul are essentially the same; to facilitate easier understanding these are the three names given to the three aspects of the principle that we come to realize at different stages of the spiritual journey. In order to conceptualize *Īśvara*, we must first understand *Purūṣa* as a unique principle or a concept. The entire universe is considered a single continuum extending from gross to subtle. If our everyday world is gross and seen as finite, changing, and mortal, it is logically inevitable to have something beyond that which is infinite, never-changing, and immortal as its source, by whatever name it may be called. In the given context of this framework, let us call it *Purūṣa.*

Is our world finite or merely "seen" as finite? There is no way to be sure as long as our only tool of inquiry and witness is the sensory thinking; that's where the catch is. Thinking draws on *guṇa* (qualities), and thus objects acquire forms that are possessed of qualities. We may shift awareness from gross to subtle levels, yet as long as we are "aware," *guṇa* are present. Processes of sensing and thinking portend finiteness. The subtlest entity we can become aware of and meditate upon is called as *Īśvara*, because we cannot be "aware" of *Purūṣa*, which is infinite and imperceptible.

Īśvara and *Purūṣa* are difficult concepts and to get even a glimpse of their presence you need to be in an advanced spiritual state. Especially, through our finite body-mind system, the "formless infinite" is difficult to capture in words and it can only be understood intellectually. To make it worse, these terms are used by many authors quite differently in different contexts. If you do not understand the underlying principle, the labels alone will have you completely confused.

Here we keep the definitions simple to help and not hinder your Yoga practice. We saw earlier that *Purūṣa*, the Spirit is taken as infinite, intangible and hence, inaccessible to ordinary perception.

However, *Īśvara* is a perceivable, *guṇa*-based manifestation of *Purūṣa*. Thus, though they are one and the same, *Īśvara* is the apparitional[38] version of *Purūṣa,* the hypothesis that challenges a *mahāyogī* in the making.

However, the conceptual realization of *Īśvara* is only a stepping stone towards knowing *Īśvara*. We do that by *"aligning oneself with Īśvara—that is, yoking every aspect of conscious life to the perspective of pure awareness."*—Chris Hartranft, 12.

By intense devotion to *Īśvara*, knowledge of *Īśvara* is gained (Sūtra 4.5/I.23). Does "devotion" refer to *japa* and *bhaktī*? Devotion is an essential force that keeps one firmly on the *yogīk* path, but that by itself is not enough. Even the process of such "alignment" remains primarily grounded in the body-mind system. In knowing *Īśvara*, ordinary awareness is not enough and pure consciousness is needed that Yoga practices can deliver. Hence, devotion coupled with Yoga practices becomes the right way.

Yoga-Sūtra uses generic terms and explains the process of enlightenment in distinct but universally recognizable milestones. To understand this, you must be truly secular and unlearn the language of the world's religions, which were born for a different purpose years after *Yoga-Sūtra*. The methodologies leading to each of these aspects may vary. Thus, devotion here is more a state of mind and may reflect externally in various forms, rites, or rituals—or may not reflect externally at all.

By carrying any religious baggage, a *yogī* may also struggle with a conditioned reaction to the term *Īśvara*. No amount of debate or doctrinal proofs can take you any farther. *Īśvara* is to be internally experienced and that needs no name. And once experienced, there is no need for any crutches to help stay in that realization. From that point, *Īśvara* becomes your one-on-one guru. The name you call it becomes completely inconsequential, and the form you ascribe to it becomes utterly irrelevant. The guru reveals the truth about Itself.

---

[38] *Here, "apparition" means "an act of becoming visible" because of the human perception.*

Īśvara *Is the Soul*

Ultimately, it is not possible to describe terms like *Īśvara*, *Purūṣa*, and soul in words; and worse to try to grasp them with our conditioned minds. They all represent pure energy and look different only because of a fault line in the process of our perception and our relating with them in different perceptual contexts. "Soul" is the core inside of the subtle causal/atomic body, but is distinct from it. Unlike the bodies, the soul is indestructible.

We have also been saying that *Īśvara* is that core. That creates an apparent paradox—when one looks at any individual (as a whole), that individual is distinguishable from others; but *Īśvara* at the core is not distinguishable from one individual to another. "Packaged" in perishable bodies, *Īśvara* only "appears" to be finite; it is really not. Now you will realize why, for ease of reference, the core of an individual is called the "soul." Soul does not have a personality—either of its own or derived from the enveloping bodies. It is a fragment of the divine, but any part of the infinite is infinite, too. It has no beginning and no end. It is timeless, because "time" is born as a product of mind that belongs to Existence, into which the omnipresent soul has descended only *for the time being*!

The soul appears to be entrapped in the body-mind system, but is still *Īśvara*. Again, "entrapment" is a deceptive word because it sounds as if the divine fragment is helpless. To put it rightly, the body-mind system is more a vehicle chosen by the divine fragment for experiencing the objective world. Thus, the "entrapment" (for lack of a better term)—a way of engaging with the objective world; it does not limit the soul.

Thus, *Purūṣa*, *Īśvara*, and the soul are one and the same; except for varying needs of the human perception they are respectively "imperceptible," "perceivable as one," and "perceivable as many." ***Īśvara* is the soul untouched by limitation, free from *karma* and desire** (Sūtra 4.6/I.24). When you gain knowledge of *Īśvara*, it is this that you would know *experientially*. In the presence of *Īśvara*, this is what a *yogī* realizes. Then, after such realization, you no longer need to be confined and imprisoned by the three bodies. Living on any of these planes is not by *karma*-driven incarnation, but by your own will. A *yogī* is about to realize that life is self-imposed and there is some divine purpose to it.

Only when all *karma* debts are fully understood and completely redeemed is there freedom from *karma*-driven cycles of birth and death; and only a human life has potential for such redemption. Furthermore, no new *karma* is created, because all your thoughts and actions are with a full knowledge of the results, which are completely congruent with that divine purpose. You can potentially withdraw into and function from the causal body.

Moreover, no new *karma* is created because there is freedom from desire on all the planes. There is no longing or desire except to remain in pure consciousness. Mind is no longer a source of knowledge that used to be personalized; now, all actions and thoughts are completely devoted to *Īśvara,* who is the source of infinite knowledge.

Source of Infinite Knowledge

Knowing (the process) and the known (the object) both belong in the mind. As the individual mind evolves, it slowly disengages from the thinking instrument, the brain. Progressively, the same separation of the mind occurs with brain's subtler counterparts (*mānas* and *buddhi*) as a *yogī*'s knowledge expands and graduates from the world of effects into the world of causes. In becoming one with *Īśvara*, the object-dominated world impressions must completely cease to exist, and knowledge must begin accruing from beyond even the causal plane. The purified individual mind regains its transparency and becomes the catalytic Universal Mind that it really is. However, the Universal Mind is still finite. **In *Īśvara*, the germ of all knowledge expands into infinity** (Sūtra 4.7/I.25).

So, now we need to know the Universal Mind in relation to *Īśvara.* Universal Mind that "knows all that is to know" is a challenging concept to grasp with our limited individual minds. To do so, we must approach it unconventionally.

All objects are either natural or human-made. Let us first look at the "human-made" objects. No such object of matter is born on its own. At some point in time, it is desired by a mind, and conceived and designed by some mind, along those lines. Finally, mind(s) are still at work every step of the way when it is brought into existence by the human "organs of action." So, if you can visualize all human minds forming a virtual grid as one, such a meta-mind would collectively know everything there is to know about the "human-made" objects. Let us remember that the subtle minds have amazing potential for connectivity.

There is a greater challenge in applying this interpretation consistently to the "nature-made" objects. First, let us dispose of the premise that "humans are at the center of the universe," as an inconsistent idea. That will allow us to fathom a virtual meta-mind that the human minds collectively form. In "nature-made" objects too, an ultra-human mind is at work; a mind more subtle than a human mind. All adapted minds, human or otherwise, are parts of the subtlest Universal Mind. Thus, the overarching Universal Mind knows everything there is to know about all objects, gross or subtle. And because time too is a product of the mind, also known to the Universal Mind is the past, present, and future of all objects.

A *yogī*'s knowledge is now intuitive, direct, and complete. It is not a reflex bounce-off of the predispositions, nor derived from conditioned thinking. Free from all desires and *karma*, the expanding knowledge arrives without seeking, and a *yogī* imparts the same to those who need it on the three planes. Though the soul is "entrapped" in the threefold body-mind, it is no longer conditioned by them. Soul remains infinite and wholesome.

The ever-expanding knowledge also embraces the complete spectrum of the macrocosm and its microcosm. A *yogī* knows the soul and the infinite Spirit intimately and cognizes them as one. However, the Universal Mind belongs to the universe, while *Īśvara*, as *Purūṣa*, is beyond and independent of that. Thus, any "knowledge" of *Īśvara* is yet "unborn" in the confines of the Universal Mind, though potentially it has always been there. This is a very intricate principle that can be taught only by a master teacher.

Teacher of Teachers

"All are learners and all are teachers, differing only in the degree of realization."—Alice Bailey, 53.

But *Īśvara*, being unlimited by time conditions, is (the one with infinite knowledge and) **truly the Teacher of all teachers** (Sūtra 4.8/I.26). That this Teacher actually resides within each one of us is something that is hard to fathom; and hence, weird for the skeptics, but tremendous joy for those who experience it. As long as we are outward-bound, it appears more expedient to find an external guru. Such a guru does serve a useful purpose in the initial phase, because the guru's own knowledge allows the learner to take quick strides instead of the circuitous self-help routes. The external guru helps and guides in herding the unwilling out-bound attention inward.

The learning in Yoga is essentially experiential in nature and transformational. It is qualitatively different from the pedagogy of doctrinal knowledge and the resultant incremental learning that depends almost entirely on previous knowledge. Although there is a common goal and similar milestones along the way, the teaching makes each path unique. It takes great courage and experiential knowledge to realize the limitations of your external guru. But, please remember that you are not sitting here in judgment to appraise your guru's performance. You need to remain eternally grateful to him/her. It is only incidental that, like an exhausted booster rocket falling away after the lift-off, guidance from such a guru becomes redundant at an appropriate moment. During the training, a guru appears to be god. But when a *yogī* discovers that *Īśvara* has been the guru's guru, then it becomes easier to say a gentle *adieu* to the external guru without any sense of disrespect, ingratitude, or remorse.

The concept of God is embroiled in the syntax of religions with each claiming to know its whereabouts and to have exclusive visitation rights. As a result, God has been identified by so many names and symbols, that it is impossible to take it conceptually as "infinite, omnipresent, omniscient, and formless Spirit." The moment one thinks of God, one "thinks" and then a "word" is assigned to a concept. Both are pathetically limiting. Hence, all our concepts of God or gods remain conditioned by the processes of perception. Also, since time itself is a product of sensory perception, the concepts of God/gods are limited by time conditions. But Spirit, by whatever name called, is not so limited.

Though Spirit is one, a conditioned mind perceives an appearance of "many" souls. Thus we have the plurality in the universe. From this first illusion emerge all others, creating an unending chain of causes and effects, each with its own pairs of opposites. In connecting with soul, a *yogī* only prepares for a final launch—realization that *Īśvara is* Spirit. In this endeavor, only *Īśvara* can be the Teacher with a unique mode of teaching.

The Mode of Teaching

The external guru who guides during the initial spiritual struggle easily becomes your sole anchor on the *yogīk* path. Then to extricate yourself from this passionate obeisance is easier said than done. Even such a thought sounds like a betrayal, and you feel guilty of arrogance. Dispassion is needed, and that is the next frontier.[39]

Guidance from *Īśvara* takes many forms and modes hitherto unfamiliar to you. As a *yogī* gets involved with life on the physical plane, *Īśvara* takes charge of the astral body during sleep and uses *mānas* for training through new experiences. A *yogī* learns to synchronize physical body-brain with the astral body-*mānas*, so that **steadiness of the thinking instruments can be reached through meditation on what is learned in the dreams** and this knowledge can now be passed back from the subtle to the gross (Sūtra 4.9/I.38).

At this advanced stage, dreams have quite a different texture. The ordinary dreams as we know them are out-of-control collages of unrelated images that one sees during sleep and cannot remember

[39] *The obstacle of "laziness" was dealt with in* sūtra *II.3. Now is the stage for curing the next obstacle, "lack of dispassion."*

in whole or even in parts upon waking. We also daydream a lot by engaging in fanciful thoughts. Does a *yogī* acquire new knowledge by interpreting dreams? No, because interpretation is thinking and such a wasteful exercise. This new knowledge is right there, requiring no interpretation.

Paradoxically, in the light of the new knowledge, a *yogī* finds the objective world dream-like, as *māyā*! The term *māyā* has been superficially interpreted by many. That is why it is repeatedly said in this book that unless you travel this whole *yogīk* path, a label of *māyā* does not make sense. Unless the relativity of reality is realized experientially, labeling a "real" objective world as *māyā* is preposterous.

Not just the concept, but even the nature of the dream state gets radically transformed. From chaotic dreams that make one perspire, the dreams become more sensible and life-like. Soon it is possible to remember most of them, and later, to relate with them in the context of immediate day-to-day life. After some time, one can even influence dreams and make creative choices, like a playwright, to script the course of the dreams. Eventually, as conscious sleep is achieved, conventional dreams fade away completely. There comes an ironical situation where one remembers the precious training from *Īśvara* as dreams! Though *Īśvara* is formless, it presents the *yogī* with form(s) commensurate with the stage of development, like various deities and spiritually advanced *yogīs* whose images can be meditated upon. Sleep is also used for training in out-of-body experiences for a specific purpose strictly under the guidance of *Īśvara*. It is experienced as dream knowledge but has no relevance to dreams in the conventional sense.

The Teaching

The subject matter of these teachings—the three skills of concentration, meditation, and contemplation—may be practiced first on worldly objects. Gradually, as they are refined and honed, more subtle objects are taken as targets. Eventually, another barrier is crossed. A *yogī* learns to interiorize attention completely and dwell exclusively in the subjective domain, thus transforming the same skills into *dhāraṇā*, *dhyāna*, and *samādhī*, which would become the Primary Means of Yoga.[40]

SKILL OF CONCENTRATION

A concentrated mind withdraws itself from the rest of the peripheral world and lets the train of impulses arise entirely from the perceived object. A steady posture of the bodies, rhythmic breathing, and restraint of distracting causes through *yama-niyama* help in such a process. A steady posture of the bodies facilitates the dissolution of body awareness. Rhythmic breathing considerably slows down the torrent of sensory stimuli. A *yama* and *niyama* regime creates an internally and externally purified environment conducive to actions and thoughts that are not readily distracted. Thus, in concentration you learn to devote your entire perceptive ability and the thinking process to a chosen object by simultaneously disengaging from all other objects or impressions ,which your attention would otherwise flit to.

Sage Pātañjali assures that **peace can also result through concentration upon that which is dearest to the heart** (Sūtra 4.10/I.39). On the first read, this sounds odd. How can peace result from running after everything that is dear to the heart? The mind is prone to be lured by low hanging fruits, seeking what is most pleasant and dear to it. That is what one dreams of. Like a child continuing to outgrow old toys and seeking new ones, an individual's mind continues to flit from one thing to another. Growing spiritual knowledge shows how pleasure gained from worldly objects would perish sooner or later. Running after objects in a quest for pleasure ends in realization that all objects are temporal and transient, and that removes the objects from attention and concentration by taking subtle things as the targets.

[40] Dhāraṇā *has been loosely defined as concentration; it is in fact "one-pointedness." Concentration is a concerted application of brain and mind in the objective world, while one-pointedness is when the individual mind is uninvolved and turns inward. Likewise,* dhyāna *is a meditative attitude (or a sustained* dhāraṇā*) rather than meditation implying a conscious act as popularly understood. For the same reason, different* prāṇāyāma *exercises requiring conscious efforts, though beneficial in one way or another, cannot be instrumental in* dhāraṇā *or the later states. A 24 × 7 rhythmic breathing is the only* prāṇāyāma *that does not need conscious involvement of the mind and is something that can be internalized with "slight effort," as emphasized by Yoga-Sūtra.*

"That which is dearest to the heart" in the spiritual context, is a sequel to "when the object to be gained is sufficiently valued" (Ref: Sūtra 1.14/I.14). Concentration, when directed to worldly objects, yields some pleasure but inevitably more pain. The longing creates a sense of deprivation. When the object "rises and fades away," the deprivation returns.

For the first time, a vision of *Īśvara* causes a rush of elation that is not limited by rising and fading away. And after that, everything falls into place. *Īśvara* then becomes dearest to the heart and is sufficiently valued. Total and abiding peace naturally follows. What remains next is to learn from *Īśvara* how to retain this concentration for longer and longer time. Awareness of *Īśvara* as the core of dreams now spreads over all wakeful living.

SKILL OF MEDITATION

A sustained concentration leads to meditation. A *yogī*'s horizons are continuously expanding. The synchronized ability of the harmonious bodies to concentrate is natural, sustained, and ready to be applied to subtle objects. Yet meditation is still *upon* some object, however subtle. **All this constitutes meditation with seed** (Sūtra 4.11/I.46). As long as your own awareness is recognized during meditation, the awareness itself is still an object and it is still perception of a "form." It inevitably germinates a seed, however latent the impression, and that is the "seed" referred to in the sūtra.

The use of energy in the act of concentrating and in holding on to that concentration are different, hence the latter is considered a next milestone. Some direct effort against the forces of distraction is needed to concentrate. Any effort, however, has to be slowly withdrawn and replaced by a delicate balance between thought-formation and peripheral awareness, which keep alternating and will eventually cancel each other out. While concentration ensures a mono-rail of impulses arriving uninterrupted, meditation further ensures that an exclusive direct perception of the object will prevail.

In the course of training, *Īśvara* presents itself in a manner that will not overwhelm you. A *yogī*'s mind is not yet ready to withstand a state that is purely spiritual. So, initially, *Īśvara* may be seen as different godly or saintly spiritual symbols and images, those consistent with a *yogī*'s cultural background. At times there are sudden, apparently inexplicable, physical visitations of spiritual masters, which leave lingering impressions. A *yogī* continues to meditate on these images and impressions. This progression is essential and inevitable in the inner evolution.

This is where the soul as Self (as opposed to not-Self) is discerned, experienced and interiorized. Initially, any experiencing of *Īśvara* also stands aside of self, the false "I," and becomes a not-self, as "me and *Īśvara*." Even in direct perception, perception itself stands as an intermediary. As a *yogī*, you will eventually reach a stage where the light will not be just *seen* but you will *be* light; a word/sound will not be *heard* but you will *be* sound and you will be lost in the contemplation of your pure spiritual nature. That is true meditation.

SKILL OF CONTEMPLATION

From the point when one-pointedness is achieved without any external stimuli (Ref: Sūtra 4.2/I.18), you are a true *yogī* devoted to *Īśvara*. Then there is no wish or desire to act independent of *Īśvara*; there is total surrender.

In contemplation, the train of impulses is not needed anymore, nor is there any delicate balance to maintain. You remain completely immersed in what you have been meditating upon and you are sustained only on the subtle energy of the internal stimuli.

It may be reiterated here that any shift in awareness, like everything else on the *yogīk* path, is inclusive. At no point in time do you renounce the objective world. In the new awareness, you recognize on all the planes—form, word, and the idea—all at once. No aspect alone colors the mind. This gives you an intuitive understanding beyond the three dimensions. The ordinary perception process is now clearly understood by instantly connecting the three aspects. Time and space are also recognized as the dimensions of perception.

Perception of objects is now unfailingly exact, revealing only the ultimate truth (Sūtra 4.12/I.48). There is no need any more to excavate the layers of truth by unmasking the apparent to see the buried real. There is another effect. Because only the absolute truth is perceived, only the absolute truth is conveyed. In this way the highest level of *yama*, truthfulness, is achieved.

However, the "ultimate truth" remains only a concept until a *yogī* reaches a state of no-mind. **The direct perception without mind's help is unique and reveals that which the rational mind and its tools—testimony, inference, and deduction—could not reveal** (Sūtra 4.13/I.49). A rational mind delivers only a "relative" truth, but the "I" identity mistakes it to be the only truth, as if that point in time were to be a status quo forever.

The human mode of arriving at the truth is through rational thinking. Any thinking is preceded by sensory perception of the object-oriented world, and perception in itself makes everything subjective. But a seeker's transformation brings about a huge difference. To a seeker, subjectivity was form-driven and could not present the whole truth. The form recognition depended on what was already known but in the process got colored by the stored personal impressions. The thought-forming process then was susceptible to the emotional contents of the sensory data. Sensory perception kept you glued to the **world of effects.**

It is only by liberating yourself from the senses and perceiving on the subtle planes that you dwell in the **world of causes**, and that is why now you are a *yogī.* The three harmonized bodies ensure that the realization on the subtle planes gets transmitted to the gross. The sensory data flows unhindered and creates fewer or no thoughts; mind is at rest with no modifications; direct perception is now the main source of knowledge that is not dependent anymore on the incomplete truth delivered by the churning of the impressions. At *this* level, your subjectivity is truly objective, and the inner domain is ready for launching the advanced states of *dhāraṇā, dhyāna*, and *samādhī.*

A *yogī's* direct perception (in the "no-mind" state, as described above, is unique, always reveals only the truth, and) **thus supersedes all the other impressions that are products of the mind activity** (Sūtra 4.14/I.50). However, it must be noted that a *yogī* is "there but not yet there." Direct perception is still a "perception" and has a causal veil, however pure and luminous that veil may be.

To sum up, concentration involves an effort of projecting a single thought; meditation eliminates this effort with a delicate balance between thought-formation and awareness; and contemplation is just awareness. Even at the risk of repetition, recall that *pratyāhāra* is a major step in this eight-limb practice that brings a *yogi* to a fork where objective and subjective become two distinct paths. Only then do the objective skills, like concentration, transform into subjective states like *dhāraṇa*.

Enlightenment

When the skills of concentration, meditation, and contemplation transform into *dhāraṇā, dhyāna*, and *samādhī*, and even **the direct perception itself is restrained or superseded, then pure enlightenment is achieved** (Sūtra 4.15/I.51). It is without any seed of associated desire.

> *Only when all forms and the field of knowledge itself is lost, and the knower recognizes himself for what he essentially is (being lost in the contemplation of his own pure spiritual nature), can the ideal formless, seedless, objectless meditation be arrived at. It is here that language fails, for the language deals with the objectivity and its relationship with the Spirit. Therefore this highest condition of meditation is likened to a sleep or trance condition, but is an antithesis of sleep or the trance of the medium, for in it the spiritual man is fully awake on those planes which transcend definition. He is aware, in a full sense, of his direct spiritual identity.*—Alice Bailey, 101-102.

As long as the skills of concentration, meditation, and contemplation, however refined, are targeting an object, however rarefied, the truth is still a perception, and there is awareness about it that separates one who is aware from what one is aware of. The once indulgent individual mind is now purified. Trained to stand by, and thus reincarnated as the Universal Mind to be the source of knowledge, it reflects awareness of *Īśvara*. But it transpires now that even the Universal Mind must be left behind to meet *Īśvara*. *Īśvara* does not have any desire, wish, or motive. When It leads a *yogī* to Itself, a *yogī* also starts learning how to be devoid of his or her own self and not be aware of being so devoid. No seed can thus result. In a seedless enlightenment/ illumination, the Universal Mind dissolves and a *yogī* is just aware, pure and simple. Though seedless enlightenment is an apparent end-state, it is not the end of the journey. There are many mysteries still to be solved.

A *yogī* has understood the process of perception. But that also means that in being "aware" of the perception, there is something that stands aside the process. Thus, one who is aware and one who really sees through the perception is beyond the three bodies, and that is *Īśvara,* the divine fragment. If *Īśvara* itself is without any desire, then why has this desire-less "seer" had the whole game of the objective world played out in the first place? That remains one of the most intriguing puzzles.

Īśvara is the primary cause of everything—of the three-fold bodies and the mind of all objects in the universe. In the evolution process (downward and outward), the grosser matter gets projected from the subtler. In the involution process (upward and inward), the grosser must fold back into the subtle. In evolution, the Universal all-knowing Mind projects itself into several individual minds, and the same individual minds remain the tool for the folding back as well.

As seen earlier, when the perception of a form on the physical plane reveals its innate nature on the astral plane, that object ceases to exist as such for you on the physical plane because you are no longer locked in the form. The same in turn applies to the causal plane. When from a seeker you become a *yogī*, ability is gained to perceive the form, the word, and the idea of an object, all at once. Pure awareness is thus reflected in a totally harmonized all-in-one perception.

When you achieve enlightenment with seed, it is realized that *Īśvara* has always been both the witness who looked at the form through your sensory perception but didn't "see" it, and the one who has been the sum total of all perception (physical, astral, and causal) but didn't "think." *Īśvara* is like a crystal. When any object is brought close to it, the crystal appears to be taking its color; but in essence, a crystal always remains a crystal. In this sense, *Isvara* might have seen through the mind, but it is no-mind and is not subject to any pressure from the *guṇa* that are inherent in the form-making.

***Īśvara*, the seer, is pure knowledge. In the process of perception, this real Perceiver is made to look upon the presented idea through the medium of the individual mind. Mind causes the apparent knowledge to be less than pure. But that is inevitable, and the evolution eventually sets the individual mind aside until purified. The Seer remains as pure as It always is** (Sūtra 4.16/II.20).

An essential realization that occurs here is that the Universal Mind is also matter, on the same subtle-gross continuum. No object, big or small, has come into being by its own volition. A thought, a product of mind, has always preceded an object's conception and birth. The whole objective world is a product of five essential elements of matter—earth, water, fire, air, and *ākāśa*—interpenetrated by mind. In a time frame sufficiently long, subtle perception of an object causes the gross object to come into existence. A *yogī* eventually understands how and why **all existence is for the sake of soul;** a play of mind (*prakṛti*) for the sake of Spirit (*Purūṣa*) (Sūtra 4.17/II.21).

Even when an individual person's soul is likely to appear as a part of infinite Spirit, it is still infinite. Since the individual soul resides in an objective world, the Spirit chooses to wear an objective body-mind in order to experience it. The physical body-mind presents the objective world to the perceiver as an experience. Though the physical body-mind succumbs to its bondage, the perceiver is not affected.

Now, let us see how the skills of concentration, meditation, and contemplation earned in the objective world are transformed into *dhāraṇā, dhyāna*, and *samādhī* in the subjective mode.

Primary Means of Yoga

Enabled by *pratyāhāra* the skills get transformed in the subjective domain and that leads to the primary means of Yoga, *dhāraṇā*, *dhyāna*, and *samādhī*. But what is a subjective domain?

> *The difference between common perception and scientific observation is not one of kind but only of degree of sophistication. Both are active efforts to discern presented objects by subject-framing hypotheses and trying to confirm them by correlating evidence for and against; in the first case, the process is largely subconscious, and in the second, it is deliberate and explicit. But it is the paradigm that dictates in scientific advancement, and attention is selective—what guides is interest, on one hand, and previous knowledge, on the other. What is perceived is partly what is expected and partly what is sought; it is simply never what is there.*—S. C. Malik, *Matter is Consciousness, The Nature of Matter*[41]

In the context of *Yoga-Sūtra* the difference between objective and subjective thinking is critical and subtle. Here, the term "objective thinking"[42] is a misnomer. Its intended meaning is "a process that is free from the thinker's biases, prejudices caused by personal feelings; presenting facts, not thoughts and existing independently of mind." However, no thinking process is ever free from biases and contexts, thanks to the Machiavellian predispositions at the foundation of our thinking. And no thinking is free from mind unless that is achieved through spiritual pursuits. Thus, ironically, any labored objective thinking remains essentially subjective! And any so-called "universally acknowledged normative thinking" is mostly a consensus of many subjective thoughts that are extremely similar.

---

[41] *© 1995 Indira Gandhi National Centre for the Arts, New Delhi, India. See: www.ignca.nic.in*

[42] 1. *Free of bias: free of any bias or prejudice caused by personal feelings;* 2. *Based on facts: based on facts rather than thoughts or opinions;* 3. *Observable: medicine describes disease symptoms that can be observed by somebody other than the person who is ill;* 4. *Existing independently of mind: philosophy existing independently of the individual mind or perception. (Source: Encarta Dictionary)*

The subjective perception of an **advanced** *yogī* is, however, really objective! It amounts to a direct perception of an object made possible by the subject's ability to disable predispositions, to suspend conventional thinking and to let a purified mind be a catalyst. Suspended thinking also disables *guṇa*-laden appearances from influencing and deflecting objectivity. In fact, all the perceptive tricks of form-word-idea are grasped at once, and the object is perceived as it really is. The *guṇa* no longer define what the object is, but it is seen through at the subject's free will.

Dhāraṇā

The process of being one with *Īśvara* occurs in stages and requires further practice for holding on to it once achieved. It starts with concentration. **Concentration is** (the fixing of the thinking instrument and the individual mind upon a particular external object) **when the individual mind is uninvolved and such concentration turns inward to become subjective, it is *Dhāraṇā*** (Sūtra 4.18/III.1). Concentration requires effort, and though its initial target may be an external object, the effect is for the disciple to slowly step back from "form" awareness and glide into "life" awareness, thus penetrating the object. In doing this, attention also turns inward and the objective essence turns subjective. There is an evolutionary process in such concentration that takes a *yogī* progressively from knowing the form, to cognizing what it symbolizes, to knowing what caused it to be so.

In concentration, initially the thinking instrument is fixing its attention and the memory is still participating. The thoughts are steadfastly connected to the same object. Then, an important thing happens: *pratyāhāra*, the mind is willed away from thinking, the memory pools get disconnected, and the sensory data is sent out (via *ājnā chakra*) unhindered. That's when you develop the ability to see the object purely subjectively, "as is" and not colored by anything, moving the concentration to dwell in the subtle domain of life and causation. This is *dhāraṇā*.

Dhāraṇā is creation of a stable posture of physical, astral and causal bodies as well as the thinking instruments to capitalize on the *pratyāhāra* ability of non-attachment. The new-found freedom of sensing without sense organs arrests any need for outward bound attention. All along, you have been processing images, but a constant avalanche of sense impulses would change them rapidly. Now, it is a lot easier to engage with the images on your own terms.

However, your thought-making process is still operative, and that is what you will now need to concentrate upon. Your goal in Yoga has been to restrain the mind modifications by working on their cause. You have not been able to dissect the thought process, the cause of modifications, mainly because of your involvement with it. Now, the stopping of outward orientation reduces the *guṇa* influence and you can "look at" the thoughts.

Thoughts are in your subtle domain. *Dhāraṇā* allows you to elevate your awareness of the subtle astral body. Thought-watching, thought-spacing and thought-suspension is your continued practice now. At this stage, there would be constant failures when sense organs rebel and try to return to their old game. You have to harness your energized will, keep up the fiery aspiration and rededicate yourself to the unceasing efforts.

Dhyāna

Sustained *dhāraṇā* is *dhyāna* (Sūtra 4.19/III.2).

Is the difference between *dhāraṇā* and *dhyāna* just one of *time*? No, it is also implied that sustaining *dhāraṇā* is met with different obstacles than those which make initial concentration in *dhāraṇā* prone to repeated failures only overcome with great effort.

Āsana, the body posture, must now make a *yogī* completely devoid of body awareness. Rhythmic breathing must completely harmonize with *prāṇa* and energize all the three bodies. It is important to remember that the bodies are not forgotten, but the body awareness is consciously transcended. The energized bodies vibrate in harmony to make such transcendence easier. *Yama* and *niyama* must deliver a perfect environment that is incapable of causing any mind ripple. Whenever this does not happen and you are unwittingly drawn into the normal obligations of life, it may create obstacles in sustaining *dhāraṇā*.

Another essential component is making the detachment of *pratyāhāra* "effortless" and at will, for it to be held onto, and in order to enable *dhāraṇā* over a sustained period. As mentioned earlier, any conscious effort to do so may be counterproductive. Secondly, as long as the object of concentration is not *Īśvara*, but any physical form or even a mental image, it still involves an active engagement of mind.

Dhāraṇā is sustained in *dhyāna* by transferring the knowledge of "life" over "form" down the bodily hierarchy. The knowledge that initially occurs as a flash is relayed to the body-brain system. This way, even when you are called upon by the demands of normal life to live amidst the forms, you manage to see only a veiled "life" and to be conscious of its underlying uniformity throughout the object-filled world. A *yogī* emerges as a different species of humanity—though not much different in outward appearance. Remember a time early in Yoga when we were talking about steadying and harmonizing the bodies for reaching the then inaccessible soul? Well, it is now that a *yogī* experiences the divine soul as if wearing the three bodies effortlessly.

In your introspection, you have started understanding the whole thought-making process thoroughly. In Yoga, nothing can be sustained by efforts. The initial struggle at any stage may justify efforts but sustenance will require eliminating the cause and thus, removing a need for efforts. What causes thoughts? The sensing of *guṇa*. That being substantially diffused, now you realize the mischief of old seeds sitting in the memory.

Thoughts have always been your source of knowledge, the building blocks of your reality. So, the predispositions, emotional overload and images embedded in the memory have been products of the same thought-based knowledge. You have learned to reduce dependence on memory but how would you cleanse it? *Dhyānā* would enable you to reverse the flow of knowledge. Memory will be made to receive spiritual knowledge from direct perception that will remove the debris left behind by thoughts. Knowledge of "life" over "forms" will insulate your thought-making process from agitations and thus, reduce need for efforts to stay in a state of concentration. Once you can easily glide into *dhyāna*, you will be able to maintain equilibrium between this subdued thought-generation and the subtle awareness of life within that does not depend on the thoughts anymore. In that frictionless, non-agitated mind-state (a precursor to the no-mind state) you will be able to hold on to *dhyāna*.

Samādhī, *with Seed*

When the thinking instrument becomes absorbed in that which is reality (an idea embodied in the form) **and is unaware of the separateness of the personal self, this is *samādhī*** (Sūtra 4.20/ III.3).

In *dhāraṇā*, concentration is an "act" of the thinking instrument, and though it is uninvolved, the mind is aware of the medium. In *dhyāna*, the mind is still aware of the meditating self and the subject of meditation, the not-self. This separateness is not only lost but it does not even enter your awareness in *samādhī*. This is what makes the journey between *dhyāna* and *samādhī* so long.

Using the *guṇa* concept, in *samādhī,* the absence of mind (or unawareness of separateness) catapults you beyond the form and the *guṇa* vibrations, and thus you are completely devoid of *prakṛtī*. What remains is *Purūṣa*, the effulgent light, and you become that light, unaware that you are anything else. *"He is however intensely alive and alert, positive and awake, for the brain and mind are held by him in a steady grip and used without any interference on their part."*—Alice Bailey, 249.

Thus, eventually, the efforts of *dhāraṇā* and the delicate balancing of *dhyāna* between thoughts and awareness are no more required for settling in the *samādhī* state in which you don't remain aware of even the awareness. You are still a few steps away from zero mind modifications as long as there is some object of *samādhī,* even if subtle.

The breakthrough of *pratyāhāra* is a pivotal happening for a *yogī*. It not only opens a door to the Primary Means of Yoga bringing enlightenment on the horizon, but also signifies *Īśvara*'s acceptance of the *yogi* as an eligible candidate for those higher studies. That acceptance makes you a truly initiated *yogī*. In *dhāraṇā*, a *yogī* reciprocates *Īśvara* with full cooperation, and in *dhyāna*, the communication link with *Īśvara* is firmly established. In *samādhī*, there is a total loving and willing surrender to *Īśvara*. You are now becoming transformed into a *mahāyogī*.

Nature of Transformation

By following the *yogīk* path, do all *yogīs* transform alike? No; each *yogī's* path is distinct and the transformation itself, unique. The milestones are similar, but the way they are reached and the manner in which the obstacles are encountered do differ. **The choices made in the underlying process of healing the psyche cause the difference in the pace on the *yogīk* path and the nature of the transformation** (Sūtra 4.21/III.15). But, let us first look at the generics of change itself.

Animate or inanimate, all objects change. Though we can grasp it only as discrete snapshots, change is a continuous process. The sensory perception, with which such a change is ordinarily cognized, works within a limited, perceptive bandwidth (range). Any change falling beyond the two extremes of the band is not perceptible to the body-mind. However, change *does* take place on all the three planes. Together, the object presents itself through a series of dynamic "perceptions," each providing a seemingly "stable and real" experience for the perceiver that defines his/her reality for the time being.

You, as *yogī,* are no exception. As a "changing object" yourself, your perception of the path and of the change is intricately interwoven with the change itself. At each perception, alongside a frozen snapshot of form, word, and idea, any number of potential but unborn possibilities exists. Through the "underlying process" of perception and thinking (thought as well as action), you end up making choices in life that keep shaping the potential course. Thus, from the potential generalities emerge individual possibilities that would put you on a unique course of change.

As a seeker, you have made several choices along the learning curves of *āsana*, *prāṇayāma*, *yama*, and *niyama*. Right at the outset Sage Pātañjali told us that, "Yoga is a process of healing of the psyche and the calming of the thinking instrument" (Ref: Sūtra 1.2/I.2). *That* is the underlying process, with a steep learning curve strewn with limitless potentialities. Moreover, the initial choices cause innumerable seeds to form, and the seeds return to redeem as *karma* on the *yogīk* path. Hence, where you stand in the process of transformation at any point in time depends directly on the extent and quality of your efforts.

At the end of the process, when the ultimate Yoga is accomplished, a *yogī* knows the ultimate reality. This is the transformation:

- *From* the relative reality arising from ever-changing perception in various awareness modes
- *To* the unchanging ultimate reality that is in pure consciousness mode.

Even after acceptance by *Īśvara* for advanced training, your efforts must remain steadfast, if not even more intense, now that the rewards are more and the tests are harder. The rewards to boost the process of transformation are granted on all the three planes.

Knowledge of Past and Future Forms—Physical Plane

A concentrated meditation upon the triple nature of every object reveals to a *yogī* that which has been and also that which will be (Sūtra 4.22/III.16).

The three-pronged changing nature of an object—the *state* of the form, the defining *context* of time and space, and the essential idea or *span of life*—becomes known to a *yogī*. With a three-way concentration upon an object or a person, just one glance reveals everything. An object is not only perceived on the three planes but a complete bitmap of the trajectory of its evolutionary process is understood. The law of causes and effects is seen reflected in this evolutionary unfolding. What is seen now is only a result of what has been, and that which is yet to come will be a result of the causes seeded in the present.

A *yogī* does not actively seek the knowledge of the past and the future; it is simply revealed to him or her. It is intuitive. Usually, such powers are intended to foster further *yogīk* progress and a *yogī* is burdened with walking a thin line—between its judicious use and a possible indulgence. On a continuum of past and the future, a form appears as a frozen and limited impression.

Power of Word (Sound)—Astral Plane

The perception of a frozen form instantly triggers a thought, and we tend to equate the form with the thought, which is a verbalized expression. However, contrary to our expectation, even the worded thought does not completely embrace or precisely represent its essence/ meaning on the causal plane. In fact, in our world, all three get lumped together or appear interchangeable. For example, when we are thirsty, the thirst itself is an unarticulated desire. But a thought arises with the word "thirsty" and is almost instantly followed with a culture-specific image of water or Coke, depending on where you live.

Now firmly anchored on the astral plane and aware of the spiritual Self, you start unraveling the astral plane of perception. "Expression," an act of ascribing a "word" to the form happens on the astral plane. The word symbolizes all that the form means to us, and that association becomes our only handle on objects in the world. In fact, "uttering" the word on the astral plane (*vaikharī-nada*) creates an image of the "form" with its *guṇa* (qualities) manifesting accordingly. Our personal vocabulary is not limited to just the functional meaning of a word, but in our memory pool it is loaded with associated impressions and sentiments from past thinking.

Thus, a word gets caught between a lower level form and higher level idea, able to cope with neither. Then, in the mind of the perceiver, a word is usually confused with the form of an object as well as with its meaning. **Now, with a concentrated meditation on these three aspects comes an intuitive comprehension of the sound uttered by all forms of life** (Sūtra 4.23/III.17)**.** The word gets liberated. It does not appear to a *yogī* merely as a string of syllables; it becomes a sound, with unique vibrations. With greater and deeper awareness comes intuitive understanding of the vibrations of the form, word and idea. As the physical body gets more and more synchronized with the astral, *guṇa*—the mother of forms—is also understood as vibrations. In turn, one starts understanding the power of sound vibrations as the creator of forms.

A word is seen as an incarnation of an idea that descends from the causal plane, and its limitations are also realized now. When put in words, the idea, purpose, or the meaning on the higher causal plane does not remain foggy and nebulous anymore, but, a mere word seems unable to contain it either, and a *yogī* realizes that a word is a poor embodiment of meaning. Gradually, this insight cultivates an intuitive understanding of the three bands of vibrations that separate the physical, astral, and causal planes.

This is an important aid to your training. All along as a seeker and as a disciple, you had used different symbols, images, and concepts to label *Īśvara*. They were poor yet inevitable substitutes. Now, training in sound as the creator of form gets you initiated in the primordial word/sound (AUM) thus connecting with the presence of *Īśvara.* It is possible to untangle yourself from all the symbolic forms in which *Īśvara* had to be perceived.

This delivers two profound skills for the future studies:

- How not to feel overwhelmed by the world of words and to appreciate silence, eventually learning the "vibrations of silence."
- How to go beyond sound—the form maker—and to "experience" breath as a precursor to sound.

Span of Life—Causal Plane

After knowing the triple nature of the object and after understanding the astral plane of sound, the concentrated meditation can now be elevated to the causal plane to realize that everything exists for a purpose. The idea behind any object, its whole purpose, is finite, and that purpose determines its span of life. Put differently, it is known how long the soul of an object will continue to experience through the three bodies, at the end of which the purpose will be over and its term will expire.

The *karma* seeds are the main drivers of life experience. The law of causes and effects dictates **which *karma* seeds warrant immediate redemption in the current lifetime and which might be deferred to a future life. With perfectly concentrated meditation on the repeating patterns of redemption *yogī* can see the term of own experience in the three worlds** (Sūtra 4.24/III.22). It becomes possible to be aware of the seeds that are yet to be redeemed and to know whether the redemption is due in the present life or a future one.

By practicing *pratyāhāra*, you have ceased to generate new seeds through any act, thought, or intent during that state. But, there is no question of evading redemption, even at the feet of *Īśvara*. The power of the omnipotence of *Īśvara* is for encouraging and expediting redemption and not for interfering with it or condoning it.

However, at this juncture you, a *mahāyogī*-in-the-making, are no longer the old self who would worry about karmic consequences or even dread the knowledge of impending death. You have traveled enough on the *yogīk* path and been sufficiently transformed to look up to the redemption or ensuing physical death as a moment of liberation. It is not a terminal event but just a milestone. This knowledge comes intuitively as well as through the ability to read spiritually. An instant knowledge of forms, words, and ideas offers clues to what is in store from a variety of signs that appear to a *yogī* as different vibrations.

It is a delicate state, though. You find the so-called powers falling in your lap, and the temptation to use them is enormous. But if this temptation test is passed, the "moment of grace" arrives. Like still water can reflect the moon, the still mind reflects *Īśvara* whose grace is sought. "When the disciple is ready, the Master appears." Guidance from *Īśvara* intensifies, and by the sheer resplendence of the indwelling teacher's presence, a *yogī* is deeply devoted to the higher learning process. Now the goal of Yoga is "sufficiently valued" and earnestly pursued. The material self has completely surrendered to the spiritual Self, and the material world is no longer seen with colored eyes and through imperfect senses that become staple food for a contaminated thinking process.

However, the best body structure is still a body. The same is true of the mind. As long as the seeds of past *karma* are not fully redeemed and new *karma* is not prevented from arising, a possibility always exists that a latent seed may germinate into a thought and indulgence may follow. When this happens, the brain still oscillates and the mind does fluctuate, and you are at risk of getting overwhelmed.

Beyond the Emotional Intelligence

On the threshold of becoming a *mahāyogī*, now bridges are needed—first, between the bodies and the spiritual Self, to reach beyond the causal state; and second, between your own soul and that of others, to realize soul connectivity. The emotional intelligence has helped so far, yet the purely spiritual domain requires that you transcend both the emotions and the intelligence. This can only be achieved by elevating the three harmonized bodies to such a level that they could be synchronized with the soul. Then, you are closer to realizing *Īśvara* as the real Perceiver.

Art of Synchronization

A *yogī*'s repertoire of experiences is immensely enhanced with the new discovery of breath as a predecessor to sound. Sound precedes everything else. Rhythmic breathing, when perfectly synchronized with *prāṇa*-breathing, energizes the astral and the physical bodies. Then a *yogī* starts realizing the power of breath and sound. This new awareness brings about a profound change. The astral self is now supple enough to co-vibrate with other beings in earnest compassion, and this resonance creates empathy. Thus, you can completely vibrate with others and suffer with them, if required.

The self-centered actions give way to tenderness. Unselfish and heartfelt desire makes thoughts and actions compassionate, and these are helpful to others. That's Yoga too. Such "union" with others extends on the causal plane as well, in the form of dispassion, the desiring of nothing for self. Thus, **the union with others**

is gained through concentrated meditation upon the three states of feelings on the three planes—tenderness, compassion and dispassion, and still a *yogī's* thoughts or actions generate no *kārmik* seeds (Sūtra 4.25/III.23). (Remember the "four-way" practice of "sympathy-tenderness-steadfast joy-dispassion" prescribed in Chapter One to combat the obstacles? That practice becomes an effortless way of life now to preempt all the obstacles).

Such a union is achieved through synchronization of your own breathing with that of others. Your three bodies are already in a higher state of harmony with vibrations under the control of the spiritual will. That is why you can quickly restore your own harmony even after temporarily aligning with a cacophony of emotions in others. Thus, a *yogī* transcends the emotional intelligence. With the anatomy of emotions known, it is now possible to co-vibrate with the emotions of others and yet rise above them.

You learn to use your breathing like a stethoscope and realign it, in sync with the causal state of others, to generate a harmonious response on your own three planes. Thus, dispassion, compassion, and tenderness go hand in hand. Any thought, deed, or intent so accorded helps others in their *kārmik* redemption without inviting any residue back to a *yogī*. This merciful disposition is a gifted ability for you; but of course would use it only when a merciful act is needed in your own redemption of *karma*. However, there is another and more valuable kind of "union with others" that is gained at this stage. At the feet of *Īśvara* and with Its consent, a *yogī* can experience the presence of other advanced souls as co-travelers. It is difficult to recognize true Yoga masters (*ParamaYogī*) outwardly. Most of the Yoga masters will not be seen wearing exotic robes and preaching to public congregations unless their "less fortunate" *kārmik* redemption so requires. Usually their work is quiet and anonymous. Their teaching is usually one-on-one to the chosen and the eligible. They avoid donning any public profile. It is only after a *yogī* attains a similar ability to co-vibrate with compassion that such an interaction with advanced Yoga masters is granted. And this happens under *Īśvara's* watch, now recognized by you as the real Perceiver.

Īśvara*, the Real Perceiver*

Who is the real perceiver? It is a realization that happens in stages. Ordinarily, when we perceive, we say, "I perceive." We don't realize that we cannot "see" what we perceive until we examine it. At that time, **brain is the lord**. We are so hypnotized by what we perceive that it never occurs to us that something besides our own "self" is watching it to make us aware. When the seeker becomes a disciple, the machinations of the mind are recognized. Then **mind is taken as the sole anchor** and the perceiver. Eventually, the causal body seems to take charge with its intellectual prowess and, for a while, that is assumed to be a perceiver. When a *yogī* is sufficiently advanced on the *yogīk* path it is known that *Īśvara* is and has been the real Perceiver all along. But, that happens in a **"no-mind" state**.

WHEN BRAIN IS THE LORD

In the initial stages, the brain is the "lord" and we are so engrossed in the thinking process that any independent perceiver is not even recognized. To be vibrant and unsettled is the nature of mind, whether individual or Universal. The mind's involvement reinforces the supremacy of the thinking instrument, and the two appear as one. (This view concurs with the prevalent scientific knowledge that mostly revolves within the self-created boundaries of neurology, taking the brain as an autonomous organ with the mind as its intangible proxy.) It is, therefore, an important turning point for you to look inward and recognize something else as *the* perceiver. It is not easy. The restless individual mind repeatedly obliges the brain to sense outward, and every time that occurs, you have to use your will to return inward.

However, recognition of a "behind-the-scenes" perceiver does not happen at the exclusion of the brain. It is neither possible nor desirable to silence or to deactivate the brain. Hence, pressing yourself into wasteful attempts at forced meditation ends up harming the brain cells. *Dhyāna* as a true practice of meditation commences after *pratyāhāra*, when mind is not attached to the brain, which is thus consciously kept away. Then, in *dhyāna*, the mind-induced thought-making process is suspended, and yet the brain remains fully active and alert. This is the reason why all the successes on the *yogīk* path are achieved through awareness rising from gross to subtle, and a subsequent reverse knowledge transfer from subtle to gross. A perceiver has to experience through the three harmonized bodies.

Eventually when a *yogī* comes to recognize *Īśvara* as the Perceiver who keeps watching through the active mind, it is realized that the mind also keeps It independent of itself. **The Perceiver is ever aware of the constantly active mind, the main effect-producing cause of *karma*** (Sūtra 4.26/IV-18). This is the Perceiver, as "no-mind." With this realization, a *yogī* is even more devoted to *Īśvara* and can keep the mind only as a catalyst, aloof from the brain, thus eliminating new causes seeking effects.

Those who approach *Yoga Sūtra* without an experiential orientation always get baffled by the "no-mind" state. Through long and intimate association, the mind is a key player in gaining, retaining, and using knowledge to enable living in the object-filled world. Making it neutral appears akin to taking away all life-support. To tackle this apprehension, a key is provided now.

WHEN MIND IS THE SOLE ANCHOR

Our brain is an excellent tool for use in initiating human actions by means of knowledge. The mind tricks it into becoming a "knowledge creator" too, which results from faulty sense data and a solitary confinement imposed by the "I" awareness. The very fact that the mind can be separated from the operations of the brain, and observed, makes it independent of the brain. One realizes that even when the brain creates "knowledge" it does not know or think by itself. A single thought is independent of its components (sexual, emotional, intellectual), which reside in various parts of the brain as signals or memory patterns. The separateness of the brain (the thinking instrument) from the mind is experienced when you turn inward.

As awareness of the subtle bodies grows, thinking brings about an involvement of the mind with each of the brain's counterparts (*mānas* and *buddhi*), and as long as your identification remains with one of these bodies, the mind is mistaken as the knower.

Only when a *yogī* recognizes the Perceiver is it realized that the mind, however fine it is, can still be watched and *is* watched by the Perceiver. The opaque individual mind is an instrument and nothing more. It is reflective, for that is how it creates perception and understanding. But it is yet incapable of perceiving or understanding by itself and only works as a "go-between." It collects vibrations emanating from the *guṇa* of the three worlds and offers the Perceiver an experience. **The Perceiver is the illuminator; the mind is only a reflector** (Sūtra 4.27/IV-19).

From knowing the mind as the "sole anchor" to knowing the mind as the "intermediary between the soul and the tangible world" is a revealing experiential journey that you would undertake as a *yogī*. You must make the mind purer and finer so that it vibrates in tune with the soul rather than with a chaotic, ever-changing *guṇa*. A purer mind becomes a repository of more real knowledge that is then transferred to the brain. Then its association with the brain is useful. Thus, not using the sense data and disengaging a refined and stilled mind from the thinking process is not "non-sense"!

NO-MIND STATE

How do you know the real state of the mind? Knowing this is an inevitable but the most difficult step. You are condemned to use your mind to understand the mind unless you come to understand it experientially. **The mind cannot know two things simultaneously, itself and that which is external to it**; like the physical eyes that can see the universe but not an inch within (Sūtra 4.28/IV-20).

Ironically, if mind could know itself and also all that is external to it, there would be no need for Yoga. These are two distinct modes: one, when knowing needs cognitive perception to precede, and the other, when knowing is simple awareness. The mind plays in the first mode, whereas the Perceiver plays in the latter. When there is no sense-perception, there is no coloring of the mind, and with the mind thus staying away to just stand aside, what prevails is pure awareness. Unless this is known experientially, it is difficult to grasp how this phenomenal world is a ground (field of knowledge) for both experience and liberation. Liberation can be attained only when you focus your attention on the process of consciousness itself, thus recognizing its source. A "process of being aware" at this stage still binds brain, *mānas, buddhi*, and mind, howsoever refined. Directing such dualistic and limited awareness to the process of enlightenment at best makes you aware of being aware. Such awareness still produces dualistic cognition that breeds predispositions and consigns them to memory. **This creates a bottomless pit of mind knowing mind, as it would infer an infinite number of knowers** (Sūtra 4.29/IV.21). This is why it is essential to set the mind aside to immerse in pure consciousness. This is a *yogī*'s final struggle before stabilizing in the "no-mind" state.

If the "no-mind" state still baffles you, consider this. We are talking about a mind that was once contaminated, colored and opaque. But thanks to a lot of internal and external purification, a purer mind is delivered to act as a wonderful catalyst in knowledge creation, and not as an indulgent team player. As a catalyst it is at its best, standing by. Secondly, it absorbs knowledge arising from direct perception and spiritual reading and converts it into actionable wisdom for which the brain is an excellent partner. This is a preparation for the "no-mind" state.

One step away from the "no-mind" state your new awareness is elevated to the causal level. Yet, the soul connection is guiding the intelligence that is no longer emotional, but has become spiritual.

Intuition, the Spiritual Intelligence

Giving up thinking and reliance on mind in favor of an intuitive reliance on the spiritual intelligence alone is difficult to accept. It appears to be risky, if not disastrous, given our conditioned living in the material world. But the cultivated power of intuition has to be experienced to be able to trust it. The initial hesitation of a first-time "swimmer" in these new waters fades away when the spiritual intelligence serves as superior to physical or emotional intelligence, and keeps you afloat even without your previous forms of knowing.

> *Intuition has a fourfold power. A power of revelatory truth-seeing, a power of inspiration or truth-hearing, a power of truth-touch or immediate seizing of significance, which is akin to the ordinary nature of its intervention in our causal intelligence, a power of true and automatic discrimination of the orderly and exact relation of truth to truth,—these are the fourfold potencies of Intuition. Intuition can therefore perform all the action of reason—including the function of logical intelligence, which is to work out the right relation of things and the right relation of idea with idea—but by its own superior process and with steps that do not fail or falter.*—Sri Aurobindo, *The Life Divine*, Pondicherry: Sri Aurobindo Ashram, 1919, 949.

This is a wonderful description from a great authority on Yoga. Spiritual intelligence is not "thoughtless"; not a substitute for normal logical intelligence; it subsumes it to deliver an instant and unfailingly exact truth. The truth so revealed, harmoniously unifies the three dimensions of form, word and idea. Ordinary intelligence bloats the "self" and makes it occupy the center of your objective world. **When the spiritual intelligence, which stands alone and free from objects, reflects itself in the mind, then comes awareness of Self** (Sūtra 4.30/IV.22).

If the vessel containing water is kept out in the moonlight, the moon reflects itself in the water, provided the water is not in turmoil. The water does not have to "pull" the moon in, in order to reflect it. An individual mind, now a catalyst again, helps the brain in "knowing" as if by throwing light. But the mind does not know itself and is not self-illuminating. So once it is stilled, the Perceiver itself is reflected in the mind to create spiritual intelligence in the brain. Thus, the Perceiver may not be actively making the mind and the brain aware of its presence; but by sheer experience of the Perceiver and the stilling of the mind, the same brain can acquire that spiritual intelligence.

The realization of the real Perceiver is an important milestone in Yoga training. This is the only way a *yogī* can comprehend how the world does not change and yet everything changes. As a seeker, you had a concept of such a paradox but wondered how could it ever happen! This realization also answers for a *yogī* a few fundamental questions: If the Perceiver is the one who perceives through the three bodies, why is the world perceived initially as "object-centric"?And why is the whole *yogīk* path traveled to reach a point of realization that the Perceiver, the all-knower, has been only a witness to all along?

Yoga, the union, occurs at many stages and among many elements, until the final union takes place between the *Prakṛti* (your bodies, the Mind-matter) and the *Purūṣa* (your soul, the Spirit); then, realization follows that both are really one.

But such a union between the Mind-matter and the Spirit has to be preceded by your ability to intuitively discern their presence in each and every object of matter. Then, as the mind becomes purely and completely reflective of the Perceiver, you decipher another cryptic principle: *Purūṣa* (beyond *guṇa)* has all along been the Perceiver, and the very process of perception made it look like *Īśvara, Purūṣa*'s *guṇa*-based version. An intuitive knowledge of this apparition (*māyā*) completes all that the mind should be knowing. But how does this happen?

The mind reflects both—the knowable physical world (the field of knowledge) and the Perceiver itself (the knower); this is how the mind acquires all knowledge and becomes omniscient (Sūtra 4.31/IV.23). The brain and the mind are in tune with the Perceiver, and while the brain still dwells in the objective world, it not only perceives the form, the word, and the life-essence all at once, but it knows all that is worth knowing. In due course, intuition replaces the mind-driven perception. This is an important stage because the mega-door is now open for a direct enlightenment/ illumination. Total devotion to *Īśvara* and intuition as the source of knowledge is the only way to proceed towards the ultimate goal of Yoga.

How Is Your Yoga Practice Now?

Your life is radically different. The *prāṇayāma* of continuous rhythmic breathing ensures a sustained supply of *prāṇa* energy. With mind-modifying hindrances overcome and obstacles removed, the body-mind posture (*āsana*) is rock-steady. *Yamas* and *niyamas* have become second nature now, thereby eliminating the causes of mind modifications. Object-oriented memory is exiled, and memory is replenished with impressions of spiritual reading that are sustained by high spiritual energy.

Dhyāna and *samādhī* often invoke an image of sitting cross-legged with eyes closed. Such body postures certainly help. But they are external aids and achieve nothing by themselves. Similarly, breathing exercises only prepare the ground for real Yoga. There comes a point on the *yogīk* path when you realize that *dhyāna* is all about normal consciousness. Once, *dhyāna* or *samādhī* appeared totally disconnected with day to day life. What you learn is that they are such rich and potent states that, once mastered, you can be in those states while going through your daily chores. And thus all life becomes Yoga. "*All life is Yoga. In the right view of life and of Yoga all life is either consciously or subconsciously a Yoga.*"—Sri Aurobindo, *The Synthesis of Yoga*, Pondicherry: Sri Aurobindo Ashram, 1914-21, 2).

From a *yogī* you are transformed into a *mahāyogī* as the knowledge of the entire past and future becomes accessible on the physical plane, the power of word/sound is acquired on the astral plane, and the idea and the evolutionary path of life itself is unfolded on the causal plane.

The spiritual-reading ability takes a *mahāyogī* beyond emotional intelligence. It becomes possible to synchronize the whole multilayered body with the bodies of another object in order to perceive it directly, without any mediation of the thinking process. The individual mind becomes its original self, the Universal Mind, flowing freely and indulging in no sensing.

It is experientially realized that *Īśvara* is and has always been the real Perceiver. With this, dissolution of your "I"-identity is complete, and the intuitive spiritual intelligence is firmly established in you; now a *mahāyogī.*

***Book Four: Rearranged Sūtras*:** (Numbers in the brackets are from the original text)

4.1 (I.17) **वितर्कविचारानन्दास्मितानुगमात्सम्प्रज्ञातः ॥**

vitarka-vicārānandāsmitānugamāt saṁprajñātaḥ

One becomes fully aware of an object by concentration on its fourfold nature—the form, through examination; the quality (or *guṇa*s), through discriminative participation; the purpose, through inspiration and the soul, through identification.

4.2 (I.18) **विरामप्रत्ययाभ्यासपूर्वः संस्कारशेषोऽन्यः ॥**

virāma-pratyayābhyāsa-pūrvaḥ saṁskāra-śeṣo " nyaḥ

The further stage of concentration is achieved when the one-pointed thought no longer depends on external stimuli and is responsive only to the (subjective) latent impressions.

4.3 (I.19) **भवप्रत्ययो विदेहप्रकृतिलयानाम् ॥**

bhava-pratyayo videha-prakṛtilayānāṁ

However, even the stilled bodies take the seeker only to the door of the soul's realm, as he still stands bound to the phenomenal world.

4.4 (I.20) **श्रद्धावीर्यस्मृतिसमाधिप्रज्ञापूर्वक इतरेषाम् ॥**

śraddhā-vīrya-smṛti-samādhi-prajñā-pūrvaka itareṣāṁ

The other Yogīs (not stagnated in the psychic powers) proceed to the state of *Samādhī* and arrive at a discrimination of pure spirit through belief, followed by energy, memory, meditation and right perception.

4.5 (I.23) **ईश्वरप्रणिधानाद्वा ॥**

Iśvara-praṇidhānād vā

By intense devotion to *Īśvara*, knowledge of *Īśvara* is gained.

4.6 (I.24) क्लेशकर्मविपाकाशयैरपरामृष्टः पुरुषविशेष ईश्वरः॥

kleśa-karma-vipākāśayair aparāmṛṣṭaḥ puruṣa-viśeṣa Iśvaraḥ

Īśvara is the soul (divine fragment) untouched by limitation, free from *karma* and desire.

4.7 (I.25) तत्र निरतिशयं सर्वज्ञबीजम्॥

tatra niratiśayaṁ sarvajña-bījam

In *Īśvara*, the germ of all knowledge expands into infinity.

4.8 (I.26) स पूर्वेषामपि गुरुः कालेनानवच्छेदात्॥

sa pūrveṣām api guruḥ kālenāna-vacchedāt

Īśvara, being unlimited by time conditions, is the Teacher of the teachers.

4.9 (I.38) स्वप्ननिद्राज्ञानालम्बनं वा॥

svapna-nidrā-jñānālambanaṁ vā

Steadiness of the thinking instrument can be reached through meditation on the knowledge which dreams provide.

4.10 (I.39) यथाभिमतध्यानाद्वा॥

yathābhimata-dhyānād vā

Peace can also result through concentration upon that which is dearest to the heart.

4.11 (I.46) ता एव सबीजस्समाधिः॥

tā eva sabījaḥ samādhiḥ

All this constitutes meditation with seed.

4.12 (I.48) ऋतंभरा तत्र प्रज्ञा॥

ṛtambharā tatra prajñā

Now a *yogī's* perception is unfailingly exact and reveals only the truth.

4.13 (I.49) श्रुतानुमानप्रज्ञाभ्यामन्यविषया विशेषार्थत्वात्॥

śrutānumāna-prajñābhyām anya-viṣayā viśeṣārthatvāt

This particular perception is unique and reveals that which the rational mind and its tools: testimony, inference and deduction—cannot reveal.

4.14 (I.50) तज्जः संस्कारोऽन्यसंस्कारप्रतिबन्धी ॥

taj-jaḥ saṁskāro "nya-saṁskāra-prati-bandhī

It is totally different from or supersedes all other impressions.

4.15 (I.51) तस्यापि निरोधे सर्वनिरोधान्निर्बीजः समाधिः ॥

tasyāpi nirodhe sarva-nirodhān nirbījaḥ samādhiḥ

When this state of perception is itself also restrained or superseded, then pure *Samādhī* is achieved.

4.16 (II.20) द्रष्टा दृशिमात्रः शुद्धोऽपि प्रत्ययानुपश्यः ॥

draṣṭā dṛśimātraḥ śuddho "pi pratyayānupaśyaḥ

Īśvara, the seer, is pure knowledge. Though it looks upon the presented idea through the medium of the mind that is inevitable for the evolution and the Seer remains as pure as it is.

4.17 (II.21) तदर्थ एव दृश्यस्यात्मा ॥

tad-artha eva dṛśyasyātmā

All that is, exists for the sake of the soul.

4.18 (III.1) देशबन्धश्चित्तस्य धारणा ॥

deśa-bandhaś cittasya dhāraṇā

Concentration is the fixing of the thinking instrument upon a particular object and when such concentration turns subjective, it is *Dhāraṇā*.

4.19 (III.2) तत्र प्रत्ययैकतानता ध्यानम् ॥

tatra pratyayaikatānatā dhyānaṁ

Sustained *dhāraṇā* is meditation, *Dhyāna*.

4.20 (III.3) तदेवार्थमात्रनिर्भासं स्वरूपशून्यमिव समाधिः ॥

tad evārthamātra-nirbhāsaṁ svarūpa-śūnyam iva samādhiḥ

When the thinking instrument becomes absorbed in that which is reality (the idea embodied in the form) and is unaware of separateness or of the personal self, this is contemplation, or *Samādhī*.

4.21 (III.15) **क्रमान्यत्वं परिणामान्यत्वे हेतुः॥**

kramānyatvaṁ pariṇāmānyatve hetuḥ

As the underlying process is of "subjugation of the psychic nature" the choices that a Yogī makes causes the difference in the pace and the nature of his/her transformation.

4.22 (III.16) **परिणामत्रयसंयमादतीतानागतज्ञानम्॥**

pariṇāma-traya-saṁyamād atītānāgata-jñānaṁ

Through concentrated meditation upon the triple nature of every object, comes the revelation of that which has been and of that which will be.

4.23 (III.17) **शब्दार्थप्रत्ययानामितरेतराध्यासात् संकरस्तत्प्रविभागसंयमात् सर्वभूतरुतज्ञानम्॥**

śabdārtha-pratyayānām itaretarādhyāsāt saṁkaras tat-pravibhāga-saṁyamāt sarva-bhūta-ruta-jñānam

The word is usually confused with the form of an object and its meaning in the mind of the perceiver. By concentrated meditation on these three aspects comes an intuitive comprehension of the sound uttered by all forms of life.

4.24 (III.22) **सोपक्रमं निरुपक्रमं च कर्म तत्संयमादपरान्तज्ञानमरिष्टेभ्यो वा॥**

sopakramaṁ nirupakramaṁ ca karma tat-saṁyamād aparānta-jñānam ariṣṭebhyo vā

Karma is either for immediate redemption or future and by perfectly concentrated meditation on these, the Yogī knows the term of his experience in the three worlds. This knowledge also comes from signs.

4.25 (III.23) **मैत्र्यादिषु बलानि॥**

maitry-ādiṣu balāni

Union with others is to be gained through concentrated meditation upon the three states of feeling: tenderness, compassion and dispassion.

4.26 (IV.18) सदाज्ञाताश्चित्तवृत्तयस्तत्प्रभोः पुरुषस्यापरिणामित्वात्॥

sadā jñātāś citta-vṛttayas tat-prabhoḥ puruṣasyāpariṇāmitvāt

The Perceiver is ever aware of the constantly active mind, the effect-producing cause.

4.27 (IV.19) न तत्स्वाभासं दृश्यत्वात्॥

na tat svābhāsaṁ dṛṣyātvāt

As it can be seen or recognized, it is apparent that the mind is not the source of illumination…. (contd.)

4.28 (IV.20) एकसमये चोभयानवधारणम्॥

eka-samaye cobhayānavadhāraṇaṁ

….neither can it know two objects simultaneously, itself and that which is external to itself… (contd.)

4.29 (IV.21) चित्तान्तरदृश्ये बुद्धिबुद्धेरतिप्रसंगः स्मृतिसंकरश्च॥

cittāntara-dṛśye buddhi-buddher atiprasaṇgaḥ smṛti-saṁkaraś ca

… because alternatively, if the mind is presumed to be known by another mind, it would infer an infinite number of knowers and the resulting sequence of memory reactions would simply implode.

4.30 (IV.22) चित्तेरप्रतिसंक्रमायास्तदाकारापत्तौ स्वबुद्धिसंवेदनम्॥

citter apratisaṁkramāyās tad-ākārāpattau sva-buddhi-saṁvedanaṁ

When the spiritual intelligence, which stands alone and freed from objects, reflects itself in the mind stuff, then comes awareness of the Self.

4.31 (IV.23) द्रष्टृदृश्योपरक्तं चित्तं सवर्थिम्॥

draṣṭṛ-dṛśyoparaktam cittam sarvārthaṁ

Then the mind stuff, reflecting both the knower and the knowable, becomes omniscient.

Chapter Five: *ParamaYogī* (Yoga Master) and Illumination

5th Milestone

The soul connection ushers you into a state of bliss that is beyond ordinary mind-assisted awareness on the physical, astral or causal planes. You stand blissfully isolated even in a crowd. But the grooming still continues. Concentration, meditation and contemplation, whether in an objective or subjective mode, are still individual states that you move in and out of. You have to reach a state purely contemplative (instantly and not progressively) and stay in it uninterrupted.

As a *mahāyogī* now you enter the final phase. All answers to all the seeking are now to be found. The practices have now completely blended and become a part of life. A spiritual state is now becoming a steady state. Separateness of any kind, even in the highest spiritual experience, is next to be given up. The cause of all causes simply shows up in each and every object when you witness that object's desire for experience triggering a union between the Spirit and the mind-matter; but now you have to make the final discovery that the two are really one. You have to let the matter alone and remain in the consciousness of the Spirit in everything. In the end, there can be no desire, not even of the bliss of an ultimate union.

At this stage, you are able to alternate in two different states of awareness at will—a normal householder's life or a state of *samādhī*. You have free access to the Universal Mind that abounds everywhere without getting "individualized." Your Yoga practices have changed completely. The need for conscious Yoga practices has come to an end because all living is now Yoga. You can interact directly with the gross-to-subtle elements that are under your control. Still, you have to remain unflustered by these powers.

The last and the most challenging test comes at this point. In the no-mind state, the entities of time, space and awareness disappear, since they are only products of mind. It is yet to be realized how *Īśvara* is a perceivable version of the Spirit. The last Yoga hypothesis is that the Spirit and *Īśvara* are not really separate, but only appear to be so because they are *seen through the screens of time, space and causation.*

In the end, you have to contemplate without being aware of it. "Being aware" creates separateness and even that has to dissolve for the total isolated unity with *Īśvara*, the Spirit. *That* unity is enlightenment/ illumination proper, and makes you a *ParamaYogī*, a Yoga master. You have reached your final milestone.

In this phase: transition from Mahāyogī *to* Paramayogī

Yoga hypothesis	The universe is apparitional: it is the Absolute (*Purūṣa*) seen through the screens of time, space and causation (*Māyā*)
Know through experience	The fourth state (beyond physical, astral and causal)
Involuntary control	Secondary *saṃyama* (with seed)
Achieve Voluntary control	Primary *saṃyama* (without seed)
Become	An intensely tested *mahāyogī*
Be	A *ParamaYogi* (The Master)

New words used in this chapter

Bindu	A chakra located very close to *sahasrāra*. In metaphysical terms Bindu is a point at which begins creation and the unity becomes the many. Also described as "the sacred symbol of the cosmos in its unmanifested state."
praṇavaḥ	Primordial soundAUM
saṃyamaḥ	Reaching *dhāraṇā*, *dhyāna* and *samādhī* all at once
antardhānaṃ	Being invisible
Pradhāna	State of equilibrium between gross and subtle
pratiprasavaḥ	Involution; opposite of the process of birth

The Spiritual State

Is the spiritual state so completely cut off from the other three states? No, it cannot be. Gross to subtle is a single continuum. Vibrations, with only their intensity varying, are common among all the states. Vibrations cause sound and thoughts verbalize it.

Is "word" a cord connecting the gross-to-subtle states? A word holds a middle ground between a deceptive form on the physical plane and its unarticulated purpose on the causal. If sound is the subtlest sense of the subtlest element of *ākāś,* we need to understand the essence of "word."

In the process of articulation, an idea or a concept descends from its nebulous cloud on the causal plane onto the astral plane in the form of a word. In that very process, we scramble words to immure the meaning. On the astral plane, words enable a thought, and feed into and emerge from the thinking process. Words and thoughts are inseparable; external, and internal aspects of each other. Thought is generic, while word is clothed in the culture and in its contemporary usage. Word—phonetic or scripted—is a symbol whose connotation becomes meaningful only in a given community. Outside the community, that word is a mere sound.

Words also make it possible for the thoughts to continue to carry an image of an object even when the object itself is not present. Words come to symbolize objects and define an individual's world. Consciousness thus projects from behind the causal plane into the physical plane via words. Words range from an exclamation to a verbiage. New words evolve continuously, in order to cope with change, because words can only approximate and never fully contain the world of ideas.

Words have their own legacy and hierarchy. In their most potent form, they are sounds. If ancient human history is traced, words became currency when the cultural requirements could not be fully addressed through mere sounds.

The primordial sound, the first word, is "AUM."

AUM, a Bridge to the Soul

The import and potency of the sound of "AUM" is enormous. But let us see what it is even at a mundane level. When the mouth is opened to let the breath (air) in or out, it creates a sound of a syllable "A" ("o" in *come*). The sound of "M" ("m" as in *jam*) emerges when the lips slowly close from a fully open mouth, and "U" is a complete trajectory of sounds of "A" expanding into "O" (as in *foam*) and fading back into "M." It is a basic human sound and, hence, closest to the idea that it symbolizes. It does not differ from person to person, culture to culture, or age to age. That is one of the reasons why it is an external symbol of *Īśvara*. It is also the *prāṇava*, the primordial sound of all conscious life and hence is regarded as the root sound of all sounds.

Though apparently simple, AUM needs volumes to convey its hidden meanings and properties. Suffice it to say here that it takes a long Yoga practice before *Īśvara* trains a *mahāyogī* in properly pronouncing AUM, because it creates incredible vibrations. An internal purification of a *mahāyogī's* body accrued through Yoga practices ensures that the body is now ready to sustain these vibrations.

AUM IS THE WORD OF *ĪŚVARA*

The "word" of *Īśvara* is AUM and hence it is to be learned from *Īśvara* only (Sūtra 5.1.1/I.27). The chanting of AUM has been sometimes distorted in the hands of inexperienced practitioners. AUM is an extremely powerful sound, and the enormous significance of why it is one of the important teachings of *Īśvara* deserves your earnest attention.

In Vedic texts, the scale of sound vibrations is mentioned. In its true state, AUM creates *para-nād*, with vibrations unsustainable in this existence. That vibration, when reduced to a quarter, is *paśyanti-nād*, which the causal state can sustain. A quarter of *paśyanti* is *madhyamā-nād*, which the astral state can sustain, and a quarter of *madhyamā* is *vaikharī-nad*, which we ordinarily sustain in the physical state. That should explain how powerful "AUM" is and why only *Īśvara* can guide in its proper recital.

At this stage, you have understood the principles underlying the concept of *Īśvara* and are ready to give up that or all the other symbols and words to address It. This also helps you to get rid of a struggle with the conventional wisdom about "God," either of the theists or the atheists. In AUM, *Īśvara* externalizes itself when it is soon realized how AUM illuminates even in silence.

SOUNDING OF THE WORD AUM

Through the sounding of the word and through a reflection upon its meaning, a way is found to further oneself on the *yogīk* path (Sūtra 5.1.2/I.28). Sounding AUM through your mouth is an important but really a small step. It is not hard to experience how the overt spoken word is always preceded by its covert appearance in the thought form, and even a thought is preceded by an idea. Thus a link exists between idea, word (the expression), and an object. This threefold link is ordinarily disjointed. Isn't it common to fumble for words because we never feel an idea is adequately articulated? Aren't we verbose sometimes and still find that an object is not described completely? It is evident that the "mother" bodies of form, word and idea, vibrate at different and discordant frequencies until purified.

Yoga practices bring about purification that releases and elevates awareness. As you become aware of the spiritual Self, and start perceiving all the three aspects, the three bodies start vibrating instantly in harmony. Then it becomes less significant to say AUM overtly, and you start learning how to listen to AUM in silence instead. That is when *samadhī* becomes a real state of silence or stillness.

AUM EMANATES FROM EACH ATOM

Any gross object, whether small or as massive as stars and planets, is an ensemble of atoms each vibrating at its own rate. AUM is the primordial sound of that vibration born within an atom from the time the atom manifests out of the omnipresent *ākāśa*. *Īśvara* teaches a *mahāyogī* about *this* AUM and how to listen and to co-vibrate with it in the total stillness of mind and with an absolute focus on it. These are much more subtle, finer, and powerful vibrations of AUM than chanting it verbally. Hence, a lot of care is needed and the bodies require preparation to endure that task.

While AUM is chanted and listened to on the causal plane, this vibration is communicated to the physical brain via the astral plane. This forms a "silver cord" linking all the three planes. The subtle AUM also annihilates the subtle kārmik seeds that lay latent on the causal plane and make their fruition redundant.

A *yogī*'s shift from a recital on the physical plane to the rendering on the causal makes the silver cord of AUM extend inward. This completes the process of interiorization.

> *Interiorization is a shifting of perspective away from externality toward an interiorized point of view... More specifically, it is the growing sense that awareness is not seeing an object per se but instead observing a consciousness representing an object.*—Chip Hartranft, 12-13.

This, however, is an extremely gradual process. It is fostered by purification brought about by the Yoga practices. A strict yet effortless adherence to *yama* and *niyama* ensures that the obstacles erupt no more. But the obstacles do not go away without a mutiny every day, and only perseverance and fiery aspiration would help you to stay on such a course that is replete with battles. However, the rewards *are* extraordinary too.

To a disciple, the initial vision of *Īśvara* appears in flashes. But it inspires you to try to hold that vision. Now *Īśvara* teaches AUM to you, and thus hands over a key for accessing that vision at will. Then you could live in the objective world and still perceive only *Īśvara* in everything by extending the silver cord of AUM within or without. **Thus *Avidyā*, the sum total of all obstacles, is dissolved in the realization of the soul** (Sūtra 5.1.3/I.29).

Until now, though you have experienced a lot on the subtle planes as a *mahāyogī*, you have understood many advanced things in a mostly intellectual fashion naturally and inevitably. But, intellectual activity is still a mind activity, and the mind's compulsive "thought-form making" now becomes an obstacle. Through a devoted and uninterrupted practice you have earned the ability for one-pointed concentration. Earlier, there wasn't enough care taken to check the occurrence of thoughts. But, the ordinarily flitting mind is now largely in control. Now the stage is set to remove the last obstacle, "carelessness" (Ref. III.13.).

AUM, THE OBJECT OF MEDITATION

While practicing AUM, a *mahāyogī* begins to have *Īśvara* as the only "object" of meditation, realizing that **the meditation upon light and radiance** is only an intermediate step **in the knowledge of the Spirit,** as they are images left behind by the visions of *Īśvara*. Images are objects processed by thinking and **non-duality can be reached for achieving peace only by transcending the thinking process** (Sūtra 5.1.4/I.36). Thus commences the first experiment on the threshold of subjective objectivity. Having *Īśvara* as an object is really not having any object for meditation at all.

Meditation on AUM offers to you a real glimpse inside. But the beauty of Yoga is that in the very process, the same "silver cord" is extended in everything else. By knowing yourself, you know the world. The outward *guṇa*-dominated appearance of the forms dissolves and in its place emerges a subtle world of force-fields and energy. As you grow acutely aware of your own three bodies, the molecular and electronic sheaths inherent within all the external physical forms are perceived as well, adding two more virtual dimensions to the "new" world.

Gradually, your direct perception deepens and expands. The divergent physical forms melt, and you become aware of the generic essence of all the forms, and thus of their essential oneness. You have reached such a *sāttvik* state that forms reveal *guṇa*, *guṇa* reveal vibrations, vibrations reveal the binding forces and convey why and how a form is composed, and finally the life-force reveals itself as its core energy. From infinitely minuscule to infinitely massive, this essential "form- *guṇa*-vibrations-life-force" hierarchy is scale-invariant; it is the same across all objects. Then it is also realized that, in this entire spectrum of life, a beholder of this realization, the human being, stands right in the middle. **As an accomplished *mahāyogī,* your knowledge is perfected when you can telescope your vision into the universe as well as microscope it into an atom** and find the same pulsating energy at the core (Sūtra 5.1.5/I.40). Thus, this all pervading energy is recognized firsthand to be *Īśvara*, no longer needing any name or label.

Now, the whole spectrum of the universe can be seen without any external aid. The boundaries of Existence are seen. The role of an individual mind is understood in contrast to the Universal Mind, and it is understood how mind is instrumental in creating a make-believe, subtle-to-gross kaleidoscope by projecting its energy into the physical forms. *Īśvara* teaches AUM so that you can begin experiencing the no-mind state, and so that your causal body may get some idea of what the Creation process must be. The mind-created linearity of experiencing becomes apparent, and it is known how it creates continuums of time and space in Existence. Here it is possible to get some idea of an absence of time-space that leaves behind an "eternal now" where everything simply *is*, in the un-created state before Existence.

In sensing the eternal now and the fourth state, a *mahāyogī* is still using the three bodies as a vehicle. How, you wonder, in these harmonized bodies, do the subtle (causal) and the gross (physical) still co-exist? How is this vehicle capable of experiencing anything spiritual?

Pradhāna, *the Balanced Spiritual State*

It is often mentioned that the Spirit and matter form the first pair of opposites which come together to create this dynamic world of objects. The time to grasp a complex but fundamental concept of *pradhāna,* a balanced state, when the Spirit meets the matter, is currently at hand. The process of cognition senses the *guṇa*-created vibrations explicit in the form of an object. As a seeker, when the physical body was yet not tuned, you used to receive these vibrations distorted by the dominance of *tamas* or *rajas guṇa.* That cognition used to be further obscured by your colored structure of predispositions. The perception used to remain trapped at the physical level because the astral body was still disjointed and you were not even aware of this fact.

However, further on the *yogīk* path, your physical body got refined and the astral body started vibrating in sync with it. This allowed reception of the true vibrations of a form followed by their recognition at a mature, emotional level. Then the personality-defining structure of predispositions started dissolving and the coloring stopped. Eventually, the causal body also got in sync with the other bodies to make it possible for you to realize that awareness of pure consciousness was the whole purpose of these bodily forms.

SPIRITUAL AWARENESS

When a *mahāyogī* reaches a no-mind state in pure consciousness, the processes of cognition and perception do not change. What changes is the awareness. In touch with all the three bodies at will, at this juncture you can vibrate with the corresponding three bodies of any other object. The omnipresent Universal Mind constitutes the field of knowledge to which all the objects of matter belong. Saved from getting individuated, now Universal Mind itself flows undiminished through the bodies. Since there is nothing to color, condition or corrupt the brain's processes of cognition, the resulting knowledge is the same as the field of knowledge. And since a *mahāyogī*'s three bodies co-vibrate with the corresponding three bodies of the object, the bodies (the "matter") collectively balance and withdraw from awareness to bring you directly in touch with the life within, the knower (the real Perceiver) itself. **Thus,** in the no-mind state **where mind modifications are completely stilled, the field of knowledge (the "knowable"), the knowledge, and the knower become one. There eventuates a state of identity with and similarity to *Īśvara* as that which is so realized** (Sūtra 5.1.6/I.41).

Those who have not actually walked on the *yogīk* path may imagine that at this stage you become a little wacky, rendered incapable of living a normal object-centered life. The truth is the contrary. Since the gross and the subtle life are seamlessly homogeneous, you can engage in everyday life with full gusto and no distracting strings attached. Your actions may not seem culturally valid or fashionable, but they are perfect in the larger context of humanity and the natural environment. *To be eligible to become one with Īśvara, it's really all or nothing.*

SUBTLE SUBJECTIVITY

A *mahāyogī* thus becomes a subtle self. How does it happen? Recognition of the objective world is a direct function of self-realization. In the beginning, when your own *guṇa* were not in balance (when *sattva* was overpowered by *rajas* and *tamas*), the concern was with calming the thinking instrument and healing the psyche. To achieve this, Yoga methods and practices were rigorously followed. Then, there came *pratyāhāra*—the ability to detach the mind from the brain, followed by concentration, meditation, and contemplation in the objective world.

As a *mahāyogī*, you have arrived at another breakthrough point—you have realized that object sensing has its subjective counterpart. Though pure consciousness is known as the generic core of all objects, the connection between an object and the senses has remained elusive. For example, the physical atom of earth has a subtle element of odor, water has of taste, light has of color, air has of touch, and *ākāś* has of sound. When water is sensed as an object, why does a subtle sensing of taste occur?

Here is the secret. The Spirit meets matter during the process of perception when the senses meet the *guṇa* of the object. You realize for the first time that, in the subtle sensing during perception, **the gross leads into the subtle and the subtle leads into progressive stages of a spiritual state called *pradhāna,*** where in the no-mind state, matter meets Spirit and creates an undifferentiated state of equilibrium of *guṇa* (Sūtra 5.1.7/I.45). It also explains how, ordinarily, the mind-driven sensing ends up exciting *guṇa* and throwing its three components off-balance; a difficult concept only vaguely understood before being experienced. This is a crucial breakthrough in understanding the delicate balance between "gross" and "subtle" and how a balanced *pradhāna* resolves the pairs of opposites. Turning inward and experiencing *pradhāna* is a prerequisite for commencing *dhyāna*, *dhāraṇā*, and *samādhī* (with seed) on the subjective plane.

PERMANENT MEDITATIVE STATE

Because the purified individual mind has withdrawn into a catalytic role and the thinking instruments are calm and quiet, now a *mahāyogī* has a pure spiritual realization and is in a permanent meditative state; a perennial *samādhī* with eyes wide open (Sūtra 5.1.8/I.47). (This is the fourth state, or the "yet another way" as described earlier in Sūtra 3.2/I.22). With *rajas* (activity) and *tamas* (inertia) under control, the *sattva* (revealing/illuminating) prevails and holds the three *guṇa* in their highest equilibrium. *Pratyāhāra* has progressed into *dhāraṇā*, *dhāraṇā* into *dhyāna*, and *dhyāna* into *samādhī* with seed.

Clarity of perception comes instantly and fluently without requiring linear cognitive processes. It is also without any limitation, and you see the formless in all the forms. This pure spiritual knowledge is transmitted to *buddhi*, to *mānas* down to the physical brain. You go through the normal chores and obligations, but do not indulge in sensual perceiving, and never lose the meditative attitude.

> *He has pierced the great Maya (illusion) and passed behind it into the light which produces it and for him mistake is impossible, his sense of values is correct, and sense of proportion exact.*—Alice Bailey, 104.

A formless perception brings an end to *karma*.

Freedom from Karma

When you live in this uninterrupted meditative state where a thought has no coloring of the past emotions but arises immersed in the spiritual wisdom, *karma*—past, present, or future—has lost all power over the individual. **"With this,"** the Sūtra says, **"pain which is yet to come can be warded off."** (Sūtra 5.1.9/II.16). There are several threads of interpretation possible here. Warding off pain is central to all human endeavors. Pain-producing elements exist on the physical plane, but pain itself is a product of the mind. Unless you learn to bring the mind under control while dealing with the world of objects, there is no real solution to pain. The pain-producing seeds are far more subtle than any physical solution, and their legacy across lives makes even death inconsequential in ending the pain.

A *mahāyogī* attains a state in which the structure of predispositions is completely dissolved. Actions are no longer prompted by the vagaries of the mind but stem from the Universal Mind's pure knowledge of objects, in which the now marginalized mind does not meddle. You are left with no fears, anxieties, desires, or longing. Thus, the seeds of *karma* are burned in their causal state, and no seeds are left behind to germinate in the future to cause any pain.

However, the past seeds could still be latent. One of the canons of the law of *karma* is to continue to present the seeds in newer circumstances so that you can redeem them by living through them, and thus learning in the process. The *guṇa* are now brought in equilibrium and rhythm through balanced *pradhāna*, the structures are ennobled, the textures are purified, and thus pure knowledge is obtained under the auspices of *Īśvara*. There is no need, furthermore, to learn from some of the cycles of *karma* redemption, because they are rendered redundant. If redemption is still needed, a *mahāyogī* is now capable of fully understanding its nature and import even independent of redemption. So a redemption process is no longer painful, because one lives it out with equipoise.

There is another way to look at it. **The preventable cause of all pain is the illusion that the perceiver** (depending on one's level of awareness) **and that which is perceived is one and the same**

(Sūtra 5.1.10/II.17). This illusion ordinarily results in *avidyā* and an attachment to the objects, ultimately leading to pain.

All objects are manifestations resulting from the interplay between *Purūṣa,* the Spirit, and *Prakṛtī,* the mind-matter. Though *Īśvara* is the perceivable version of *Purūṣa*, awareness of *Īśvara* as the real Perceiver was forever lost in the false "I am"-awareness. This bred the structures of predispositions (worldview) and of personality (self-view). When one becomes aware of *Īśvara* as the perceiver, a realization occurs that the "I"-identification was an illusion. You see how this illusion created a series of pain-producing effects all along.

> *The great objective of Raja Yoga (as expounded in Yoga-Sūtra) is to free the thinker from the modifications of the thinking principle so that he no longer merges himself in the great world of thought illusions nor identifies himself with that which is purely phenomenal. He stands free and detached and uses the world of the senses as the field of his intellectual activities and no longer as the field of his experiments and experience-gaining endeavors.*—Alice Bailey, 152.

Again this is a fundamental change—to stand free and detached while engaging with the world. Rooted in the "I"-centric world, it is impossible to see anything else. Erasing "I"-awareness sounds catastrophic until you realize, firsthand, how the resulting forms captivate awareness, and how that becomes the main cause of all pain.

However, pain is an effect of *karma* that leads to existence, birth, and death. Having exiled memory; having made the effect-producing cause—the incoming impulses—powerless; and seeking only the guidance from *Īśvara*; all the causes are now set aside. After a seeker-disciple-*yogī-mahāyogī* transformation, you are ready to die consciously, ready to be born again if needed, and ready for enlightenment, to become a true master.

A few other practices need to be done carefully and only under able guidance, beyond this point. The practices themselves do not *make* anything happen, but with their help the inner evolution makes balanced progress. Where there is fiery aspiration, the needed guidance arrives. It can take any form—a dream, a friend, an event, a book, an external teacher. But as the practices advance, one goes beyond the popular "health, fitness, and feel good" domain, and the risk of damage grows sharply. Trustworthy help arrives not only in response to one's aspirations, but also only to the qualified. That is why if *Īśvara* does not assume an external form to guide, you are advised not to proceed further.

In such situations, one is well served by introspecting and examining honestly if a "holier-than-thou" attitude has crept in, or if the ability of spiritual reading has been misused as a stunt of eavesdropping into the privacy of others, or if the devotion to Īśvara is not total. Sage Pātañjali has repeatedly warned at different stages and urged us to adopt "a passionless attitude toward any spiritual attainment and soul powers." Even a subtle bondage would disable a *yogī's* entry into the isolated unity. At this advanced stage, the master-to-be has to walk a thin line between dispassion and fiery aspiration.

A subtle formless perception in the spiritual state is possible with awareness located in the causal body that has been purified by Yoga practices. With that, a *mahāyogī* reaches a stage where the practices can now target the subtle bodies in preparation for a sustained spiritual state. That needs sustained *prāṇa* energy directly controlled through a practice of advanced *prāṇayāma.*

Advanced *Prāṇayāma*

In our earlier discussion about *prāṇayāma*, we touched upon a unique point, an intimate relationship between breathing and *prāṇa*. With the exhalation of air, *prāṇa* gets drawn from the cosmic energy—with the centrifugal force of *samāna*)and vibrates inward; with inhalation, it gets deployed into the physical body (with *vyāna*); and in the motionless states in between, it is sitting expectantly waiting.

It takes years of practice to realize experientially that *prāṇa* drives breathing and not the other way around, and that there is a subtle umbilical cord connecting *prāṇa* inside your dense body with the life-force that abounds in the cosmos. It is also essential that the three bodies, which are both generators and consumers of energy, are regulated, aligned, and synchronized to work as one. Only then can they become a durable vehicle for the finer energy to transit back and forth. A rigorous practice of various rhythmic breathing methods is mostly preparatory. When AUM recital reaches a proper resonance, it signifies that a *mahāyogī* is now ready for the fourth stage of *prāṇayāma*.

There is a fourth stage of *prāṇayāma* which transcends those dealing with the internal and external phases (Sūtra 5.1.11/ II.51). Once *prāṇa* is set into motion, the breath can be totally kept out, thus *external* breath is totally separated from the *internal prāṇa* and that is the fourth stage of *prāṇayāma*. Then *prāṇa* is circulated within the three bodies in such a way that the power points (*chakras*) in the finer bodies are activated and nourished. If the physical body is not yet ready to carry this powerful force, it is likely to get damaged. Through sustained practice, it has to rise up to endure the higher rates of vibrations. Such practices should be undertaken only with able guidance and can never be correctly understood by just reading about them.

For the preliminary *prāṇayāma* practices, there were stipulations of "place, time, and number" that we dealt with earlier. However, in the fourth stage of *prāṇayāma*, regular breathing is totally suspended. Hence there are no conditions of place, time, and number. Breath is either held inside the lungs or kept completely out, while the inside *prāṇa* is moved with focused concentration. You should remember that *prāṇa* is being accessed here consciously. To a practitioner at this stage, *prāṇa* should be as perceptible as the air that is breathed. Exercising a mere imagined and vague *prāṇa* leads nowhere. If you cannot perceive *prāṇa*, you are simply not eligible as yet and need to have patience.

The finer bodies are both generators and carriers of finer energy. They radiate when properly attuned and vibrate in concert when in equilibrium. This intrinsic luminosity is perceptible now. The radiance comes from the *sattva* element that predominates as the *rajas* and *tamas* are tamed. *Prāṇa* is energy, and the essence of consciousness is energy, too. By practicing the fourth stage of *prāṇayāma*, a *mahāyogī* perceives light directly radiating from the astral and causal bodies. It no longer remains a visualizing exercise as in the initial stages.

It is essential that the subtle bodies are actually perceived. During the initial stages on the *yogīk* path, many times you experience an image of light which often is just that, an image! The mind plays endless tricks. In the early stages, the achievement-oriented psyche is eager to see the much-anticipated "light" and "aura," and anxious to reach the popular legendary signposts. Mind is always there to oblige. But that remains a futile exercise as long as it is "I"-centric. *Yoga-Sūtra* is no spiritual fiction, and hallucinations and gimmicks have no place in it. A qualified *mahāyogī* who practices the fourth stage of *prāṇayāma* literally sees the luminous astral body that is enveloped by the dense and opaque physical body. Later, you can see the causal body that is even more luminous. At times these extraordinary experiences can lure you into mistaking them for illumination itself. But a true *mahāyogī* is now focused entirely on realizing *Īśvara* and avoids any such mirages.

Did you once believe, as an aspiring *yogī*, that Yoga practices alone could bring illumination, and hope that light would be brought unto the mind's eye from somewhere? As you are so far ahead on the *yogīk* path, you would realize how naïve that idea was. The mistake was similar to our reflex belief that the sun dawns on the eastern horizon to bring light to us. Eventually, we realize that the sun is always there and we, riding on the planet Earth, only return to it. Similarly, it is realized that all bodies are essentially divine but veiled in ignorance. Yoga removes ignorance. **Through this, that which obscures the light is gradually removed** (Sūtra 5.1.12/II.52) and illumination shines forth. That is why Yoga is called a process of self-realization.

An individual mind colored by past impressions is no longer a source of knowledge. A refined mind is now ready to do its primary function of transmitting knowledge. It is able not only to withstand the "light" but is ready and able to carry it through to the physical plane. A *mahāyogī* is truly in a position to do away with the methods and practices for internal and external purification (the Secondary Means of Yoga) that were the hallmark of the initial Yoga journey. The state of meditative attitude can be maintained now, where there is no need for conscious practice and control. The identification with *Īśvara* is complete and stable, never to slip away. Mind stands squarely as a catalyst and as a repository of all knowledge, and the light is never obstructed.

The fragile personality structures are demolished and in their place a meditative attitude dawns. A *mahāyogī* enters and exits the states of *dhāraṇā*, then *dhyāna*, and then *samādhī*, during the *yogīk* practice. This makes you adept at gliding into the householder's role in the objective world and back into the meditative attitude in the subjective world with élan. Now you *use* mind instead of *being used by* the mind and **it is prepared for holding an uninterrupted meditative attitude** (Sūtra 5.1.13/II.53).

But, even the states of *dhāraṇā*, *dhyāna*, and *samādhī* need not be entered and exiled in succession when a *mahāyogī* masters the next stage.

Saṃyama, the End of Yoga

So far, concentration, meditation, and contemplation have been practiced on external objects in the early stages, and later, *dhāraṇā*, *dhyāna*, and *samādhī* in the subjective or direct perception mode. The Universal Mind, as the mother of all, is an indispensable source of knowing what matter is, what it is composed of, what the *guṇa* are, and how mastery over them could be achieved so that the senses and emotions, the drivers of the thinking process, can be quieted. Some understanding of all this is gained through the states of *dhāraṇā*, *dhyāna*, and *samādhī* which, in turn, have drawn strength from that understanding. However, even this part of Yoga has been mostly preparatory.

Saṃyama

The final goal of Yoga is achieved in ***saṃyama*, one sequential act of *dhāraṇā-dhyāna-samādhī*** that is not directly aimed at any object (Sūtra 5.1.14/III.4). When *saṃyama* is achieved through communication with the Universal Mind, it is the secondary *saṃyama*, and when achieved through communication with *Īśvara* alone, it is the primary. (This distinction is explained by Tavariaji and is not explicitly mentioned in the *Yoga-Sūtra*; both the states are of a very advanced nature and the difference can be explained only by a guru). Secondary *saṃyama* is performed while remaining aware of all the bodies, while the primary *saṃyama* is performed in the causal body alone.

Before being guided toward *saṃyama* a *mahāyogī* is thoroughly tested whether real mastery has been achieved over the mind modifications, emotions, and memory as well as whether the physical and astral bodies can be set aside such that you can remain only in the causal body. When *saṃyama* is consciously practiced, it is "*samādhī* with seed." But when it becomes a permanent meditative attitude, not disturbed even during the waking hours by the normal life of a householder, it is "*samādhī* without seed."

Saṃyama does not occur as a natural progression after *samādhī*. It must be earned, almost like a reward. To qualify for this, you, the master-in-the-making, have to truly disengage from the three worlds; neither attracted to nor despising them. And yet, you should be able to stay rooted in the consciousness as separate from the mind and the three bodies, regarded as mere vehicles. What is experienced through the bodies is not the biased objective world, but an unveiled, pure, subjective reality; and what is transmitted back to the physical brain is this perfect knowledge. You should be able to concentrate mind and train it steadyily on anything at will for any length of time.

Saṃyama is a critical milestone. A *mahāyogī* has come a long way since the first vision of *Īśvara* and since practicing *dhāraṇā*, *dhyāna*, and *samādhī* as exercises. Now everything has to fall into place. *Samādhī* has been interpreted variously, depending on the interpreter's experience. The "light" seen during the state of *samādhī*—is it "experienced," or is it something else? Regardless of whether it is seen or experienced, it is still matter.

An important factor in *samādhī* is *prajnyā*, a high type of pure awareness, almost consciousness itself, resulting from a proper communication with the Universal Mind. But before *saṃyama* begins, even this communication is also to be snapped. A *mahāyogī* has experienced *Īśvara*, and there is no need to enlist more information *about* it. **So, as a result of *saṃyama* comes the shining forth of "light"** though you are much ahead of just "seeing" light (Sūtra 5.1.15/III.5).

In *saṃyama* culminate several states of being. The awareness of *Īśvara* results in pure knowledge. The awareness itself works like a searchlight that when directed to any object reveals the real nature of it intuitively and instantaneously.

This pure knowledge does not stay as just awareness but "shines forth" as illumination and is transmitted to the brain. A *mahāyogī* is thus in a position to impart this knowledge to others. As long as *avidyā* is symbolized by darkness, realization that dissolves *avidyā* is taken as enlightenment. Otherwise, the enlightened Yoga masters say, "*Īśvara*'s abode, the fourth state, is the same as an inky, black darkness." Light, as we understand, is a material object; *Īśvara* is not. As a *mahāyogī,* you have come a long way.

Yogīk *Path in Retrospect*

Sage Pātañjali brings home an important caution that **this illumination is gradual and is developed stage by stage, plane by plane** (Sūtra 5.1.16/III.6). The powers gained in the attainment of certain Yoga states encourage many seekers to rush the efforts. Rushing is inconsequential at best, if not patently dangerous at worst. It must be remembered that there is no outward change in a *mahāyogī. Everything changes within.*

And only when changes take place in the very core of one's being does illumination dawn and slowly become a state by itself.

As a seeker you might have often fantasized about various "achievements" in Yoga. In spiritual infancy, what meets the eye are the powers, and one tends to paint fanciful images of favorite spiritual heroes superseding the not-so-favorite ones, like in professional wrestling! Such a shallow view is likely to deliver only ill-prepared Yoga "experts." What expertise in Yoga could be expected of a person who, after years of Yoga practice and teaching, may still be greedy for personal glory, bask in half-knowledge, and crave for recognition? From the forms to the form-less is a long journey; but essentially an ennobling expedition.

When the mind is purified and stands aside as a catalyst, the knowledge that accrues cannot even be imagined (with a mind!). That's why *pratyāhāra* is such an important breakthrough. However, even beyond that, the *yogīk* path is not one sequential progression. There are innumerable trials and errors, and the path to perfection at each stage is to be covered with millions of tiny steps. Similarly, synchronization of the physical body with the astral and then, of the two together with the causal, is an excruciatingly gradual process.

In *pratyāhāra*, a *yogī* learns to withdraw the outbound awareness and to interiorize it completely. Still, a total detachment from the objective world does not come easily or overnight. In the early stages, one practices concentration, meditation, and contemplation largely in relation to the objects in some form. Even *Īśvara* is held *in* contemplation, and the light of the soul is still an object.

But progressively, *dhāraṇā*, *dhyāna*, and *samādhī* are achieved in the subjective mode, increasingly devoid of relation with any objects or symbols, when compared with the first five means of yoga (Sūtra 5.1.17/III.7). This subjectivity draws you ever closer to *Īśvara*. The secondary *saṃyama* with the Universal Mind and the primary *saṃyama* with *Īśvara* are even more intimate encounters. To be able to sustain the force and the vitality of this intimate tête-à-tête with pure energy, a *mahāyogī*'s bodies stand totally overhauled through external and internal purification, ready for the experience of *saṃyama*.

Such is the depth of its "intimate" subjective effect that **even these three—*dhāraṇā*, *dhyāna*, and *samādhī*—are external to the true seedless *samādhī*** (Sūtra 5.1.18/III.8). With *Īśvara* known, no duality is needed now.

In the early stages of Yoga, during the process of turning inward, a *yogī* becomes aware of the knower, the field of knowledge, and the thinking process or the instrument of knowledge. In *pratyāhāra*, the thinking process is rested, and with an increasing awareness of *Īśvara* as the real knower, purer knowledge accrues. Eventually, with direct perception the whole objective world turns subjective, and knowledge is an instant awareness of *Īśvara* reflected in everything. Thus, all that is contained in the Universal Mind is instantly accessible and, now, awareness is pure consciousness.

But that is still duality. Sage Pātañjali considers *dhāraṇā*, *dhyāna*, and *samādhī* with seed as external because they are seeded with a motive. These three states, though quite advanced, are prompted by a motive of experiencing *Īśvara*. Now in *saṃyama*, there is neither motive nor desire. (In illumination, brain and self-mind do not interfere for a moment because they have identified with *Īśvara* completely). This is why *dhāraṇā*, *dhyāna*, and *samādhī* with seed are states that are reached by a *mahāyogī* in the inward subjective world with one's own efforts, while the final *saṃyama* is only by the grace of *Īśvara*.

Some interpreters try to oversimplify the *yogīk* path to make it appear like just another occupation in life. The process is admittedly one of unlearning, but it is a massive task when accumulation dates from far back in our infinite past. Besides, unlearning requires change that is so hard. Our ego has an iron-clad grip over us and it makes us believe that from here on life will just maintain a happy *status quo*. Ego's most adamant stance is to deny the inevitability of our own death in spite of its unfailing presence all around. To let ego melt away to facilitate surrender to *Īśvara* is a huge challenge.

The state of just "being One" (since even "union" implies two) is the ultimate objective of Yoga and the ultimate state to be reached. But for the same reason, it is almost impossible to express it in words, howsoever lucid. The sphere of Existence can only be imagined, because we are bound by it. But *saṃyama* takes the master-to-be beyond it to be able to understand the purpose and process of Existence, and *that* is beyond worldly expression. What lies beyond words?

Subtle Coded Patterns

A *mahāyogī* sees everything only as coded patterns variously manifesting the omnipresent core energy, just as different electrical appliances use the same electrical energy but manifest differently based on their configurations.

Though we can connect with the world only through words, and even thoughts appear in a verbalized form, a word is only a symbolic representation of the world of matter. Just like the meaningful text and graphics appearing on a computer screen have only bits and bytes at their core, the incoming sense impulses, too, are actually in certain coded patterns. They get associated with a series of similar patterns from the memory pools, and when the thoughts are formed they acquire their own codes. The shallow memory contains codes of present life, and the deep memory contains codes of many previous lives. The memory exists in subtle form and gets transferred from one life to the next.

Human memory contains residual traces of thought images that are diligently stored in the seed atoms in your causal body. A *mahāyogī* learns to read these digital images in order to know his or her own past and present as well as that of all others. Instant knowledge is gained of how the seeds were born through the actual experiences of past lives. **Thus, knowledge of previous incarnations becomes available when intense *dhāraṇā* or *dhyāna* on one's memory reveals the code and shows thought-images** (Sūtra 5.1.19/III.18).

Thoughts merely depicting mind games can be distinguished from those that bear an actual experience.Then, one can read a series of experiences unfolding the enactment of the *kārmik* seeding and the fruition that happened or is to happen—the interplay of causes and the effects. At this advanced stage of realization, you can choose to review these codified past events of a person or an object strictly for a valid purpose that in some way furthers your own or another's spiritual progress.

All thoughts have existence. Thoughts are not waves that rise and fade away in oblivion. Rather, thoughts exist and *create* waves in the subtle astral body. All thoughts are now seen as images that instantly reveal intent and idea from behind their emotional cloaks. Thoughts are not visible to the ordinary eyes, but a *mahāyogī* now acquires the ability to see them in the form of coded patterns. **Through concentrated meditation, the thought images in the minds of other people become apparent** (Sūtra 5.1.20/III.19).

Thoughts precede any action or coming into existence of anything on the material plane. In that sense they are the causes that set in motion certain manifestations. Through concentrated meditation, a *mahāyogī* is able to see the thoughts and know where they have come from, as well as what they would lead to.

There is, by necessity, some strict discipline connected with this ability. It is to be used only for gaining knowledge or furthering spiritual progress. It cannot be practiced for any other gain and can never be used to tamper with anybody's *kārmik* balance sheet. In this context, it is considerably different from the mind-reading or telepathy that usually occurs by a simple alignment of two minds, and which is most often a smart speculation or an expert extrapolation.

Here is a caveat: A *mahāyogī* sees thought patterns through intense meditation, but is not interested in the specific objects that cause the thoughts or those which will become effects thereof. For reading the code there is no need to run the full course of the thought process or engage with scenarios on the physical plane. That is not one's realm anymore. **Thus the object of those thoughts is not apparent and *mahāyogī* sees only the thought and not the object; meditation excludes the tangible.** (Sūtra 5.1.21/III.20).

Knowledge of the object is not required either. First, a *mahāyogī* is in a position to know what would unfold through the knowledge of cause and effect. The thoughts are known as coded patterns and not in a verbalized form. The eventual manifestation of the object in a particular form is caused and conditioned by the coding embedded in the thoughts. In this sense, a form is potentially present in thoughts in an "uncreated" state, and the moment the mind is taken away from the object, thought ends, thus ending the form.

Secondly, an engagement with the forms is only for the purpose of redemption of any *kārmik* legacy. If the will is directed to other objects for any other reason, that is only an indulgence. In this case, even a *mahāyogī* would be straying from the path (though a true *mahāyogī* would not).

Saṃyama *on self*

What can be done to other objects can also be done to your own self. **Through concentrated meditation upon the distinction between a form and a physical body, those properties of the body that make it visible to the human eye are negated, and a *mahāyogī* can become invisible to others** (Sūtra 5.1.22/III.21).

Unless a *mahāyogī* has advanced this far, such a feat is not possible, and unless the reader has understood the true process of "seeing," even its possibility cannot be fathomed. It is common knowledge that eyes are mere lenses and the act of "seeing" is actually image-processing (decoding) by the brain. Image-processing is a function of the astral body. The reason eyes do not see in total darkness is that eyes need to collaborate with some luminosity for the image to occur.

Visibility is relative. You are visible to another perceiving person. Ordinarily, perception yields *guṇa*-based form for visibility. A *mahāyogī* can elevate self-awareness at will into a pure *sāttvic* state by eliminating the *rajas* and *tamas* activities, thus making the physical form disappear in the physical eyes of others.

A concentrated meditation enables a *mahāyogī* to center the awareness in the astral body and will its complete withdrawal from the physical body. This results in a loss of luminosity, depriving the eyes of the beholder from forming any image. In other words, a *mahāyogī* chooses to remain located only in the coded patterns, and others do not know how to decode these. Obviously, it is dispersion of energy not visible to the untrained eye. The physical body can be unseen, yet continue to exist otherwise, since a *mahāyogī* can return awareness from the astral to the physical at will.

Technically, a body (a form) manifests the energy of consciousness. This manifestation brings into prominence the *sattva* (energy), *rajas* (forces), or *tamas* (matter). The eyes of the beholder are equipped to sense certain bandwidths of vibrations of the objects of matter. A *mahāyogī*, through a long practice of refining and purifying bodies, acquires the ability to make the physical body vibrate with *sattva* predominantly, which lends the luminosity. The vibrations can be raised even higher to render the astral body out of bandwidth for ordinary eyes to sense.

It is needless to add that this ability requires significantly responsible use. History contains abundant examples of individuals who reached this far but were felled by temptation, relegating *Īśvara* to a position of a mere observer and no more as a guide. This and other powers are products that occur because of the very nature of the relationship between Spirit and the mind-matter. But when power is what you seek, the future of your Yoga journey is held in abeyance.

Grooming the Master

Having explained the final phase of Yoga and how illumination occurs via *saṃyama*, Sage Pātañjali now prescribes specific exercises to create and sustain *prāṇa* energy of a very high grade in order to culminate the on-going process of mutation. The conditions required for mutation are now present, and various chemicals and elements are released in the body-brain system, causing quicker and more conscious biological evolution conducive to the most advanced Yoga practices. A *mahāyogī*'s three bodies undergo expedited mutation, which requires release of certain purified chemicals. In general, the process involves:

1. Empowered will is used to concentrate purified and potent mind energy on certain parts of the bodies where the chemical-producing glands are located so that mind's *prāṇa* energy is directed to them, and
2. *Prāṇa* is rotated in a certain manner like a scalpel to purify, activate and energize them. (Note*: Obviously, the*

instructions here are given by Sage Pātañjali in a cryptic and symbolic form. Any understanding of it at face value will be of no effect, and any intense practice can be done only by Īśvara's consent and under Its guidance.)

With the ability to perceive *prāṇa,* a *mahāyogī* earns eligibility to control it. *Prāṇa* is energy. Controlling it and using it during further Yoga practice (*sādhanā)* mandates able guidance, a strict watch and help when needed. These exercises are much more advanced than those seen so far as they prepare a *mahāyogī* to sustain pure energy of the fourth state. It involves a particular technique of rotation, linking, and circulation of *prāṇa* within the bodies. With an abundant sense of responsibility this author has thought it expedient not to deal with it in this book beyond an informative broad-brush narrative, sincerely hoping that the reader will kindly understand why. The reader is also assured of a spiritual truth that "when you are ready, the help arrives," which guarantees an access to such advanced exercises when your time comes.

Siddhī, the Spiritual Powers

At one time, you used to distinguish between the personal self and the world, and that resulted in the experience of the pairs of opposites, a confusion that is clarified by *saṃyama* on *Īśvara* (Sūtra 5.2.5/III.36). All along, the pairs of opposites have caused the brain's tumultuous thinking and created mind fluctuations. Ironically, it is the human perception and thinking process that makes "one" to look like "many." Until the connectivity among all objects, living or seemingly inert, is recognized, our thoughts push them apart as "distinct" objects. This duality and relativity is further compounded by human memory that stores all experiences with reference to the time and space contexts.

The sum total of all these errors is *avidyā* and the common result is any number of pairs of opposites. Essentially the opposites are the same, but there is a difference of degrees. This self-imposed wrong view of the world makes the thoughts swing between two opposites, creating a defective reality, and in turn generating ten-

About Advanced Exercises

A brief overview of these advanced exercises is provided in Appendix 5. Since this training has to be earned at the feet of Īśvara, Who would make the details available to the eligible ones in Its own way. These exercises are highly advanced and are aimed at a complete alignment of the hidden energy within the physical body, the energy centers in the astral body, and the enlightened soul. No powers are sought, but a **mahāyogī** *is advancing now to attain a perfect equilibrium of* **guṇa**—*the ultimate frontier. It may be reiterated that progress is going to be as gradual as ever, and the real ability at each stage is painstakingly earned in order to build the next one. Any shortcuts will only result in a practice based merely on visualizations and imagined abilities; not the real ones. It is also imperative that the bodies are sufficiently purified through the continuous rhythmic breathing, the corrective exercises, the upgrading of awareness, and a sincere practice of the means of Yoga. With this, a* **mahāyogī's** *life undergoes a complete transformation, and* **yama, niyama, āsana,** *and* **prāṇayāma** *no longer remain just the behavioral scaffoldings but become an integral part of the very way of life. Exercising* **prāṇa** *is regulating energy itself, and the channels must be strong enough to withstand the force. Having achieved this, you need a nod from Īśvara to proceed with the practice of* **saṃyama**.

sion and instability. That is the fundamental deception promoted by the "I"-consciousness, the false perceiver.

Saṃyama reveals to you that *Īśvara* has been the only witness, even ever since as a *yogī* you were struggling through the early phases of realization. Thus, reflex judgmental thinking towards the opposites is now discernible, and the shrewd deception of "I" is realized as the awareness of *Īśvara* grows.

But there is still some confusion. *Sattva guṇa*, *Purūṣa*, the soul, and Universal Mind still continue to exist separately in a *mahāyogī*'s perception. Only a focused meditation on *Īśvara* can resolve this confusion. Unhindered meditation is made possible by the completion of the pathway of *prāṇa* rotation (as explained in Appendix 4) because the entire circuit is contained within, the incoming impulses are easily blocked away from entering during such practices. As *ajna*, the gateway of outbound thoughts is also sealed; the pathway is now a closed circuit and *prāṇa* circulates freely without interruption.

Earlier, hindered by the pairs of opposites and negated by the self-proclaimed sovereignty of the conscious brain and the individual mind, *Īśvara* was silent and only a witness. This illegitimate sovereignty dissolves gradually and the opposites appear as one. From a mere witness, *Īśvara* is experienced as the "lord of the mind," and the physical brain does not *create* knowledge any more, but rather *receives* it. Yet the final threshold is still ahead. *Īśvara* is about to assume Its true status as the Spirit.

The dissolution of the pairs of opposites puts you face to face with the absolute truth with no opposites and signifies the end of the road, where all duality ends. In learning to be one with *Īśvara*, a master learns how to anchor consciousness in *bindu* even during wakeful hours and even while fulfilling worldly obligations. The individual mind is now permanently reduced to "no-mind." It becomes an effortless grace of just "being."

Senses Are More Profound

As a result of the experience from the meditative state, more profound hearing, touch, sight, taste, and smell are developed that produce intuitive knowledge (Sūtra 5.2.6/III.37). Perception is a function of sense-impulses and their processing. The sense organs such as the eyes and ears are the physical end of this chain. They are also its grossest link. Hence, normally, any perception is not complete unless the grossest transmits the sense impulses to the subtler counterparts on the astral plane to create "cognition" of the senses in *mānas*.

A *mahāyogī* needs to sense the interior body now as opposed to sensing the outside objects. To be able to do the *prāṇa* rotation exercises the back-end processing centers of the senses are to be directly activated on the astral plane by *mānas*. *Chakras* are in the astral body, and in order to concentrate on them, a *mahayogi* needs to sense them first. Earlier, the subtle senses used to merely back up the physical senses. Now able to function on their own, these subtle senses operate without the physical precedent, and that creates a vital difference. On the astral plane, sensing is a thousand times sharper and extends over unimaginable physical distances.

The depth, nature, and potency of "sensing" change radically. In its subtle-gross lineage, sensing is a need that arises on the causal plane, gets articulated as senses on the astral and becomes sense impulses on the physical. When senses operate free from the impulses they become powerful.

> *This results in siddhī, the spiritual powers. A sense of hearing blossoms into clairaudience and progressively into instant comprehension; touch turns into a process of healing; sight transforms into clairvoyance and progressively into a divine vision; taste metamorphoses into imagination and discriminative knowledge; and smell, the ātmik sense, becomes all knowledge itself.* (Author's synthesis; for detailed discussion see Alice Bailey, 322-325).

The development of the sensing ability on the astral plane enables a *mahāyogī* to carry out the higher practices on the astral plane even while fulfilling the worldly obligations on the physical, by separating the two.

And the Caveat

Sage Pātañjali warns us that **though this serves as magical powers in the objective world, it is an obstacle to the highest spiritual realization.** This is a clear caveat (Sūtra 5.2.7/III.38).

Any power is a product of the earlier practices, designed to be a handy tool for the next. However, the powers can become obstacles when a *mahāyogī* forgets to control them and instead lets them control. The powers relate to the path already traveled and left behind. Any indulgence in them locks you into what you are trying to get ahead of.

It is a natural desire for any aspirant to assess where they have reached on the *yogīk* path. The flashes of spiritual vision, fluency of thoughts, hypnotic power of comprehension and expression, out-of-body experiences, improved health and vigor, ability to read thoughts, to make oneself invisible, and many other fruits on the way, make you aspire for more. And at that point some *yogīs* think they have "arrived," with so many psychic powers at their command. When this conceit is overwhelming, a desire for *saṃyama* takes a back seat, drawing them into a new whirlpool of seed generation, and thus spiritual progress is stalled.

Some regard such stalling as a punishment. But *Īśvara* is not tainted with any such human weakness. By indulging in the power play, an exceptional *mahāyogī* strays from the main course and loses sight of the ultimate goal. *Īśvara*, as always, keeps lovingly waiting. The rest continue with their intricate training.

Synchronization and Transference

The entire science of Rāja Yoga (as in *Yoga-Sūtra*) is based upon an understanding of the nature, purpose, and the function of mind. The basic law of this science can be summed up in the words "energy follows thought," and the sequence of activity can be stated as follows:

> *The thinker on his own plane formulates a thought embodying some purpose or some desire. The mind vibrates in response to this idea and simultaneously produces a corresponding reaction in the kārmik, desire, or emotional body. The energy body or the etheric sheath vibrates with synchronicity and thereby the brain responds and energizes the nervous system throughout the dense physical body so that the impulse of the thinker works out into physical plane activity.*—Alice Bailey, 327.

Progressive liberation from the causes of bondage is the principal theme of Yoga. Earlier, a *mahāyogī* was liberated from the bondage of emotion-soaked memory by exiling and freezing it. Now one needs to avoid the bondage of the psychic powers. **By liberation from the causes of this bondage as well as through the weakening of the causes themselves, *mahāyogī* would learn the mode of transference** (transfer, enter and synchronize) **with**

another body using the skill of withdrawal and entrance (Sūtra 5.2.8/III.39)

The thinking instruments (brain, *mānas* and *buddhi*), the mind, and the nervous system (two-way carrier of senses and instructions), all work together on all the three planes. A *mahāyogī* has reached a stage where there is control over mind. It is also understood that *all experiencing is a transference of vibrations, from the gross to the subtle.* A *mahāyogī* evolves biologically through the Yoga practices when new channels or passages are opened up in the brain to allow bypassing of memory and curtailing mind's unnecessary thinking. The physical brain works in total harmony with *mānas* and *buddhi*. Now the nervous system is calibrated to carry gross-to-very-subtle vibrations back and forth without any distortions.

This total control allows synchronization of your own vibrations with another person's, to make them resonate as if a *mahāyogī* has entered their body-brain system. This is the mode of transference called "synchronization and entering." However, this trespassing occurs when the power is used only for healing and helping, and without transgressing or interfering in the framework of the *kārmik* law of cause and effect.

When the bondage from *yogīk* powers is sufficiently weakened, *Īśvara* commences the education in "*saṃyama* without seed" also through the mode of "synchronization and entering." But how would you sustain those high frequency vibrations?

Sound: Spiritual Hearing

We have noted earlier that there are four grades of sound, or vibrations. In the physical world, we remain in the *vaikharī* band/range of vibrations. It extends from the spoken word to all other sounds that we can hear and decipher. Yoga practices and exercises tune in one's senses to hear and sustain *madhyamā* (astral) and later, *pashyantī* (causal) bands/ranges of vibrations. *Para-nāda* (which does not belong to Existence) is the highest range of vibrations that can potentially disintegrate the three worlds, and hence a *mahāyogī* is trained in *para-nāda* only by *Īśvara*. Sensing of higher vibrations enables understanding of the astral and the causal worlds.

A continuous change in each organism is a result of vibrations. These vibrations exist in the universe and in all the forms. With the ability to sense them and decipher them, a *mahāyogī* can pierce the sound of a veiled word and understand the essence of any form. This gives an insight into the energy fields operating within all physical entities.

A baby is born into life with its first breath, which is immediately followed by the sound . . . of a cry. What is true about the birth in the microcosm may also be true about the universe, the macrocosm. Breath, the cause of life and the initiator of the vibrations comes first and is followed by the "word" of *Īśvara*, "AUM," which is the sum total of all sounds. Spiritual hearing is the ability to hear the entire range, from the mundane words to this primordial sound.

In perception, images of objects trigger words that are essentially sound. Words (implicit or explicit) make you aware of the forms that keep all of us glued to the physical plane. While turning inward, there is an increasing awareness of the images rather than the objects they symbolize. You realize that the words are a symbolic representation of the objects. The words get tagged onto the images, and that draws you closer to the meanings, concepts, and ideas.

This is when your vocabulary starts optimizing as you become aware of more powerful words to express the ideas effectively. Our vocabulary is not as clean and to the point as are definitions and explanations in the dictionary. Our words are enmeshed in past associations and their emotional cobwebs. With the cleansing of memory comes freedom from the strings and more clarity. You access these words intuitively.

On the spiritual path now you are less verbose and more silent. The vast meaning embedded in the words of wisdom is unfolding before you. The mesmerizing brevity of truly great people is no longer a mystery. The potent power of *mantrās* and the scriptures is now realized. This is how you, a master-to-be, understand the real phonetics and acquire the ability to hear spiritually.

Thus, by means of one-pointed meditation upon the relationship between *ākāśa* and sound, ability for spiritual hearing is developed (Sūtra 5.2.11/III.42). *Ākāśa* is like a nucleus that everything is born out of, with vibrating energy causing the medium (*ākāśa)* to vibrate. Vibrations travel as longitudinal waves and sound is its first manifestation. The wavelength of each vibration has a finite curve of ascent, climax, and descent that represents a lifespan. A map of the vibrations then unfolds in the phases of birth, growth, and death. The more subtle a substance, the higher are its vibrations. *Īśvara* is the subtlest entity with the highest vibrations.

All the Yoga practices are for synchronization and establishing various communication links:

- between the primary and the secondary bodies
- between brain and individual mind as catalyst
- between brain—*mānas*—*buddhi* and Universal Mind, and
- with *Īśvara.*

Purer energy vibrates at a very high frequency. Higher and higher communication requires the ability to vibrate and sustain at that frequency. Such knowledge is best imparted by word of mouth from a teacher, because higher frequencies can damage any ill-prepared body instruments.

Traveling in Space

Whether dense and ordinary, or subtle and extremely refined, the core of the three worlds is matter. It is only when the matter is in an uncreated state that one crosses the domain of matter. A master-to-be has now qualified for **one-pointed meditation upon the relationship between *ākāśa* and the physical body, for ascension out of all the three worlds of matter and power to travel in space** (Sūtra 5.2.12/III.43).

A physical body is in an uncreated potential form in its astral state, and the astral body is in an uncreated potential form in its causal state. So now there needs to be the ability as well as consent to go beyond the causal state. Through long and arduous efforts, ability is acquired to sustain the exceedingly high vibrations. Attunement to the no-mind state is also complete, so that even when not dwelling in any of the bodies, you can still remain alive and the bodies intact.

To manifest on a certain plane like physical, astral, or causal, a body has to vibrate within that specific band of frequencies. Though there is one single continuum from gross to subtle, these distinct bands exist due to certain critical rates of vibrations at various stages of *yogīk* development and the keys to these "ring-pass-nots" are granted by the guru to a qualified student.

These "rings-pass-not" are obviously not actual rings of matter, but represent the dynamic boundaries resulting from one's perceived limits of self-awareness and abilities. They refer to tangible and intangible, albeit temporarily impassible barriers raised by past *karma* coupled with the state of the will. They act as limits in physical, astral and intellectual spheres beyond which an individual is unable to pass until he/she evokes spiritual strength and the vision to get over those circumscribing limits. These boundaries keep fading with growing awareness and finally dissolve when the bodies are completely harmonized.

Now a *mahāyogī* has arrived at the most critical juncture. Even the causal body has to be transcended, and thus the universe of Existence is to be left behind, which is a complete roll-back amounting to a body-less state. Though the ultimate oneness with *Īśvara* is still far away, before doing this dematerializing and re-materializing of the three bodies, you are ready for two tough tests:

- whether one can do this incredible feat given the hard work, and
- whether the transcendental state will not be too alluring to make you unwilling to return to the bodily existence again.

But as you are firmly on *Īśvara*'s watch, you are under the only guidance that will take you there. Initially, there is no need to leave the bodies during practices in order to have the out-of-body experience.

Ex-corporeal Experience

The state of illumination does not arrive from outside. "Illuminated" is the essential state of any being; the opaque gross bodies only veil it. Impure bodies not only veil the illumination but create an illusion that they are real. The thinking instrument and the mind modifications are the main culprits. **Now when that which**

veils the light is done away with, a state of illumination shines through and with that one gains ability to disembody, to be "discarnate" (Sūtra 5.2.13/III.44).

"Traveling in space" is an out-of-body experience without leaving the bodies, and is called an "ex-corporeal" state. However, when the physical and astral bodies are left behind and you remain only in the causal body, it is called an "actual ex-corporeal." Eventually, a master has to prepare to destroy all the coverings of the light, when even the causal body is also left behind in order to meet with *Īśvara.*

Anytime on the *yogīk* path, and especially at this stage, each *siddhi* (power) has a definite purpose. All the successes in raising awareness, purifying the bodies and subtle sensing culminates in an out-of body experience. Soon it becomes a conscious, willed act.

This is a discarnate or disembodied state in the truest sense of the word. This state is absolutely free from all modifications, not only of the thinking instrument but from all the changing, fluctuating subtle bodies, as all of them stand transmuted through the inner evolution. This is truly total freedom, and nothing hides the light when one is outside all the bodies in transcendence.

"One is outside all the bodies" is to be understood as one's "awareness is standing aside" of all the bodies. Legitimate questions could be, "What happens to the bodies?" and "Do they decay?" It should not be forgotten that the subtle controls the gross. The transcendental awareness is powerful enough to hold the states of the grosser bodies in full rein.

A Master Arrives

The spiritual powers culminate the grooming of a master with the ability to control and sculpt the subtle in preparation to enter a state of pure consciousness.

Mastery over Elements

As a *yogī*, you could perceive any object in its form, its associated word, and the idea. Now as a master who knows the subtleties of air and sound, **with focused meditation you can dissect the object into the five essential elements—earth, water, fire, air, and *Ākāśa*. These elements are seen variously taking five dimensions: denseness, appearance, all-pervasiveness, subtleness, and functionality** (Sūtra 5.2.14/III.45).

A recall from Chapter Zero will help.

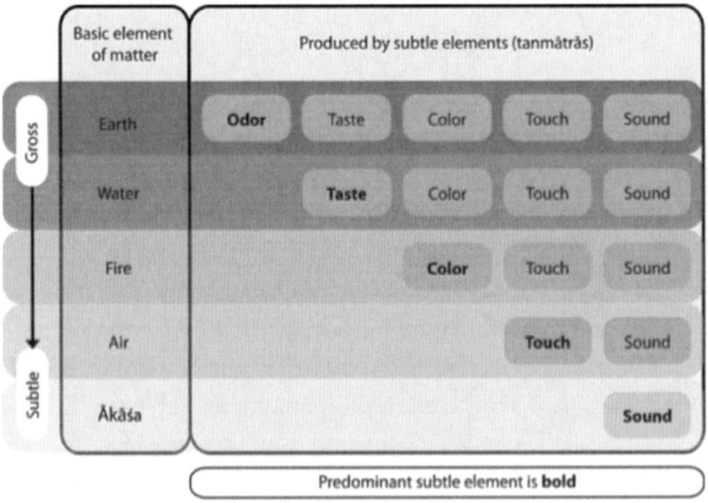

Figure 5.1: The elements and subtlety

The dynamism of the elements provides *denseness* to an object. Myriad permutations and combinations of the elements provide an object with a distinct *appearance* of its own. One or more of the five elements must be inherent in every object, and in that sense, the elements are *all-pervading*, because no object is an exception and there is no sixth element. The *subtleness* is perceptible when one or more elements are missing in an object, because the missing element(s) fail to generate the corresponding sense when perceived. Subtler objects have more elements missing, hence, *ākāśa* is the subtlest with just one element.

The gross-to-subtle evolution that cascades from the subtlest *ākāśa* to the grossest earth is neither accidental nor random. It has as its driver an underlying cause-and-effect relationship. Hence, in any object there is no absurd or irrelevant combination of the elements, because each is guided by some *functionality* or purpose that precedes its coming into existence.

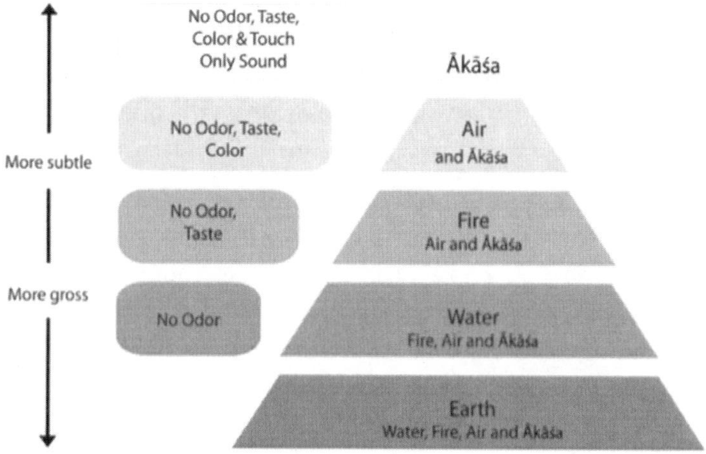

Figure 5.2: Sensing and subtlety

When these dynamic aspects become known, a master acquires a vision of the universe as never before. The minutest, the largest and everything in between are seen as myriad permutations of the five basic elements. Objects with all five of them, with earth as the most prominent element, are the most inert and at the grossest level at the foot of a pyramid that rises with more and more subtle objects that have one or more of the elements missing. The more subtle their form, the more rarified and unified they are, and the most subtle objects constitute only *ākāśa* at the peak of that pyramid. Parts of it have been seen earlier, but now a master can see a virtual elemental universe in all its simultaneous dimensions that extend from the most diverse bottom of the pyramid to its unified top, thus becoming all-knowing, like the Buddha.[43]

[43] *Yoga Master SN Tavaria has documented that the physical, astral, and causal planes, each has seven sub-stages with distinct purpose and state. The involution of humankind (causal → astral → physical) descends to its lowest point, the end of the seventh sub-stage of the physical plane. The present humanity, after hitting the bottom, is on an upward arc, the evolution (physical → astral → causal), and has just emerged from the fifth sub-stage into the fourth. One of the characteristics of this sub-stage is that each sincere seeker can reclaim the astral body and can choose to make it the primary body.*

It is important for the astral body and the associated deeper vision to gain recognition in the applied sciences. Science has reached its limits of enquiry on the physical plane. Deeper insights are needed into the mystery of the earth, the depth of the sea (water), the metabolic processes (fire), the eco-systems (air), and the inner and outer space (*ākāśa*). Simply being faster is not enough for a scientific probe; its reach has to be on a radically new scale in order to acquire the unprecedented speed afforded on the astral plane.

An important gift of *yogīk* practice is awareness that the macrocosm and its microcosm are alike in composition and are diverse only in perception. Each gross object comprises one or more of the five elements; and the five states in which each element vibrates (from gross to subtle) create those many virtual planes, rising from the physical to the causal. The higher planes are always at work and indirectly manifest in the physical domain; if they are not "seen," it does not mean they don't exist. (These may be the proverbial "curled up dimensions" lost in the initial few seconds after the Big Bang. If science probes reality and truth, these can never be fully reached without knowing the higher planes.)

After the "speed of light," the next threshold is the "speed of mind." We should stop trivializing the mind-stuff as imagination and fantasy, we can properly understand mind as a form of matter, or rather a source of matter. Mind-speed would bestow upon humankind a generous tool and a speed of enquiry that is unthinkable today. Only this would unfold to science the reality of Planet Earth, stars, galaxies, and the universes, and would facilitate unprecedented knowledge of humanity itself. In the no-mind state, *Yoga-Sūtra* shows that the last threshold would be the "speed without mind," where, true to all other apparent contradictions, you would realize that in order to know anything you do not have to travel at all. The ultimate speed is instantaneous.

An even more significant gift of *Yoga-Sūtra* is an awareness of "awareness" itself. An enquiring person is no exception to the object or phenomenon under enquiry. The tools of enquiry are matter; the process of enquiry alters the matter and the outcome of the enquiry, new awareness, provides a subtle handle over the new matter. An enquirer/observer also exists on all the gross and subtle planes. It is only by upgrading the awareness that one can learn to vibrate at higher frequencies and perceive the higher planes. *Yoga-Sūtra* shows the way.

Eightfold Powers

Everything has a purpose, and a master's journey so far has one too. Total elimination of the obstacles and hindrances empowers you to do in the physical, astral, and causal worlds what you want. Whatever is wished, happens. But ironically, by then the master has hardly any desire or wish left. Naturally, what is wished, if anything at all, is all for the common good or for helping and healing others—nothing that can generate any *kārmik* seeds. Toward this end, these powers are granted.

Through the mastery over the elements these eightfold powers are attained (Sūtra 5.2.15/III.46):

1. It is possible to be one with the minutest . . .
2. . . . or with the greatest; **scale does not limit**.
3. One can attract anything to oneself . . .
4. . . . or disperse it away at will; **gravity holds no bar**.
5. One can reach anywhere and make any element to obey a wish; no constraint whatsoever for one's will to come to fruition.
6. It is possible to create "effective causes" from any subtle element and manifest them in any form on the physical plane; **total mastery over the elements**.
7. To enable an uninterrupted work with the above powers, **bodily perfection** is also gained. It becomes easy to modulate and use any one of the bodies as a perfect vehicle for the intended work.
8. Though one continues to work with the forms, they cannot affect anything anymore because you are **free from an engagement with guṇa**.

Mastery over Senses

Mastery over the senses, (*tanmātrās*) is brought about through concentrated meditation upon their nature, peculiar attributes, egoism, pervasiveness and the useful purpose (Sūtra 5.2.16/ III.48). Sensing comprises the external/front-end sense organs and *tanmātrā*, the subtle back-end counterparts that enable sensing. A master understands the fine distinction between a sense organ and the sense itself, by deciphering how and why each sense organ is designed to cater to a particular type of sensing. The peculiar attributes of the senses are understood by the way they work and with aspect of the macrocosm they interact. Knowledge of soul as distinct from the self allows a master to understand how the sense data creates an "I"-sense when it collaborates with the self-mind, and how egoism continues to reinforce itself through sensing.

In the process of knowing this, it is also realized how the senses work in all other objects. You understand how the senses can be teleported or projected over great distances, and how the nature of sensing can dramatically change from gross to subtle, with ability to control the elements. Above all, your focus is no more only on the sense organs, which could mistakenly have lead you to conclude that sensing happens by itself; rather, you understand how the purpose of sensing is experiencing. By realizing the purpose and being able to consciously watch the *tanmātrā*s, you gain mastery over the senses. You also get connected to the unifying principle that pervades all sensing throughout the universe. The object-level (gross) and the subjective (subtle) mastery together enable a great ability to heal and help.

A mastery over the senses is ably explained thus:

> *Saṃyama directed at the perceptual process itself means interiorizing to the point at which the subtle aspect of sensing, the tanmātrās, become visible in consciousness. To grasp this conceptually, consider the chain of perception that occurs as we hear a sound. The object, an audible vibration in the air, reaches an organ of perception (the ear) that transduces the vibration into another medium, the sense of hearing; this surfaces as an impression*

in consciousness, where it is stratified and brought into coherence with all the other sense inputs by the sensory mind in concert with the other components of consciousness—intelligence and the ego. As the sensory mind collates these inputs, conditioned reactions arise in intelligence and ego that welcome certain input, filter others, and produce the organized causal representation we experience as sound. As intelligence and ego color the sensory projection, the subtle internal sense (tanmātrā) evokes the hearing experience, or soundness, of the phenomenon. Tanmātrās are always present in the perceptual chain but ordinarily cannot be contemplated in isolation, since they fuse with the other cognitive aspects of perception. Only in the transparency of Saṃyama can the causal overlay be seen through and the subtle essence of hearing be observed. The tanmātrā of hearing is now "free from the constraints of its organ"—that is, the other, bodily links in the auditory sequence.—Chip Hartranft, 57.

Mind-Speed

Please have a second look at Sūtras III.44, 45, 47 and 48 together, for a concerted meaning. They mention a culmination of all that has been done progressively during the seeker-to-master evolution. **As a result of this perfection there comes a rapidity of action like that of the mind, perception independent of the organs and mastery over the root substance** (Sūtra 5.2.17/III.49).

What is the net effect of acquiring eightfold powers (*siddhī*), perfection of bodies, and mastery over the sense organs, senses, and the root substance? The net effect is rapidity of action at the speed of mind, which is almost instantaneous; even the speed of light is much slower! What is happening "now" is known along with what will trigger it in the future anywhere in the universe.

Because *dhāraṇā, dhyāna* and *samādhī* are not piecemeal stages anymore, they form one integrated action. Perception is always independent of all senses or sense organs, and now it is perfected into a meditative attitude.

> *With him the intuition has been developed into [a] usable instrument, and direct apprehension of all knowledge, independently of the reasoning faculty or rationalizing mind, is his privilege and right. The mind no longer [will] be used to apprehend reality, the senses need no longer be employed as mediums of contact.*—Alice Bailey, 353-354.

A master reaches a climax of sorts with the ability to reverse the sensory process. After reining in the outbound senses, now, with them under full control and consciousness firmly anchored in *Īśvara*, the mind and the senses are used to transmit inner knowledge outward. Matter and all the forms are rendered helpless in front of a master, because energy can be projected through the mind and the senses. Any manifestation can simply be willed without being affected by *guṇa*.

Uncommonly Common

It is noteworthy that *Yoga-Sūtra* does not distinguish anything as good or bad in terms of a value judgment. What is explained here is only the cause-and-effect relationship, and we are shown what leads to the ultimate goal and what doesn't. Thus, even a master is warned that he/ she is not beyond law, since the psychic powers have "seeds of bondage." **It is only by growing passionless towards the spiritual achievements evidenced in the powers that a Master can remain free from the seeds of that bondage and attain the condition of isolated unity** (Sūtra 5.2.18/III.51).

A shift from self-awareness to Self-consciousness has to be made permanent, and that is the last barrier to cross. With consciousness anchored in the spiritual Self, the only purpose of existence in the material world is to carry out *Īśvara*'s directions. Even *sattva*, the now-predominant *guṇa*, with all its luminosity and perfect rhythm and balance, needs to be distinguished from pure awareness and to be left behind. The isolation has to be total from anything that belongs to the material domain.

Seen superficially, this may present a wrong idea that a master in this state becomes unfit for normal human life. First, the definition of "normal" needs a review, because it is so relative. Secondly, such a person is overwhelmingly ordinary and completely free of any deceit, desire, or design. Isolated from the material aspects of life, a master is the most fitting person to be around, as everyone else stands only to gain either knowledge or a healing touch. A true master is passionless about everything, even the achievements. The "miraculous" powers shine more in deference than in their use.

How isolated does a master have to be? There should be total rejection of all allurements from all forms of being, even the celestial, because the recurrence of *guṇa* remains possible. It is easy and probable to get lured into spiritual happiness and to refuse to return to the material life for the residual *kārmik* redemption.

It is admittedly tough. There are so many on the *yogīk* path whose journey has stalled thanks to a false air of having arrived. It takes tremendous patience and perseverance to stay put and to accept nothing except the blessings of *Īśvara* alone. Especially in the early stage of flashing visions, and later with the arrival of *yogīk* powers, many aspirants develop a sense of complacency. They are overwhelmed with their own uncommon achievements. Their spiritual façade not only fools others but becomes self-hypnotizing. The institutionalized religions provide an alluring tableau of spiritual decorations and a hierarchy of powerful offices that imprison the spiritual masters just short of their real destination.

Hence, Sage Pātañjali warns again and again that **there should be an entire rejection of all allurements from all forms of being, even the celestial, for a possibility always remains of recurrence of seed-causing contacts** (Sūtra 5.2.19/III.52). A master has to realize that even the celestial beings, which were revered and followed in the early days, are forms and need to be left behind. In fact, anything and everything that has been achieved on the *yogīk* path is to be disowned now in order for you to become uncommonly common. At the doorstep of the total isolated unity, one is walking a very thin line. Even a scent of pride in such a magnificent experience with *Īśvara* can create waves that can rock the boat and germinate *karma* seeds. A caution is needed so as not to vibrate with any vibration that is even a wee bit lower than the most exalted state of being.

Walking such a thin line is the ultimate test. *Īśvara* challenges the candidates before finally accepting the accomplished disciple in one great spiritual embrace. The really great masters do not fall. They remain true custodians of the *yogīk* powers and not the owners. The isolated unity with *Īśvara*, then, is just a state of being; waiting to happen.

Intuitive Knowledge

Intuitive knowledge is developed through the use of the discerning faculty when there is focused concentration that pierces through even the moments and their continuous succession (Sūtra 5.2.20/III.53).

This beautiful sūtra is enormously deep in its meaning. Time is an entity that belongs to Existence and is a product of mind. But "time" is also a created label for something that is perceived but does not really exist. (Just as the boundary of our physical vision results into a "horizon," or a limit of our perceptive ability gives us a "sky," yet none exists). Time is experienced linearly. Time is the moment-to-moment arising and passing of modifications that make us conscious of events, distances, and interactions; thus, we are made "aware" of time. When modifications cease and awareness is held in itself, the linearity ends. Only in an isolated unity does this possibility arise, where the focused concentration is from moment to moment, and its continuous succession can be held virtually still.

The mastery over the root substance is now complete because even the non-subsisting factor, like "time," stands dematerialized. A master has known that an atom or a particle exists as such only when it is so perceived. Now, another seemingly paradoxical achievement is possible: By *saṃyama* on the notion of time, comes knowledge of—something so vital, which has no real existence—the Nothingness!

By definition, time and space create relative duality;[44] where there is no duality, where there are no pairs of opposites, where there are

[44] *In 1905 Einstein noticed that space and time are a pair of opposites, so that the time interval between two events must be subtracted from the space interval to get the total space-time separation that stands at zero if the space and time intervals between the two events are equal.*

no modifications because there is no mind, no senses, and no objects—there can be no time. A master witnesses the universe not simply as a multi-dimensional image but also as a still holograph of frozen motions, an eternal "now."

From such intuitive knowledge is born the capacity to distinguish between all beings and to cognize their genus, qualities, and position on the evolutionary ladder (Sūtra 5.2.21/III.54). But the way the spiritually-enhanced discerning faculty works is diagonally opposite to that of ordinary discrimination. In the objective domain, the forms differ in their appearance. Even forms within the same species or classes differ individually. Thus, one understands the surrounding objects-filled world only by fragmenting and separating.

Spiritual insight makes one aware of the subtle and the generic aspects behind the forms. A perception of differentiated forms gets replaced by an understanding of their unifying genres. Awareness grows about the distinction between the generic and the phenomenal. You also understand why, in spite of inheriting the common qualities of a genre, the varying degree of imbalance between the *guṇa* (qualities) makes the individual manifestation so different. A classic example is us, the billions of human beings, who come across individually so different. The imbalance in *guṇa* is a result of the object's particular position on its evolutionary ladder.

Thus, a master becomes aware of the unifying subjective sources of the disparate objects and in turn becomes aware of the discrimination between the subjective and the objective. Ultimately, there is an experiential understanding (not just intellectual) that the Spirit, beyond elements, is the only "simple" and "basic" cause from which the five elements (*ākāśa,* air, fire, water, and earth*)* emerge; everything else is a manifested compound of two or more of these elements. Only this enables discerning between the bodies and the soul.

To such an accomplished master, everything about anyone on any of the sub-stages of the three worlds of Existence, whether on the involutionary or evolutionary arc, is now accessible.

Essence of Consciousness

It has been a long expedition! At the beginning, you were entrenched in the midst of hundreds of distinct objects, completely unaware of the very entrenchment. As a *seeker*, you began to recognize the mistake of engaging with the appearances instead of the objects themselves, and how tentative the engagement was. In the long process of becoming a *disciple*, you started learning about the mind and its tricks—which sum up into an autocratic ego that creates and thrives on the appearances. Then the awareness started rising to the subtle levels, and you went through an arduous journey of a *yogī* in sorting out the forms as distinct from the thought-embroiled words as well as from the essential idea embodied in the object. You became a *mahāyogī* after what appeared to be an endless journey to be able to recognize life pulsating at the core of all the objects, living or seemingly inert. Unaware, you had developed kinship with the near and dear objects. But, behind all their exciting divergence, to realize that there was one single consciousness, was indeed a long journey. Now, the pivotal question confronting you, a *master,* is how that *one* becomes *many* and why.

Real Discernment

It is time now to see *Īśvara*, the soul (the divine fragment), as distinct from everything else, a real discernment. In doing so, a master grasps the fact that everything else is a product of mind but *Īśvara* is not. Mind belongs to Existence.

This realization leads to an important distinction. When we look at fellow human beings and consider that each one has a soul, the divine fragment, we make a fundamental mistake of thinking of many souls. The divine fragment does not constitute multiplicity. The divine fragment is a part of the infinite but remains as wholesome and infinite as its origin. On the other hand, in the manufacture of human bodies, the Universal Mind collaborates with the elements of matter and becomes many localized individual minds as it takes the form, color, and shape based on the individual structure of predispositions. A form or an appearance is needed to participate in Existence. The individual mind promotes a separateness of "I" and infuses a sense of artificial distinction between "I" and everything else.

As long as *karma* seeds create and sustain your structure of predispositions, the world remains full of "many." It is a state of ignorance, *avidyā*. Only when awareness finally anchors in the subtle consciousness is the whole world seen as **one life, one state of illumination, one consciousness that produces the varied forms of the many** (Sūtra 5.2.22/IV-5). A master understands how one creates many, but many reflect one; how microcosm, the atom, reveals the nature of the macrocosm, the universe. It becomes known how *Īśvara*, the soul, created the causal, astral, and the physical bodies so that by experiencing the many and the varied, a "self"-realization process would roll you into seeker-disciple-*yogī*-*mahāyogī*-master back into the one consciousness, that is, *Īśvara*.

Consciousness Is One, Many Is the Perception

Why many forms? It is a closed loop from a desire to the forms. First, there is a causal desire that stirs up a medium of expression in the astral body. The expression is outbound and initiates a process of perception. Sense perception reaches out to an object and excites *guṇa* that generate forms. Thus, a desire ushers in a law of cause and effect; a form is the effect. A desire reaches out to meet the form and anchors the awareness there. As the forms are seen and experienced, attachment results and awareness stays confined. The forms are liked or disliked, owned or disowned, depending on your structure of predispositions, which is a function of *guṇa* resident in the perceiver's own self. Those likes and dislikes create actions and reactions across physical, astral, and causal domains, leading to *karma*. Over eternity, the resultant *karma* necessitates resolution and closure, and the "concept" of one life leads to the conception of a variety of "organs" in the bodies to carry that concept out. The cycles replicate and multiply, resulting in innumerable forms. *Karma* always perpetuates forms for its fulfillment.

However, not even latent *karma* is generated when the three *guṇa* in a master's own self are in absolute equilibrium and balance each other out, and are thus incapable of generating any form in any object. **Among the forms which consciousness assumes, only that which is the result of meditation is free from latent *karma*** (Sūtra 5.2.23/IV.6). When totally absorbed in consciousness, the outgoing awareness is pure, with no adulterous desire to bind the self-mind to the thinking instruments, thus preventing any mind modifications induced by *guṇa* and inciting action/reaction. *Karma* is such an inevitable presence that an attitude of concentrated meditation alone makes you free of *karma*.

> *He dwells on the plane of mind, persists in meditation, creates by an act of will and not through the helplessness of desire, and is a "free soul," a master and a liberated one.*—Alice Bailey, 389.

Now, Sage Pātañjali approaches another tricky question. If each individual has as consciousness the same infinite divine fragment from which everything else is derived, how come the forms are so varied?

Those two, consciousness (*Īśvara*) and the form, are distinct and separate; though the forms may be similar, the consciousness (diminished into individual awareness**) may function on different levels** (Sūtra 5.2.24/IV.15). Unless and until the self-realization process upgrades the awareness into pure awareness and then into consciousness itself, the pure consciousness (as *Īśvara*) remains distinct from the complex human structure, the form. The functioning ability of each individual human being is different because it is based on the individual's thinking instruments, self-mind, the structure of predisposition, and their collective choices. As a result, the consciousness is camouflaged by awareness as its proxy, and that awareness functions at different levels. So even when all human beings look similar as a species in the eyes of the beholder, they take different forms corresponding to their levels of awareness.

Just as awareness follows a path of evolution so does each form. There are seeds latent in all bodies, and they follow their own cycles of redemption and the paths of evolution. A master develops an understanding of this process as the awareness gets refined. But you have to realize that the forms have to still follow their own evolutionary paths, and they appear to be different to you only because of your upgraded and now changed awareness. This idea is crucial in dealing with your fellow beings, and a master must avoid the temptation of feeling "holier than thou."

If the form disappears, you wonder, how do objects of the world present themselves to a master now. The object is not seen as if disintegrating, or like a mist without denseness. A *mahāyogī* brings under conscious control the ability to switch awareness so as to see objects with or without spatial dimensions. A yoga master can select an object as a target for direct perception by making the unwanted clutter of other objects disappear in plain sight. The selected object is also seen in an additional seven virtual dimensions, five—by its constituting elements; and two—by past and future spatial-temporal progressions. Again, this act is completely willed, and a master can see the object in the ordinary perspective any time, if the circumstances so require.

This also touches another profound question: Do objects of matter exist independent of the mind and awareness? They certainly do, as they present themselves again and again for our perception. Each object is independent of the individual mind(s) that created it. But as long as cognition of an object has to be through an individual mind, it always remains "subjectively" experienced. A generally accepted "objective" version emerges from many shared subjective experiences of a concerned community. Though it is a confluence or a common denominator of many shared perceptions, it is believed to be the true nature of the object. Scientific objectivity is born similarly, but it represents a painstakingly refined and closely unified confluence. Thus, the reality of an object is always relative and subjective, because it inevitably changes from one individual to another and from this moment to that.

As we have seen before, the Universal Mind present in the thinking instruments of all individuals is supposed to be acting only as a catalyst; instead, it gets involved and becomes a self-mind, and that creates an impression of many "minds." In a way, it is the self-mind that makes us see "many." We remain entrenched in it because we depend on it as our only source of knowledge connecting us to the living world. The no-mind state enables direct perception to relieve the mind of a misplaced task—that of conjuring individuated knowledge by reflecting on an array of impressions. Instead, now the mind assumes its real role of reflecting on reality. The mind is self-reflective and makes you aware of its own working. Even when one begins to realize the mind games and starts setting the mind aside, the mind does not stop its mischief. It creates false impressions of spiritual experiences too, and even pretends to be working for *Īśvara*.

Unity of Body, Mind, and the Soul

When a master has succeeded in bringing the modifications to an end, the self-mind reincarnates as the Universal Mind. The mind "learns" that the soul needs no accessory for perceiving reality, and then it willingly surrenders to *Īśvara*. The roles are now reversed. **The mind also reflecting on the infinity of mind impressions, now becomes the soul's instrument** and starts reflecting pure awareness to the brain—awareness that "many are really one." **Thus, the brain, mind, and the soul stand unified** (Sūtra 5.2.25/IV.24).

This completely reverses the body-mind system. The sense organs and the bodies are no longer the source of knowledge; now they serve as the instruments of action to bring about what *Īśvara* directs. Senses don't feed the mind, but mind conveys to them what *Īśvara* conceives. As mentioned earlier, with no desire for the self, you use the body-mind only for healing and helping as a part of the greater scheme of things.

With such a completely metamorphosed body-mind system, a master approaches the world. A life is lived, the world is experienced, you move along with fellow beings, and the duties and obligations are fulfilled; yet a master is *in* the world and does not *belong* to it. In the truest sense of the term, the mind is used as an instrument and is not affected by itself at all. Now a master is close to the final state, a state of isolated unity (withdrawn into the true nature of *Īśvara*), which will soon be granted.

Becoming and Being

The last threshold to cross is the sensation of "I" being one with *Īśvara.* At-one-ment with *Īśvara* is a *state of being* and not an accomplishment that can be recognized by creating, in effect, a subtle duality. Thus, even the awareness of spiritual illumination is now to be set aside. By becoming conscious as a knower, you are completely devoid of the field of knowledge and the knowledge itself, as nothing is needed anymore. The Yoga practices, meditation, and all other means, now a part of life, can be and must be transcended as the end is reached.

The time has arrived for a discernment of the highest order, not just relative to your quality of awareness as it always was, but proper discernment. The mind, now reincarnating as Universal Mind, is to be recognized as separate. That makes the understanding of the power and independence of *Īśvara* more and more *impromptu*, not derived with any help from the mind. **Then, the state of isolated unity (withdrawn into the true nature of Self) comes as a reward for making this final discrimination** (Sūtra 5.2.26/IV.25). A master moves to a state of being simply conscious.

A master has still to live the remainder of the *kārmik* life. Some of the last *sūtras* are specifically aimed at conveying that, even after the realization of truth and experiencing the state of isolated unity, you have to live until the moment of bodily death, when freedom from form and Existence arrives. As said earlier, the dissolution of the desire to live does not mean ending life. An act of deliberately ending life is fundamentally contrary to Yoga (see: *Yama*), but a desire to do so is still a mind's selfish engagement. In fact, the at-one-ment is going to happen only because the three bodies have carried a master to this point. Death is also accorded now a relaxed indifference.

Now *samādhī* is a state fully of a master's own volition. When leading life as a normal human being, a master can lower the awareness to the state of a *yogī*; in the company of other illuminated persons become a *mahāyogī*; and when alone, be a master, totally immersed in *Īśvara*. **Then the mind also tends to abide by the discrimination against itself to remain withdrawn in the true nature of the one Self with increasing illumination** (Sūtra IV-26).

Bear in mind that the realization of the true nature of the soul is pure and complete awareness, not a suspension in oblivion. The illumination brings in knowledge, and you are face to face with the ultimate reality. This knowledge, then, is conveyed to the brain, and all bodies work seamlessly in the illuminated state. During the initial experience of withdrawal from sensuous perception, sometimes meditation does lead into a seemingly similar state of peace, but the subject-object duality remains. That peaceful state is more akin to deep sleep, in which the latent desires merely remain dormant, awaiting reawakening. *Becoming* one with *Īśvara* has still a hint of some awareness; *being* in a state of illumination is not an experience anymore.

Mind Still Vulnerable

Here comes another warning from Sage Pātañjali. **Through force of habit, however, the mind will reflect on other causal impressions and perceive objects of sensuous perception** (Sūtra 5.2.28/IV.27). Even at such a late stage, when there is no room for error, the all-powerful laws of nature, the illusion-inducing object-oriented world, and some traces of the almost indestructible *saṁskāra*, can prevail.

Whenever engaging with the world in the lowered-down state of a *yogī*, a master remains relatively more vulnerable. "Force of habit" stays in the thinking instruments and the thinking process. In a *yogī*'s state, memory is not bypassed as in a *mahāyogī*'s or exiled as in a master's, so while fulfilling the householder's duties and obligations, the mind is still used, and subtle mind modifications may still occur. The mind is now clean, but because it has to make use of memory patterns, the incoming impulses may yet dig out a far distant, improper memory pattern in an unguarded moment.

This is one reason why people on the *yogīk* path prefer to lead an isolated life. But doing so also makes them vulnerable, because total isolation is increasingly not practicable in today's world, unless you have access to the Himalayas, for example. A householder *yogī*, on the other hand, cultivates "spiritual" muscles and sustains them against the resistance of the material world.

However, these rare reflections are of the nature of hindrances that a master has been overcoming through the means of Yoga, and the method of their overcoming remains the same (Sūtra 5.2.29/IV.28). Thus, should a stray memory pattern still inflict the mind, the Yoga practices (*yama*, *niyama*, and so on), now a way of life, should quickly take care of it. A master can also quickly switch to a *mahāyogī*'s state in which a steady submission to *Īśvara* and a greater use of discrimination removes all such hindrances and obstacles.

When spiritually advanced people are seen suffering from bodily diseases, many seekers feel cheated and disillusioned with the spiritual path itself. They wonder why the magical wand of spiritual powers (*siddhī*) is not used to ward off one's own ailments. That should be a lot easier than helping someone else, they think. It needs to be understood that when their time arrives, some cycles of distant *karma* do not let even sages alone. A master would usually prefer to go through with the events that visit upon him, and thus be done with them. While enduring them, however, the sting is gone since all the *pain* is now "warded off," as awareness can be shifted away from the physical.

Dharma-Mégha

In these final stages of transformation a master approaches what Sage Pātañjali calls the "cloud of irreducible experiential forms," *dharma-mégha*, an ultimate state of human experience that is awesome even to a keen intellect.

> *It is observing things at their most basic level, in the briefest increments of knowable time. It is reality, stripped of the drama with which the guṇas saturate ordinary perception.*—Chip Hartranft, 70.

In order to understand this *sūtra*, you have to grasp the concepts of Existence and Creation, which are reiterated here. In Creation, there is no mind (not even Universal Mind), and the subtlest world of Existence, the causal world, is still in an uncreated state. Thus, even the causal forms need to be completely destroyed before entering Creation.

Master's non-attachment meets its final test after experiencing the bliss of illumination and the isolated unity, when there is a need for staying non-attached even to the "overshadowing cloud of spiritual knowledge" (Sūtra 5.2.30/IV.29).

More specifically, a sense of reaching the exalted state of isolated unity, and the earnestness of aspiration in doing so, must also be discarded. We have seen earlier that each world has a band or a range of vibration frequencies, and that each band is circumscribed by critical points acting as a "ring-pass-not." A huge ring-pass-not surrounds Existence and holds in custody the three permanent seed atoms connecting the causal body to the astral and physical. These atoms need to be destroyed too.

During one of the sojourns through this ring-pass-not, Creation welcomes a master bearing this "over-shadowing cloud of spiritual knowledge" that must be penetrated before entering the Celestial Home. This state of waiting is to be endured without any earnestness or desire. Ironically, the bliss that a master has experienced in the earlier stages is now gone, for bliss, too, is an experience and one has passed that. A master has only to remain in suspended animation and wait.

Samādhī Without Seed

All Hindrances and Karma *are overcome*

Dharma-mégha is the final experience of a master. At this stage, **there is no vestige of any kind of hindrances or *karma*** around such a powerful entity, and a complete freedom from them is evident (Sūtra 5.2.31/IV.30).

> *All that hindered, veiled, or prevented the full expression of the divine life has been overcome; all barriers are down, all obstacles removed. The wheel of rebirth has served its purpose and the spiritual unit which has entered into form, carrying with it potential powers and latent possibilities, has developed them to their full extent and unfolded the full power of the soul. The law of cause and effect as it functions in the three worlds no longer controls the liberated soul; his individual* karma *comes to an end...*—Alice Bailey, 426.

But, up to the last moment of existing, which you know and await peacefully, you have to live your remaining life like a normal person. You are ready for the final disintegration of the "I am," the form. That such individuals, though extremely few, carry a very low profile and do not exhibit any signs of spiritual prowess may be a surprise to many. They are not the spiritual celebrities with mega-audiences that we are habit-prone to recognize. Their work is known only to the trusted disciples and is carried out anonymously in the most serene ways.

Totality of Knowledge

All objects in Existence are the condensates of Universal Mind, a reason why all knowledge about all objects is not beyond it. When all three bodies—physical, astral, and causal—are completely pure, they are not only in total synch with each other but are also in total synch with Universal Mind. Since neither life nor any form is necessary anymore, the three material bodies can roll back and merge in Universal Mind. **Thus, through the removal of hindrances and a complete purification of the bodies the totality of knowledge becomes available through Universal Mind.** Now all that distorts and brings in impurity has been left behind **and nothing further remains for a *yogī* to do** (Sūtra 5.2.32/IV.31). This sums up all Yoga.

The duality of the pairs of opposites that undergirds life has run its course. A master is aware of the omnipresence and the unity underlying all that lives. Everything is known but it is not affected by the field of knowledge anymore.

> *Once all the layers and imperfections concealing the truth have been washed away, insight is boundless, with little left to know.*—Chip Hartranft, 70.

Guṇa *Come to an End*

A tuning fork once struck takes a long time to be still again. The astral and causal worlds are a trillion times more subtle than the tuning fork. Once the *guṇa* are thrown off-balance, it takes a series of cause-and-effect sequences running across several lifetimes for the equilibrium to restore. But now the near impossibility of stilling them back into balance and rhythm has been overcome. Only now, the "I am" and the self-form can disintegrate and become one with Universal Mind, from which they once originated. **The modifications of the mind through the inherent nature of the three *guṇa* have come to an end, for they have served their purpose** (Sūtra 5.2.33/IV.32).

> *Through the veiling power of tamas, we have been failing to see the changeless, the infinite, the undivided; through the projecting power of rajas, we have been seeing the changing, the finite, the divided, by mistake (avidyā.) But through the revealing power of sattva, you are now seeing the changeless in the changing, (inertia), the infinite in the finite, (electricity), and the undivided in the divided, (gravity).*—John Dobson, from article entitled "Einstein's Geometry," 2008.

With *guṇa* coming to an end there is only changeless, infinite and undivided Spirit.

Eternal Now, Time Terminates

Time persists only as long as the mind modifications do. With the master in perpetual *saṃyama* with *Īśvara*, there is no mind or thinking instruments to note or observe the sequential sense impulses that create a sense of time (or space). In contrast to the ordinary perception that perceives the deceptive "rain shower" in motion, a master is now at once aware of all the individual raindrops in all their states. **Time—a product of serial mind modifications—terminates when modifications are put to rest, thus completely dissolving the past, present, and future, leaving only the "eternal now"** (Sūtra 5.2.34/IV.33).

The ordinary perception inevitably brings the screens of time and space between the perceiver and the perceived Universe to create a pair of opposites. Now, with the perceiver and the perceived identified as one, in Einstein's paraphrase—the time separation and space separation collapse into zero. This lets in an experience of infinity and wholeness that was all along mistaken to be limited by time and divided into space.

State of Isolated Unity

The fundamental error finally stands corrected. All the transformation (*pariṇama*) known to cause a constant change is experienced as secondary and as an apparition (*vivarta*); "taking the changeless as changing" is realized as the primary error.

Now, an uninterrupted isolated unity is possible when the three *guṇa* no longer exercise any hold over Self. With the screens of time, place and causation completely removed, **pure spiritual consciousness withdraws into One; that is Yoga** (Sūtra 5.2.35/IV.34).

In the eternal now, the state of isolated unity is the state of nothingness, apparent emptiness. This nothingness is different. Like the value "zero," it appears to be empty, but without it, everything collapses and becomes meaningless. All three body sheaths are now redundant, all three permanent atoms are disintegrated, the causal body holding the seed atom itself is disintegrated—now, all births and deaths end. A master penetrates the final ring-pass-not, and steps into the Celestial Home that was always there. This homecoming is the true purpose of Yoga, and life.

***Chapter Five (Part 1): Rearranged Sūtras*:** (Numbers in the brackets are from the original text)

5.1.1 (I.27) तस्य वाचकः प्रणवः ॥

tasya vācakaḥ praṇavaḥ

The Word of *Īśvara* is AUM. This is the *Prānava,* the primordial sound.

5.1.2 (I.28) तज्जपस्तदर्थभावनम् ॥

tajjapas tad-artha- bhāvanaṁ

Through the sounding of the word and through reflection upon its meaning (the way is found).

5.1.3 (I.29) ततः प्रत्यक्चेतनाधिगमोऽप्यन्तरायाभावश्च ॥

tataḥ pratyak-cetanādhigamo "py antarāyā-bhāvaś ca

From this comes the realization of the Self and the removal of all obstacles.

5.1.4 (I.36) विशोका वा ज्योतिष्मती ॥

viśokā vā jyotiṣmatī

By meditation upon Light and upon Radiance, knowledge of the Spirit can be reached and thus peace can be achieved.

5.1.5 (I.40) परमाणुपरममहत्वान्तोऽस्य वशीकारः ॥

paramāṇu-parama-mahattvānto "sya vaśīkāraḥ

Thus, the Yogī"s knowledge is perfected, as his realization extends from an atom (infinitely small) to Atman (infinitely great).

5.1.6 (I.41) क्षीणवृत्तेरभिजातस्येव मणेर्ग्रहीतृग्रहणग्राह्येषु तत्स्थतदञ्जनता समापत्तिः ॥

kṣīṇa-vṛtter abhijātasyeva maṇer grahītṛ-grahaṇa-grāhyeṣu tatstha-tadañjanatā samāpattiḥ

To him whose mind modifications are completely stilled, the knower, knowledge and the field of knowledge become one and there eventuates a state of identity with and similarity to that which is realized.

5.1.7 (I.45) सूक्ष्मविषयत्वं चालिङ्गपर्यवसानम्॥

sūkṣma-viṣayatvaṁ cāliṇga-pary-avasānam

The gross leads into the subtle and the subtle leads in progressive stages to that state of spiritual being called *Pradhāna.*

5.1.8 (I.47) निर्विचारवैशारद्येऽध्यात्मप्रसादः॥

nirvicāra-vaiśāradye "dhyātma-prasādaḥ

Pure spiritual realization follows through the quiet mind-stuff.

5.1.9 (II.16) हेयं दुःखमनागतम्॥

heyaṁ duḥkham anāgataṁ

Pain which is yet to come can be warded off.

5.1.10 (II.17) द्रष्टृदृश्ययोः संयोगो हेयहेतुः॥

draṣṭṛ-dṛśyayoḥ saṁyogo heya-hetuḥ

The preventable cause of all pain is the illusion that the Perceiver and that which is perceived is one and the same.

5.1.11 (II.51) बाह्याभ्यन्तरविषयाक्षेपी चतुर्थः॥

bāhyābhyantara-viṣayākṣepī caturthaḥ

There is a fourth stage of *Prāṇayāma* which transcends those dealing with the internal and external phases.

5.1.12 (II.52) ततः क्षीयते प्रकाशावरणम्॥

tataḥ kṣīyate prakāśāvaraṇam

Through this that which obscures the light is gradually removed.

5.1.13 (II.53) धारणासु च योग्यता मनसः॥

dhāraṇāsu ca yogyatā manasaḥ

And the mind (the thinking instrument) is prepared for the meditative attitude.

5.1.14 (III.4) त्रयमेकत्र संयमः॥

trayam ekatra saṃyama ḥ

When *dhāraṇā*, *dhyāna*, and *Samādhī* form one sequential act (the meditative attitude), then is Saṃyama achieved.

5.1.15 (III.5) **तज्जयात् प्रज्ञालोकः ॥**

taj-jayāt prajñālokaḥ

As a result of Saṃyama, comes the shining forth of the light.

5.1.16 (III.6) **तस्य भूमिषु विनियोगः ॥**

tasya bhūmiṣu viniyogaḥ

This illumination is gradual, it is developed stage by stage, plane by plane.

5.1.17 (III.7) **त्रयमन्तरङ्गं पूर्वेभ्यः ॥**

trayam antaraṇgaṁ pūrvebhyaḥ

These last three means (steps) of Yoga have a more intimate subjective effect than the previous five.

5.1.18 (III.8) **तदपि बहिरङ्गं निर्बीजस्य ॥**

tad api bahir-aṇgaṁ nirbījasya

Even these three—*dhāraṇā*, *dhyāna,* and *Samādhī*—are external to the true seedless Samādhī.

5.1.19 (III.18) **संस्कारसाक्षात्करणात् पूर्वजातिज्ञानम् ॥**

saṁskāra-sākṣātkaraṇāt pūrva-jātijñānaṁ

Knowledge of previous incarnations becomes available when the *Yogī* chooses to use his ability to see thought-images.

5.1.20 (III.19) **प्रत्ययस्य परचित्तज्ञानम् ॥**

pratyayasya para-citta-jñānaṁ

Through concentrated meditation, the thought images in the minds of other people become apparent.

5.1.21 (III.20) **न च तत् सालम्बनं तस्याविषयीभूतत्वात् ॥**

na ca tat sālambanaṁ tasyāviṣayī-bhūtatvāt

As, however, the object of those thoughts is not apparent to the perceiver, he sees only the thought and not the object. His meditation excludes the tangible.

5.1.22 (III.21) कायरूपसंयमात् तद्ग्राह्यशक्तिस्तम्भे चक्षुःप्रकाशासंप्रयोगेऽन्तर्धानम्॥

kāya-rūpa-saṁyamāt tad-grāhya-śakti-stambhe cakṣuḥ-prakāśāsaṁprayoge "ntardhānaṁ

By concentrated meditation upon the distinction between form and body, those properties of the body which make it visible to the human eye are negated and the Yogī can render himself invisible.

(Begin)------------ (Reference in Appendix 4, from 5.1.23 to 5.2.4).

5.1.23 (III.25) बलेषु हस्तिबलादीनि॥

baleṣu hasti-balādīni

Concentrated meditation on mūladhāra center will awaken great force and light.

5.1.24 (III.26) p,वृत्ति आलोकन्यासात् सूक्ष्मव्यवहितविप्रकृष्टज्ञानम्॥

pravṛtti-āloka-nyāsāt sūkṣma-vyavahita-viprakṛṣṭa-jñānaṁ

Perfectly concentrated meditation on the *swādhisthāna* center (at the base of reproductive organs) will produce the pure awareness of that which is subtle, hidden and remote.

5.1.25 (III.27) भुवनज्ञानं सूर्ये संयमात्॥

bhuvana-jñānaṁ sūrye samyamāt

Through meditation, one-pointedly fixed upon the sun, will come a consciousness (or knowledge) of the seven worlds.

5.1.26 (III.28) चन्द्रे ताराव्यूहज्ञानम्॥

candre tārā-vyūha-jñānaṁ

A knowledge of all lunar forms arises through one-pointed meditation upon the moon.

5.1.27 (III.30) नाभिचक्रे कायव्यूहज्ञानम्॥

nābhi-cakre kāya-vyūha-jñānaṁ

By concentrated meditation upon the solar plexus, comes perfect knowledge as to the condition of the body.

5.1.28 (III.29) ध्रुवे तत् गतिज्ञानम्॥

dhruve tat-gati-jñānaṁ

Concentration upon the Pole Star will give knowledge of the orbits of the planets and the stars.

5.1.29 (III.35) हृदये चित्तसंवित्॥

hṛdaye citta-saṁvit

Understanding of the mind-awareness comes from one-pointed meditation upon the heart center.

Book Five (Part 2): Rearranged Sūtras**:** (Numbers in the brackets are from the original text).

5.2.1 (III.31) कण्ठकूपे क्षुत्पिपासानिवृत्तिः॥

kaṇṭha-kūpe kṣut-pipāsā-nirvṛttih

By fixing the attention on the throat-well center, cessation of hunger and thirst will ensue.

5.2.2 (III.32) कूर्मनाड्यां स्थैर्यम्॥

kūrma-nāḍyāṁ sthairyaṁ

By fixing the attention upon the tube or nerve below the throat center, equilibrium is achieved.

5.2.3 (III.33) मूर्धज्योतिषि सिद्धदर्शनम्॥

mūrdha-jyotiṣi siddha-darśanaṁ

This power is developed in one-pointed meditation.

5.2.4 (III.34) प्रातिभाद्वा सर्वम्॥

prātibhād vā sarvaṁ

All things could be known in the vivid light of intuition.

(End)-------------- (Reference in Appendix 4, from 5.1.23 to 5.2.4).

5.2.5 (III.36) सत्त्वपुरुषयोरत्यन्तासङ्कीर्णयोः प्रत्ययाविशेषो भोगः परार्थत्वात् स्वार्थसंयमात् पुरुषज्ञानम्॥

sattva-puruṣayor atyantāsaṁkīrṇayoḥ pratyayāviśeṣo bhogaḥ parārthatvāt svārtha-saṁyamāt puruṣa-jñānaṁ

Experience of the pairs of opposites comes from the inability to distinguish between the personal self and the Spirit, a confusion that is clarified by *Saṃyama* on self.

5.2.6 (III.37) ततः प्रातिभश्रावणवेदनादर्शास्वादवार्ता जायन्ते॥

tataḥ prātibha-śrāvaṇa-vedanādarśāsvāda-vārtā jāyante

As a result of his/her experience and meditation, a more profound hearing, touch, sight, taste and smell are developed, producing intuitional knowledge.

5.2.7 (III.38) ते समाधावुपसर्गा व्युत्थाने सिद्धयः॥

te samādhāv upasargā vyutthāne siddhayaḥ

These powers are obstacles to the highest spiritual realization, but serve as magical powers in the objective world.

5.2.8 (III.39) बन्धकारणशैथिल्यात् प्रचारसंवेदनाच्च चित्तस्य परशरीरावेशः॥

bandha-kāraṇa-śaithilyāt pracāra-saṁvedanāc ca cittasya para-śarīrāveśaḥ

By liberation from the causes of bondage and through their weakening and by an understanding of the mode of transference (withdrawal and entrance), the mind stuff (chitta) can enter or synchronize with another body.

5.2.9 (III.40) उदानजयाज्जलपङ्ककण्टकादिष्वसंग उत्क्रान्तिश्च॥

udāna-jayāj jala-paṇka-kaṇṭakādiṣv asaṇga utkrāntiś ca

By subjugation of *udāna vāyū* there is liberation from water, the thorny path and mire and the power of ascension is gained.

5.2.10 (III.41) sमानजयाज्ज्वलनम् ॥

samāna-jayāj jvalanaṁ

Through subjugation of the *samāna vāyū*, the spark becomes the flame.

5.2.11 (III.42) श्रोत्राकाशयोः संबन्धसंयमाद्दिव्यं श्रोत्रम् ॥

śrotrākaśayoḥ saṁbandha-saṁyamād divyaṁ śrotraṁ

By means of one-pointed meditation upon the relationship between *Ākāśa* and sound, an organ for spiritual hearing will be developed.

5.2.12 (III.43) कायाकाशयोः संबन्धसं यमाल्लघुतूलसमापत्तेश्चाकाशगमनम् ॥

kāyākāśayoḥ saṁbandha-saṁyamāt laghu-tūla-samāpatteś cākāśa-gamanaṁ

By one-pointed meditation upon the relationship existing between the body and *Ākāśa*, ascension out of matter (of the three worlds) and the power to travel in space is granted.

5.2.13 (III.44) बहिरकल्पिता वृत्तिर्महाविदेहा ततः प्र काशावरणक्षयः ॥

bahir akalpitā vṛttir mahā-videhā tataḥ prakāśāvaraṇa-kṣayaḥ

When that which veils the light is done away with, then comes the state of being called discarnate (or disembodied), freed from the modifications of the thinking instrument. This is the state of illumination.

5.2.14 (III.45) स्थूलस्वरूपसूक्ष्मान्वयार्थवत्त्वसंयमाद् भूतजयः ॥

sthūla-svarūpa-sūkṣmānvayārthavattva-saṁyamād bhūta-jayaḥ

One-pointed meditation upon the five forms, which every element takes, produces mastery over every element. These five forms are gross, constant, subtle, all-pervading and functional.

5.2.15 (III.46) ततोऽणिमादिप्रादुर्भावः कायसम्पत्तद्धर्मानभिघातश्च॥

tato "ṇimādi-prādurbhāvaḥ kāya-saṁpattad dharmānabhighātaś ca

Through the mastery over the elements the *siddhis* (powers), bodily perfection and freedom from all hindrances is attained.

5.2.16 (III.48) ग्रहणस्वरूपास्मितान्वयार्थवत्त्वसयमादिन्द्रियजयः॥

grahaṇa-svarūpāsmitānvayārthavattva-saṁyamād indriya-jayaḥ

Mastery over the senses, the *tanmātrās*, is brought about through concentrated meditation upon their nature, peculiar attributes, egoism, pervasiveness and the useful purpose.

5.2.17 (III.49) ततो मनोजवित्वं विकरणभावः प्रधानजयश्च॥

tato manojavitvaṁ vikaraṇa-bhāvaḥ pradhāna-jayaś ca

As a result of this perfection there comes a rapidity of action like that of the mind, perception independent of the organs and mastery over root substance.

5.2.18 (III.51) तद्वैराग्यादपि दोषबीजक्षये कैवल्यम्॥

tad-vairāgyād api doṣa-bīja-kṣaye kaivalyaṁ

By a passionless attitude towards his attainment and towards all soul powers, the one who is free from the seeds of bondage attains the condition of isolated unity.

5.2.19 (III.52) स्थान्युपनिमन्त्रणे संगस्मयाकरणम्पुनरनिष्टप्रसङ्गात्॥

sthāny-upanimantraṇe saṇga-smayākaraṇaṁ punaḥ aniṣṭa-prasaṇgāt

There should be entire rejection of all allurements from all forms of being, even the celestial, for the recurrence of evil contacts remains possible.

5.2.20 (III.53) क्षणतत्क्रमयोः संयमाद्विवेकजं ज्ञानम्॥

kṣaṇa-tat-kramayoḥ saṁyamād vivekajaṁ jñānaṁ

Intuitive knowledge is developed through the use of the discriminative faculty when there is one-pointed concentration upon moments and their continuous succession.

5.2.21 (III.54) जातिलक्षणदेशैरन्यतानवच्छेदात् तुल्ययोस्ततः प्रतिपत्तिः॥

jāti-lakṣaṇa-deśair anyatānavacchedāt tulyayos tataḥ pratipattiḥ

From the intuitive knowledge is born the capacity to distinguish between all beings and to cognize their genus, qualities and position on the evolutionary ladder.

5.2.22 (IV.5) प्रवृत्तिभेदे प्रयोजकं चित्तमेकमनेकेषाम्॥

pravṛtti-bhede prayojakaṁ cittam ekam anekeṣāṁ

Consciousness is One, yet produces the varied forms of the many.

5.2.23 (IV.6) तत्र ध्यानजमनाशयम्॥

tatra dhyānajam anāśayaṁ

Among the forms which consciousness assumes, only that which is the result of meditation is free from latent *karma*.

5.2.24 (IV.15) वस्तुसाम्ये चित्तभेदात्तयोर्विभक्तः पन्थाः॥

vastu-sāmye citta-bhedāt tayor vibhaktaḥ panthāḥ

These two, consciousness (*Īśvara*) and the form, are distinct and separate; though forms may be similar, the consciousness (as awareness) may function on different levels of being.

5.2.25 (IV.24) तदसंख्येयवासनाभिश्चित्रमपि परार्थं संहत्यकारित्वात्॥

tad asaṁkhyeya-vāsanābhiś citram api parārtham samhatya-kāritvāt

The mind-stuff also, reflecting as it does on infinity of mind impressions, becomes the instrument of the Self and acts as a unifying agent.

5.2.26 (IV.25) विशेषदर्शिनः आत्मभावभावनाविनिवृत्तिः ॥

viśeṣa-darśinaḥ ātma-bhāva-bhāvanā-vinivṛttiḥ

The state of isolated unity (withdrawn into the true nature of Self) is the reward of the man who can discriminate between the mind stuff and the Self, or spiritual man.

5.2.27 (IV.26) तदा विवेकनिम्नं कैवल्यप्राग्भारं चित्तम् ॥

tadā viveka-nimnaṁ Kaivalya-prāgbhāraṁ cittaṁ

The mind then tends towards discrimination and increasing illumination as to the true nature of the one Self.

5.2.28 (IV.27) तच्छिद्रेषु प्रत्ययान्तराणि संस्कारेभ्यः ॥

tac-chidreṣu pratyayāntarāṇi saṁskāre-bhyah

Through force of habit, however, the mind will reflect other causal impressions and perceive objects of sensuous perception.

5.2.29 (IV.28) हानमेषां क्लेशवदुक्तम् ॥

hānam eṣāṁ kleśavad uktaṁ

These reflections are of the nature of hindrances, and the method of their overcoming is the same.

5.2.30 (IV.29) प्रसंख्यानेऽप्यकुसीदस्य सर्वथा विवेकख्यातेर्धर्ममेघः समाधिः ॥

prasaṁkhyāne "py akusīdasya sarvathā viveka-khyater dharma-meghaḥ samādhiḥ

The man who develops non-attachment even in his aspiration (after illumination and isolated unity) becomes eventually aware, through practiced discrimination, of the overshadowing cloud of spiritual knowledge.

5.2.31 (IV.30) ततः क्लेशकर्मनिवृत्तिः ॥

tataḥ kleśa-karma-nirvṛttiḥ

When this stage is reached then the hindrances and *karma* are overcome.

5.2.32 (IV.31) तदा सर्वावरणमलापेतस्य ज्ञानस्यानन्त्याज्ज्ञेयमल्पम् ॥

tadā sarvāvaraṇa-malāpetasya jñānasyānantyāj jñeyam alpaṁ

When through the removal of hindrances and the purification of the sheaths, the totality of knowledge becomes available, nothing further remains for the Yogī to do.

5.2.33 (IV.32) ततः कृतार्थानाम्परिणामक्रमसमाप्तिर्गुणानाम् ॥

tataḥ kṛtārthānāṁ pariṇāma-krama-samāptir guṇānāṁ

The modifications of the mind-stuff through the inherent nature of the three *guṇas* come to an end, for they have served their purpose.

5.2.34 (IV.33) क्षणप्रतियोगी परिणामापरान्तनिर्ग्राह्यः क्रमः ॥

kṣaṇa-pratiyogī pariṇāmāparānta-nirgrāhyaḥ kramaḥ

Time, which is the sequence of the modifications of the mind, likewise terminates, giving place to the eternal now.

5.2.35 (IV.34) पुरुषार्थशून्यानां गुणानां प्रतिप्रसवः कैवल्यं स्वरूपप्रतिष्ठा वा चितिशक्तेरिति ॥

puruṣārtha-śūnyānām guṇānāṁ pratiprasavaḥ kaivalyaṁ svarūpa-pratiṣṭhā vā citi-śakter iti

The state of isolated unity becomes possible, when the three *guṇas* (qualities of matter) no longer exercise any hold over the Self. The pure spiritual consciousness withdraws into one.

Afterword

> *He who finds in the midst of intense activity the greatest rest, and in the midst of the greatest rest intense activity, he has become a Yogi.*—Bhagavad Gita. IV. 18.

Many aspects of Yoga appear paradoxical; it keeps unfolding with the evolving truth and becomes a spiral journey. Yoga appears to constantly change directions, yet still takes you to the destination if you have patience and persistence. Only by transforming oneself and reaching the pinnacle does the whole picture open up. The last hypothesis is really the first principle of Yoga: that the Universe is apparitional, born of *avidyā*, our basic mistake. So, we have completed a typical *mandala* (circle) and need to revisit the point where we started, expecting to meet what were once foreign concepts as our innate truth now.

If the reader has reached thus far, it may be worthwhile to tackle some additional complex ideas, the elements of which were already touched upon in the preceding text. At each milestone in Yoga, a realized hypothesis remains its only testimony. However, until then, strands and fibers of synthetic personal truth continue to build a *yogi*'s self-view and the world-view; Yoga addresses both.

The Universe, (World-View)

You start in Yoga beholding the seen world as separate from your own self. In *Saṃskṛt* the word for "world" is *jagat*, meaning changing. When the world is seen as constantly changing, perceptions are deconstructed. Its unseen subtle components are sensed. However, importantly, a correspondence is seen between everything gross to subtle from within and without. If the Spirit is the subtlest and everything else is mind-matter, a new separation becomes evident between them.

Time, Space, and Causation

A world-view that embraces myriad objects can be fully understood only if we probe why everything appears to be changing. If the world is seen as changing, it must be with reference to something that does not change, an "Absolute" that is the essence. In the *Sāṃkhya* school of Indian philosophy, the universe is often described as the interplay between pure, transcendental consciousness (*Purūṣa*) and the material world of matter or nature (*Prakṛti*). This apparent duality is second-stage, preceded by and takes place within the context of a unity (*advait*) of Absolute reality, from which all things originate, all things belong, and to which all things return. The ability to be conscious of Ultimate reality beyond the dualities of ordinary perception is the inner illumination that Yoga engenders in practitioners. This enlightenment of the self is Yoga's ultimate destination. "Being one with pure consciousnesses" is therefore Sage Patanjali's departure from the *Sāṃkhya* school.

Consciousness, awareness, and perception are, therefore, the central themes in Yoga. Consciousness causes perception that creates awareness and the opposing dimensions of time and space. Yoga teaches how to understand, master and transform awareness in order to be conscious of Absolute reality, and ultimately, to exist in Absolute reality. In this process of awakening, perception becomes more penetrating and awareness gradually becomes less gross and more subtle, finally becoming consciousness itself.

Swami Vivekānanda describes the universe, as it is ordinarily perceived, as the Absolute seen through the screen of time, space and causation (*kāla, désha, nimitta*).[45] A screen (consciousness) *causes* the image (or perception) of that which is seen to be altered. Therefore, two entities result, one real and the other perceived: the Absolute, which is real, and its perceived counterpart, the universe of ordinary consciousness, which, in Absolute terms, is not real. In other words, ordinary perception of the universe is not *created* but instead *caused* by consciousness in the act of perceiving. It is a corollary of consciousness: the "I-am-ness"-producing cause, or a *causation*. As long as consciousness exists, the *perception* or illusion of duality exists as well.

The "changeless," "infinite" and "undivided" nature of Absolute reality, which exists beyond the perceptions of time, space and causation, is the fundamental and the final hypothesis that Yoga presents to the seeker, for verification through experience of *samādhi* without seed.

Since Absolute is not in time, it cannot be changing. Change takes place only in time. In addition, since it is not in space, it must be undivided, because dividedness and separation occur only in space. In addition, since it is therefore one and undivided, it must also be infinite, since there is no "other" to limit it. Now "changeless," "infinite" and "undivided" are negative statements, but they will suffice. We can trace the physics of our universe from these three negative statements. If we do not see the Absolute as what it is, we will see it as something else. If we do not see it as changeless, infinite, and undivided, we will see it as changing, finite, and divided, since in this case there is no other else. There is no other way to mistake the changeless except as changing. So we see a universe which is changing all the time, made of minuscule particles, and divided into atoms.[46]

---

[45] The Complete Works of Swami Vivekānanda, Volume 2: "The Absolute and Manifestion" *(Māyāvati, India, 1948).*

[46] *John Dobson,* The Equations of Māyā, *1993. Originally published in* Cosmic Beginnings & Human Ends: Where Science & Religion Meet *(Open Court Publishing Co., 1995), 3.*

Einstein's equation, $E=mc^2$ and the theory of relativity state the same, but stop short of explaining why.

> *The concept of mass-energy equivalence connects the concepts of conservation of mass and conservation of energy, which continue to hold separately. Both the total mass and the total energy inside a totally closed system remain constant over time, as seen by any single observer in a given inertial frame. In other words, energy cannot be created or destroyed, and energy, in all of its forms, has mass. Mass also cannot be created or destroyed, and in all of its forms, has energy.* ***According to the theory of relativity, mass and energy as commonly understood, are two names for the same thing, and neither one is changed or transformed into the other.*** *Rather, neither one appears without the other.*—"Mass–energy equivalence," from Wikipedia.

In Einstein's theory,

1. "Relativity" is "duality" caused by perception
2. Energy is Absolute (*Purūṣa*) and mass, the matter (*Prakṛti*), "two names of the same thing"
3. Mass is inevitably "seen" as *guṇa;* while it can be pure energy to you only if you transcend *guṇa*

The misperception of duality, ironically, serves a purpose in the evolution of awareness, for it creates the parallel yet opposing forces of separation and attraction and the resulting drive to return "home" to a state of Absolute wholeness. This drive binds ordinary consciousness to the Absolute in a momentum of eternal unfolding (evolution). The force of dispersion of this itself creates the force of the homing instinct (involution).

Universal Mind

The Absolute exists in perfect balance and harmony within itself. However, in becoming self-aware, there arises a "*self*" and an "*other*." Then separation is established, balance is lost, and countless chain reactions of evolution are set into motion. In the process, the infinite Cosmic Consciousness becomes finite Universal Mind.

All objects are either man-made or natural. Behind the birth of each object is a mind that conceives an idea, designs and executes it. Whether it is a human mind or nature's mind, it "knows" everything about the created object. Universal Mind can also be conceptualized as that virtual amalgam of all the minds that collectively know everything about all the objects. Thus, as the evolution rolls out, the subtle mind creates gross matter. Mind and matter form a single spectrum, with Universal Mind on the subtle end and the most inert objects on the opposite gross end. This is the second most important Yoga hypothesis.

Consciousness, Divinity, and Will

The Cosmic Consciousness that permeates all of nature pulsates as life and awareness unfolding from subtle to gross. As the force of separation rolls out, the force of attraction for wholeness (and moving from gross back to subtle) sets in, creating an ever-increasing tension. That tension appears, in its grossest form, as gravity and the "attraction between opposites, like positive and negative electrical charges."[47]

Yoga's path of transformation frees awareness from cell-level bondage and cultivates recognition of the fundamental illusion of duality. Thus, it is a powerful tool and vehicle for transcending the illusion of duality and returning to the divinity of wholeness or pure, Absolute Consciousness.

The force to return to wholeness could be called Cosmic or Divine Will. During the mind's outward journey, from subtle to gross and from one to many, Cosmic Will becomes diluted, less powerful, and eventually neutral. *Yogic* practices help to empower the individual's "neutral will" to become "intellectual will" and finally "spiritual will." The unwavering and powerful force of "spiritual will" inspires and drives an awakening to the ultimate truth. This involution relocates awareness from gross back to the subtle, and ultimately, back to original pure Cosmic Consciousness. A Yoga practitioner experiences this first-hand.

---

[47] *Dobson , 7.*

Subtle-to-Gross and the Fourth State

Universal Mind, the mother of all matter, is not "created" in the usual sense of the word. It is *apparitional* causation: *the Absolute seen as the universe, through the screen of time, space and causation*. What is perceived as matter and what the laws of physics explain as one form of matter created from another form of matter is *transformational* causation. In such creation of matter, the sum total of energy remains the same, while the configuration of the elements of matter is changed.

Hence, *Sānkhya* theory proposes that, in relation to the Absolute, the universe of mind and matter is real (when perceived) but not manifest otherwise when the three guṇas are in perfect balance, and that gravity, electricity, energy (*prāṇa*) and inertia are all examples of the same underlying, inherent consciousness, manifesting (or not manifesting) at different levels of energetic vibrations. Patanjali calls the *Sānkhyan* 'foundation of the fundamental gravitation field, the resonant vibrations, as Īśvara.

On the Absolute plane, there exists a "potent nothingness," a "sum total of potential energy" that is "one, perpetual, dynamic and not manifest" because the Īśvara field has reached samādhi, a perpetual state of existence.[48]

The "five great elements" combine in myriad permutations to produce the whole of the subtle-to-gross spectrum of the entire material plane and, through the infinite layers of subtle-to-gross roll-out, create the appearance of diversity—though in essence and in composing the core, all things are the same. It is essentially scale-invariant. On this ultimate level, therefore, as it is in the macrocosm, so it is in its microcosm. This is the third most important Yoga hypothesis. In evolution, self-awareness becomes more and more subtle to be able to witness this subtle-to-gross spectrum present within oneself and in everything else.

---

[48] *G. Srinivasan,* Sankhya: An Ancient Philosophy Unifies Science and Religion, *http://s1.webstarts.com/Sankhyakarika/index.html* and *http://s2.webstarts.com/Sankhyakarika/index.html*

The universe of mind-matter is multi-tiered. At the grossest end the "seen" universe is physical/cellular, virtually inherent to it is its subtle "unseen" counterpart, the astral/molecular universe and even more subtle causal/electronic universe. All the objects in the universe inherit the same tiers but appear to be extremely diverse owing to *guṇa*.

Guṇa

Present-day physics maintains that everything in the universe, in all physical states, is composed of the same vibratory or oscillatory force-field. The gross, seemingly static "objects" have a slower vibration, which gives the impression of solidity, while less solid, subtler elements have a more rapid vibration. That we cannot perceive the subtle vibrations inherent in all things is a reflection of the fundamental limitation of our sensory perception.

The fundamental error in the very process of perception has three aspects, called *guṇa*. Only through non-sensory, direct perception, where the duality and division of the *guṇa* is transcended, can one perceive an object as a manifestation of the perfect harmony and Oneness of Absolute life-force.

Though each *guṇa* is merely a different vibratory manifestation of the same energetic life-force, manifesting differently at different points in time, together they create the illusion of diversity. Once again, this exemplifies that ordinary perception of the universe is, on some very subtle level, an illusion of Absolute reality.

Perception mirrors the vibratory consciousness of the perceiver. All perceived things are inherently pure, illuminating or *sattvic*, it is the perceiver's (limitation of) awareness that ultimately causes the perception of *guṇa* or diversity of reality. In the instance of fully awakened awareness, where direct perception transcends the perception of *guṇa*, that which is seen is recognized in its inherent, absolute state. On the path of Yoga, therefore, transcending the illusion of *guṇa* is considered the final frontier before arriving at the Fourth State of Consciousness.

The Individual, (Self-View)

Ultimately we are the "lucky" objects, which could transform ourselves and realize that the world and the self are the same thing. We humans possess in microcosm the same subtle-to-gross spectrum that the world full of objects exhibits on the macrocosmic level.

Time, Space, and Beyond

As environment is perceived, the ordinary mind comprehends this experience linearly (one moment follows the next). Resulting thoughts progress linearly, producing a sense of time, "*now* and *then*" or "*before* and *after.*" The time separation between two events is compensated for by a sense of space, as a context for the experiences, creating spatially an object-orientation of "*here* and *there*" or "*this* and *that*."

If ordinary perception of the universe is an illusion of Absolute reality, there must be a more complete reality beyond the concepts of time and space (products of mind and perception). The *illusion* of time and space only mean that there is an Absolute reality beyond them, which is not limited by these perceived conceptualizations.

The *Yoga-Sūtra* describe that multiple dimensions co-exist within all things and all phenomena, like a multi-dimensional hologram, where the infinite instances of subtle-to-gross roll-out (evolution) and gross-to-subtle roll-in (involution) occur simultaneously; and whether an atom or a human, a planet or the universe, each perceived unit or composite of units preserves the essential undivided characteristic of "wholeness."

Awareness and Perception

Can we see or even comprehend this holographic world where all objects and phenomena are in perpetual transition from subtle to gross? Not as long as our awareness is steeped in the gross material plane where predispositions come rushing in to color, influence or drive the thought process. Can we cleanse our thinking of predispositions created by *saṃskāra*, the impressions left from all past experienced emotions? Can we raise or expand our awareness to see and perceive without thinking?

The philosophy and practice of Yoga is ultimately about elevating awareness from the gross physical plane, where human consciousness ordinarily abides, to more subtle vibrational planes. This path of transforming consciousness is an inward journey wherein the practitioner gradually illuminates the inner spiritual Self, until eventually both what *is* and what is *seen* is the divine nature inherent in all things. "As it is in the macrocosm, so it is in its microcosm" is thus experienced. In addition, this journey back into "nothingness" becomes life's mission.

Then, all life becomes Yoga.

Appendix 1: The Rhythmic Breathing

The initial control of *prāṇa* is through rhythmic breathing.

There are three aspects to this method:

- **Technique:** In breathing properly, one should use the chest and the diaphragm, which separates the lung cavity and the stomach. Due to faulty breathing styles, many people have forgotten how the diaphragm works, with the use of the upper abdomen (the upper abdomen above the navel and below the rib cage). So initially one has to carefully watch that the upper abdomen rises (comes out) on inhalation and falls on exhalation. It is simple to understand. The abdomen acts like a balloon. When it rises, the diaphragm is pulled down, thereby causing the lungs to expand. In a reverse action, the lungs contract when the upper abdomen falls. Thus, in rhythmic breathing, when inhaling or exhaling, the chest and the upper abdomen should rise or fall together. Over a period of time, this should become a natural action requiring no undue effort.
- **Volume:** One has to remember that this is a process of correct breathing and not an athletic exercise. The volume of air breathed in and out should not be too much. And ex-

cept for a slight effort required initially as a beginner, no force should ever be applied. When emotions, digestion, and general health improve, the volume will be automatically greater. And this takes its own time.

- **Rhythm:** One inhalation and one exhalation make one breathing cycle. In rhythmic breathing, one does 12 breathing cycles per minute. In a 5-second breathing cycle, inhalation takes 3 seconds and exhalation 2. Thus, count 1001—1002—1003 for inhalation and 1005—1006 for exhalation. "Four" (4) is not counted and serves as a reminder to shift from inhaling to exhaling without any gap in between. Similarly, there is no gap between two breathing cycles. In other words, there is no retention of air inside or outside as practiced in some other forms of *prāṇayāma.*

One is advised only to practice rhythmic breathing for 5 minutes a day to begin. Then add 5 minutes at a time when comfortable. Eventually, one can do it whenever one is reminded of it. Soon one realizes that rhythmic breathing happens on its own while attending to other chores of life. By then, one's thought-cacophony is greatly pacified and the emotional self is healthier.

During the practice sessions, one can use a simple aid—a wrist-watch or a wall-clock with a hand for seconds. Later on, after a long enough practice, it will become possible to hear one's own heartbeats (which by then should have settled down to the desired level of 60 beats per minute) and to align breathing to that rhythm: three beats for inhalation and two for exhalation.

Please refer to *www.3srb.org* for details.

Appendix 2: Upgrading of Awareness

Yoga is all about understanding the deeper and the subtler world that is latent in everything that meets our eyes. One perceives at the given level of awareness. If one identifies with the physical body of the self, physical objects are what one perceives externally. In Yoga one realizes one's own subtle self and in the process develops an ability to re-locate awareness to a newer depth.

The process of ordinary perception is outsourced to a thinking mechanism. Therefore, when we perceive, it brings home a tinted and second-hand version of what is seen. The thinking mechanism is so much an integral part of our being that living without it even for a fraction of a second is unthinkable.

Yoga tells us that it is not only *possible* to see directly but also *essential* to do so in the quest for the ultimate truth. Of course, it does not happen overnight. First, the mind has to be understood and the coloration of the thinking process deciphered. There are many deep-rooted obstacles and hindrances on the way that are to be cleared. At the end of this arduous effort comes the first reward, "non-attachment," an ability to disengage mind from the process of perception. Initially it is involuntary, but with further practice, it can be consciously willed. Then, progressively, this disengagement comes to stay and skills of concentration, meditation and absorption are developed.

Concentration, meditation and absorption are skills that are first directed to the "non-self" objects. From this may result material success, both monetary and intellectual. Later, as one becomes ready to withstand the demands of the advanced spiritual studies, the same skills are used in more and more subjective domains.

In order to offer an experience as well as to aid in the initial pursuit of spiritual seeking, here are some preliminary exercises for upgrading the awareness. These exercises have been inferred by the Late Shri Tavaria, from some of Pātañjali's *sūtras*. A word of caution: like everything else in Yoga, you need abundant patience and dogged but unrushed effort.

STEP 1

Spread a clean white handkerchief on a table cleared of all other objects that would distract attention, place a glass prism on the handkerchief, take a comfortable sitting position and look into the prism (it is mere looking, not "seeing" or thinking) for a period of 5 minutes. To facilitate close watching, the face may rest on the palms and the elbows on the table. In three to six months of practice the prism will disappear from sight.

How does it happen? Initially, as soon as one looks at the prism one becomes aware of the mind-drifts, since watching the prism is really watching oneself with the aid of a neutral object. In the beginning, there will be some reactions and responses to the memory-associated impulses, but these would gradually disappear leading to attention that is steady and silent. Understand that the prism disappearing is not the purpose of the practice; the purpose is to just look into the prism. If the prism remains invisible, for say 10 seconds, which is a measure of success, continue practicing until the duration reaches 1 to 2 minutes. Only then go to the second step. Do not be overanxious and do not practice these steps unless some *āsanas* or breathing exercises have been done earlier.

STEP 2

Now spread the handkerchief on the floor with the prism on it and instead of sitting in the chair, stand or lean leisurely against a wall and just look into the prism for 5 minutes. If short-sighted, sit in the chair and look on the floor. In six months of practice, the prism will disappear from sight. If the prism remains invisible for say 10 seconds, which is a measure of success, continue practicing until the duration reaches 1 to 2 minutes before going over to the next step.

STEP 3

Spread the handkerchief on the table with the prism on it. Stand nearby, a foot away from the table and in that position be aware of all that can be seen other than the prism. The prism should disappear from sight yet all else around it that can be seen should remain visible at the same time. Both the standing position and the gaze are fixed. Try to get a measure of success of duration of 10 seconds and continue practicing until the duration extends to 1 or 2 minutes.

This step means that you are aware of your immediate surroundings and yet are able to maintain the inner linkages for some time. Over a period of time, this will lead to *dhyāna* even while one is engaged in one's normal daily duties. All eagerness and haste will be inherently self-defeating—they will only create disturbances in the thinking instrument. The use of the prism is now over for it has served its purpose by teaching us a method. One can proceed to steps 4 and 5.

In ancient times, the teachers used clear water as a neutral object and the prism is only its modern substitute. Sūtra I.35 introduces the exercise for Upgrading of Awareness.

The prism practices (steps 1 to 3) are meant collectively as a method to make direct perception a controlled process. This method is a form of concentration that disengages the mind consciously so that the selected object is perceived directly, and thus, the level of awareness is elevated. Sūtra II.54 says "in *pratyāhāra*, even though the flow of sense impulses continues, the thinking instrument is withdrawn away from them." In the prism exercise, one achieves this by simply "looking" at that neutral object by suspending its perception. When the practice is correct, the thinking instrument and the individual mind would part ways; and the moment this happens the prism disappears.

No sooner does the individual mind separate or detach from the thinking instrument than the catalytic effect of the individual mind ceases, and the thinking instrument by itself is powerless to form a single thought. When the thinking instrument is humbled against its belief that it is the source of all thoughts, then as Sūtra II.55 says, "there follows the complete subjugation of the sense organs." Instead of forcibly reining in the sense organs it is easier to snap the link between sensing and thinking to make the sense organs redundant.

Sūtra II.25 explains the next step, and how to bring about "liberation" through total non-association with the things perceived. A total non-association is possible only when the memory itself is bypassed. Sūtra III.12 shows one-pointedness that is achieved through a perfect balance between the mind control and the controlling factor. What is the controlling factor? It is maintaining the individual mind as just a catalyst. In the present practice, the prism plays the part of the catalyst. What is mind control? It is the very art and practice of merely looking at the run of thoughts. At the exact point at which 1) mind control and 2) the controlling factor are balanced, the prism disappears. This is an experience of *pratyāhāra*.

In each step, holding the "disappearance of the prism" for 10 seconds is mentioned as a measure of success. Because, as explained in Sūtra III.1, it is during such time that one's will takes over and the thinking instrument's experience of the object (prism) turns subjective. This is one-pointedness, *dhāranā.* As in step 3, the mind withdraws itself from the rest of the peripheral world and lets the train of thoughts entirely devote to a particular object. The effect of this concentration is for the seeker to slowly recede from "form" awareness into "life" awareness. In this effort, she/he turns inwards. The objective essence turns subjective. The disappearance of the prism also makes one aware of the underlying process of a willed direct perception by calming the instrument, as explained in Sūtra III.15. Practices using a prism only introduce the seeker to the idea of non-attachment and concentration. But it is important. Otherwise you take a much longer time even to realize intellectually that knowing is possible without mind's control. This also helps you come in direct contact with your astral self. As explained in Sūtra II.17, it removes your illusion that "the Perceiver and that which is perceived is one and the same." Again this is a fundamental transformation. Otherwise, rooted in the "I"-centric world it is impossible to see anything else.

Most students are eager to have the prism disappear "ASAP." The disappearance has to happen only to indicate that you have done your part well in disregarding the flow of thoughts. After *pratyāhāra* and *dharana*, Steps 4 and 5 show a glimpse of *dhyāna* leading to *samādhi*).

STEP 4

Stand 3 feet from a window and look out of it. What you see outside the window is one picture, what you see of the room is another picture. Now continue to just look (not stare) out of the window till you see nothing—the view disappears completely and it will be like seeing the sky.

In the initial stages the room picture may also disappear, but you must remain aware of it. It may also happen that either of the pictures will disappear and come into view again. The window picture must disappear and the room picture be clearly seen at the same time. Get a measure of success of duration of 20 seconds and continue practicing until the duration extends to 1 or 2 minutes.

STEP 5

Walk on a footpath. Look in front of you and walk as if you are walking through a narrow passage 4 feet wide and 8 feet high (more or less) which is visible in front of you. The rest is like sky all around—it must disappear totally from your vision, yet all life in the passage in front of you for say 150 feet be clearly seen. Get a measure of success with the duration of 30 seconds and continue practicing until the duration extends to 1 or 2 minutes.

When you are through with all the five steps and have honestly succeeded in getting a measure of success with each, your thinking instrument will be finely tuned, well-trained, capable of forming and maintaining inner linkages. Your awareness would be refined and upgraded and made penetrative.

A flow from Infinite Mind via the catalyst, individual mind, to the thinking instrument is one single process—there is neither differentiation nor interference. This is perception proper or a constant meditative attitude.

Appendix 3: *Chakras* – Energy Centers Of Transformation

Chakras are psychic centers. Just as a painting cannot be described from the standpoint of lines and curves or varying shades of paints—even though these can be said to form the basic structure of a painting—similarly, *chakras* cannot be described in terms of psychology, physiology or any other physical science. *Chakras* are centers of activity of subtle, vital force termed *sūkshma prāṇa*; they are inter-related with the parasympathetic, sympathetic and autonomous nervous systems and thus the gross body is related to them.

Chakra is a Sanskrit word that denotes circle and movement. Because everything in the body is of a circular shape and is constantly in movement, the centers of those movements are called chakras. *Chakra* is a word also used for "wheel." In discussing chakras we are necessarily discussing the subtle aspects of these centers. Nerves are merely vehicles, but the message they carry is subtle and is not devoid of consciousness or self-consciousness.

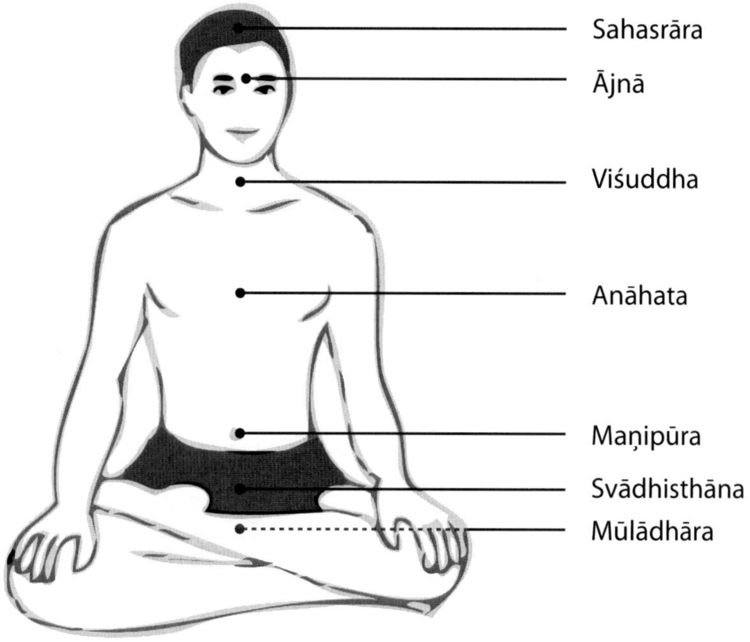

Location of the Chakras.

Seven main chakras are:

Chakra	Literal Meaning	Location
Mūlādhāra	Foundation	Pelvic Plexus; region between anus and genitals; the base of the spine
Svādhisthāna	Dwelling place of the self	Hypogastric plexus; genitals
Maṇipūra	City of gems	Solar plexus; epigastric plexus; navel
Anāhata	Unstricken	Cardiac plexus; the heart
Viśuddha	Pure	Carotid plexus; throat
Ajna	Authority; command	Medula plexus; pineal plexus; point between the eyebrows
Sahasrāra	Thousand-petaled;	Top of the cranium; cerebral plexus;

(Excerpts from *Chakras, Energy Centers of Transformation,* by Harish Johari, Inner Traditions India, 1987.)

Pre-dominant Sense	Sense Organ	Work Organ	Vayu (air)
Smell	Nose	Anus	*Apāna*- air that expels the semen; urine from both sexes; that which pushes the child from the womb
Taste	Tongue	Genitals	*Apāna* (same as above)
Sight	Eyes	Feet and legs	*Samān* – dwelling in the upper abdomen helping the digestive system; produces essence of food, assimilates and carries to the whole body
Touch	Skin	Hands	*Prāṇa* – dwelling in the chest; air that we breathe; rich with life-giving negative ions
Hearing	Ears	Mouth (vocal cords)	*Udāna* – dwells in the throat; carries air up to the head helping production of sound

Appendix 4: How Do The Refining Exercises Work?

Many disciples of Shri Tavariaji have created a website *http://3srb.org/refining-exercises.html* where detailed guidance is available about the refining exercises using a particular method of breathing called, 3-Step Rhythmic Breathing (3SRB). In this Appendix we will address how such exercises work.

The subtle body sustains itself on fine energies or *prāṇa*. That is why negative emotions can create blocks (*granthī*) that act like knots in the smooth flow of subtle energies. The negative emotions also contaminate energy. *Granthī* are the main obstacles to Rhythmic Breathing because they act as deeply embedded negative patterns that keep repeating in our reflex actions. The *granthī* form at certain specific places in the subtle bodies that are connected with energy centers or nerve plexuses (*chakra*) affecting the corresponding physical area and induce diseases.

In our effort to synchronize the physical with the subtle, these *granthīs* must be removed or dissolved. The quality of *prāṇa* must be upgraded, and *chakras* must be able to work in a steady rhythm, at the right speed, and to produce the correct amounts of fine energies. The *chakras*, with their upgraded energies, should become the primary factor promoting the proper functions of the physical body. When this happens, the subtle body becomes the primary body in the real sense.

Each refining exercise involves a particular area of the physical body, and this area in turn is connected to a *granthī* and plexuses (*chakras*) at the subtle level. So when the *granthī* and the emotional debris is cleared at a particular area, only then can the fine energies relevant to that area be upgraded.

The refining exercises are performed at a certain rhythm that is faster than the normal rate of breathing, for a threefold effect:

- The rapid rhythm shakes up and dissolves the *granthī.*
- The high rhythm extracts higher energies or *prāṇa* from the environment.
- The rhythm is transmitted as waves to activate the subtle body functions.

Apart from the faster rhythmic breathing, many practitioners perform *naḍī shodhana, kapālbhātī prāṇāyāma, bhastrikā prāṇāyāma, ujjayī prāṇāyāma* etc., as very effective refining exercises.

Stages in a Seeker's psycho-physical transformation

To become	Energies				Impulses travel thru "radi"	Thalamus	Impulses flowover	The flow	Flushed out at "ajna"	Prominent thinking instrument	Seed atoms active	Knowledge	Chakra activated	Hypothesis
	Prana (the life force)	Essence of Consciousness	Will	Awareness										
Seeker	3rd grade	Crude	Neutral	self (Physical)	Ida & Pingala	Open	Top of the brain	Ends in Thought formation	Tamasic Thoughts	Brain	P1	Thought-based	Muladhara & Swadhisthana	Spiritual Self exists
Disciple	2nd grade	Little refined	Emotional	Emotional Intelligence	Ida & Pingala	Open	Top of the brain	Ends in Thought formation	Rajasic Thoughts	Manas	P1	Refined thought-based	Manipura	Mind unfolds as matter
Yogi	1st grade	Refined	Intellectual	Spiritual Intelligence	Ida & Pingala	Open	Top of the brain	Ends in Thought formation	Sattvic Thoughts	Buddhi	P1	Insightful	Anahata & Vishuddha	Composition of matter is size invariant
Mahayogi	Connects with Universal Mind	Connects with Consciousness at Bindu	Spiritual (merges into Consciousness)	Self (merges into Consciousness)	Sushumna	Close	Side passages of the brain	Bindu → Sahasrara → Ajna	Sattvic Manas with impulses "as-is"		P1 + A2	Intuitive	Bindu & sahasrara	Ishvara is a perceivable version of Purusha, the Spirit
Yoga Master	Pure prana (Universal Mind) - Prakṛtī	Purūṣa (Pure consciousness)					No impulses enter the system	Prana rotation: From Muladhara to Ajna → Sahasrara → Bindu → Sahasrara → down back to Muladhara	Nothing		P1 + A2 + M3	Instant		Universe is Purusha seen through screens of time, space and causation

Appendix 5: Grooming The Master

Part I: Chakras *below the diaphragm,* Karma-Yoga

SŪTRA 5.1.23/III.25

Concentrated meditation on *mūladhāra chakra* will awaken great force and light.

In the fifth practice of upgrading awareness, one can choose to be conscious of one field of knowledge and consciously fade out other fields. That ability enables a *mahāyogī* to direct *saṃyama* (concentrated meditation) to the *mūladhāra* center (in the region of the perineum) and consciously fade out the remainder of the body. This also concentrates *prāṇa* energy at *mūladhāra* and can be rotated in a particular manner and in a particular rhythm.

The centers are only symbolically indicated in the sūtra, and that has misled many. It is often overlooked that *Yoga-Sūtra* is a scientific manual. The use of symbols is to protect an ill-prepared or erring aspirants from unwittingly exposing themselves to dangers. For example, an elephant symbolizes the base of a structure, the *mūladhāra chakra* where tremendous energy remains hidden. Similarly, "light" stands for wisdom, just as elephant represents wisdom.

Many interpreters have seen this and other sūtras too figuratively, thus assuring readers that one can gain animal powers. (Example: *"Through concentration over strength, one attains to the strength of an elephant, etc."* M.R. Yardi, 216). A few other interpreters, burdened by the enormity of the endeavor, have tried to oversimplify or gloss over it and have robbed Yoga of its robust "no-nonsense" character. *("The example of the elephant is likely symbolic to represent the scale of power that is attainable through the use of* sañyama *directed at the ability of our choice—physical, causal, moral, psychic, or spiritual."* —Dennis Hill, *Yoga Sūtras,* 56*)*.

Guṇa, the way energy manifests in the objective world, is the last frontier. Only when a *mahāyogī* is able to direct his refined energy of will and consciousness to the sub-atomic level can he address *guṇa*. The aim is to bring about equilibrium of *guṇa* in order to be able to transcend it. A *mahāyogī* ha s so far been able to perceive at the atomic level; now it is time to work on it, since at *mūladhāra* the energy is created through a process of fusion.

SŪTRA 5.1.24/III.26

Perfectly concentrated meditation on the *swādhisthāna chakra* (at the base of the reproductive organs) will produce the pure awareness of that which is subtle, hidden, and remote.

The emphasis here is on awakening wisdom. When the light of wisdom is generated with a continuous practice it will bring about a link with the inner consciousness through the energy of consciousness of the first grade. This means one becomes aware of things more subtle, previously unseen, unfelt, hidden, or remote—one's vision is not obstructed now by any object or thing, physical or subtle.

An important aspect of these practices is that a *mahāyogī* is able to see the inside of the body and to locate the energy centers to manipulate. It is not a mere approximate visualization based on book knowledge. A *mahāyogī* actually *sees* the physical area as well as the parallel area in the (now) primary subtle body. Again, just like in the earlier sūtra, *prāṇa* will be first concentrated at the *swādhisthāna* center and then rotated in a particular manner.

Again, at *swādhisthāna*, the energy is created through the process of fission.

SŪTRA 5.1.25/III.26

Through meditation, with fixed concentration upon the sun, will come a consciousness (or knowledge) of the seven worlds.

A reference to "sun" here is to *swādhisthāna*. Here, both *mūladhāra* and *swādhisthāna* centers are involved. There is a rotation-cum-circulation movement between the two.

The natural circulation of *prāṇa* between these two *chakras* (*mūladhāra* and *swādhisthānaa*) begins at birth (i.e., with the first breath) and continues throughout life. But in our adult life, it is not proper and rhythmic, and needs correction just as the breathing apparatus does. There is a certain method for this circulation, which runs in a figure eight. On this circulation depends the continuous production of

- the energies of life and awareness
- the energy of the essence of consciousness
- the will.

With this accomplished, a *mahāyogī* can see all the seven sub-stages of *Bhūh*, the physical universe, and know and understand them.

SŪTRA 5.1.26/III.28

Knowledge of all lunar forms arises through focused meditation on the moon.

SŪTRA 5.1.27/III.30

By concentrated meditation upon the solar plexus, comes perfect knowledge as to the condition of the body.

These two sūtras need to be taken together. The moon has totally negative vibrations. It corresponds with the totally negative solar plexus (*maṇipūra chakra*) in the physical and the parallel primary body. Right from our most primitive days on this planet, this area has been a repository and guiding factor of animal instincts. Fear and doubt have ruled supreme here.

The solar plexus is thus a massive area full of animal memory and memories of bitter events. It needs cleansing. It is in the nature of the moon, as perceived, to be negative and constantly changing. It is thought that on the upward arc of involution present-day humanity is at the middle sub-stage of awareness of the physical world, *Bhūh*. In the earlier sub-stages and during the evolution, humanity has survived mainly on animal instincts. Now, the hostile conditions of living are fast evaporating, yet the legacy of the animal instincts persists. It is reflected in today's aggressive lifestyles of individuals, communities, and nations. The veiled ferociousness in political, religious and other divisive stances is entirely irrelevant now, but it erupts from the dreadful memory stored in the solar plexus region.

For an individual, fear is clearly expressed here (not in the heart or the brain). If not cleansed properly, it will continue time and again to distract attention during every type of practice. Only when totally cleansed can physical, psychic (emotional) and causal health be experienced. Again, by focused meditation, a *mahāyogī* can know the status of another individual's fears and doubts, so that he can help and guide them. Here, too, the process is the same—location of *prāṇa* energy through concentrated meditation and then rotation of *prāṇa* in a certain manner.

Part II: **Chakras** *above the diaphragm,* **Bhakti-Yoga**

SŪTRA 5.1.28/III.29

Concentration upon the Pole Star will give knowledge of the orbits of the planets and the stars.

SŪTRA 5.1.29/III.35

Understanding of the mind-awareness comes from focused meditation upon the heart center.

Again, these two sutras are to be taken together. The pole star is an important landmark in the cosmos due to its stable position. But

Sage Pātañjali uses the word "Dhruva" as a symbol of a great saint who by his great devotion was able to perform many miracles. Devotion arises in the heart (*anāhata chakra*).

So, focused concentration on the *anāhata chakra* is directed to regenerate it. Ordinarily, it has positive and negative half-centers that are corrected by rotating *prāṇa* in a certain manner, making it one positive center.

SŪTRA 5.2.1/III.31

By fixing the attention on the throat-well center, cessation of hunger and thirst will ensue.

SŪTRA 5.2.2/III.32

By fixing the attention upon the tube or nerve below the throat center, equilibrium is achieved.

In these two sūtras, to be taken together, the *viśuddhī* center is denoted. Like *anāhata*, it is partially negative and partially positive. Focused practice in this area slowly converts it to wholly positive. The throat center is very significant. The throat is a passage of all food and drink. Hence, focused practice on the *viśuddhī chakra* brings a lessening of hunger and thirst at first, and then a complete cessation. The esophagus tube plays an important part. As *prāṇa* rises from *anāhata* to *viśuddhī* centers, it passes through this tube and helps achieve a balance of qualities.

Sage Pātañjali differentiates between the *viśuddhī chakra* and the whole tube (the esophagus) in the throat leading to the stomach. The throat-well center is the posterior-negative half, and the nerve below is the anterior-positive half. When *prāṇa* rises to *viśuddhī* through this tube, a balance of *guṇa* is achieved. The "equilibrium" mentioned is both physical and nerve-related, but more particularly, it refers to the balance and rhythm of the *guṇa*, because we are on the way to reaching the head centers.

Taluka, at the base of the skull, is not a center in the sense of the whirling power points that the *chakras* are. But it plays a very important part in opening and closing like a valve, thus routing the sense impulses. For the practices mentioned here to be carried out effectively, it is important for a *mahāyogī* to be able to consciously open and close *Taluka* in tandem. Reasonable attention to this is needed before moving to the next *sūtra*.

Part III: Chakras *in the head,* Raja-Yoga

SŪTRA 5.2.3/III.33

Those who have attained self-mastery can be seen and contacted through focusing on light in the head. This power is developed in focused meditation.

A symbolic, unflickering, black flame representing *Īśvara* should be constantly visualized at the center of the forehead. Then we are shown by Sage Pātañjali how to direct and then to rotate *prāṇa* at *sahasrāra, bindu*, and *ajna*. A *yogī* functions at the level of pure awareness when *prāṇa* is directed in the brain centers, especially *bindu* and *ajna*. By using *taluka* as an "open-close" valve, one can stop the flow of incoming impulses during the practices.

Sahasrāra chakra, in the region of the thalamus, is indeed very important, because here the upward journey of *prāṇa* ends. This is a wholly negative *chakra*. But unlike *maṇipūra*, which had animal instincts embedded in it, this center can release great power that opens many regions not known on the three planes. Once proper practice is established, such profuse light pours down that even a supernova is dim by comparison.

An intense *dhāraṇā* or *dhyāna* on this center yields a complete dissolution of the sense of one's body, and one is instantly transported to sub-stage 6 or 7 of *Bhūh*. Of course, this is a virtual journey and not a real one that involves movement. This is both fantastic and dangerous. If not prepared and supported by proper guidance, a *mahāyogī* can lose balance, fall down unconscious, and even inflict some internal damage to his body and brain.

There is another very subtle danger. Through focused meditation, contact may be established with other Yoga masters who are more advanced in their journey. It is a land of the mighty and powerful spiritual giants. A *mahāyogī* may get tempted to accept one of them as a guru and lose contact with *Īśvara*. So *sahasrāra* is to be approached carefully. Even at such an advanced stage, one can get enthralled and attached to this center; an attachment not easy to break away from.

Essentially at this stage, a *mahāyogī* is not just aware of the light in the head, but has developed an ability to use it consciously and direct it to illuminate whatever is to be understood.

SŪTRA 5.2.4/III.34

All things can be known in the vivid light of intuition.

Bindu is two fingers in front of *sahasrāra* and very safe. Sage Patānjali is indirectly pointing to *Bindu*, because one only learns more about this through a direct teacher-student relationship. It is the soul's abode during the wakeful state. The vivid light of intuition is the light of *Īśvara*, exceedingly different than the light seen as an object in the objective world. The intuition is more in the form of divine perception and not a mere creative instinct. A divine perception is a prerequisite to performing *Saṃyama* . It is necessary that any trace of ego is gone, so that the differentiating duality would not exist.

For a *mahāyogī*, the rational thinking processes based on the theoretical and hypothetical knowledge still continue. But it is instantly backed up by the discriminating knowledge that brings home an awareness of the pairs of opposites. And even this is instantly dealt with by intuitive understanding of pure awareness. Thus, the thinking processes on all the planes are aligned and guided by the intuitive knowledge.

Prāṇa Rotation

From *mūladhāra* to *sahasrāra*, *prāṇa* rises up, but the pathway is not complete yet. Then *prāṇa* is directed to two positive half sections in the brain proper, *bindū* and *ājnā* (at the center of the forehead just above the meeting point of the eyebrows) in that order, in commencement of the downward journey. The entire remaining pathway is completed by directing *prāṇa* from *ājnā* to *viśuddhī* to *anāhata* to *kundali* (which is the positive half section of *maṇipūra*), and finally back to the loop of *swādhisthāna* and *mūladhāra.*

Part IV: Regenerating prāṇa and vāyū

Now Sage Pātañjali brings us to the subtlest elements: air and sound. We know that the internal *prāṇa* stays connected with *prāṇa,* the cosmic energy. *Prāṇa* pulsates in the universe as the cosmic impulses, the omnipresent life energy that is found everywhere in a free state as well as in conditioned states within and around all the objective forms.

My guru tells us:

The 1st grade (purest) prāṇa *is beyond Existence and thus beyond the Universal Mind. The Universal Mind itself is the 2nd grade of* prāṇa *(and the first basic element of matter,* ākāśa*). The 3rd grade of* prāṇa, *in varying degrees of potency, is found in the causal world (air). The 4th grade of* prāṇa *is found in the astral world (fire). The 5th grade is found in the physical world (water), mostly in humans. The 6th grade is found in the animal kingdom (earth). The 7th grade is found in the vegetable kingdom. (The distinction is not fine and there are crossovers).*—S.N. Tavaria

When matter forms, it envelops *prāṇa*. The trapped *prāṇa* in any form degenerates and becomes five *vāyū*:

Prāṇa - "Forward-moving", propulsive motion

Apāna – "Moves away", downward, outward

Udāna – "Moves up", upward, transformative

Samāna – "Balancing", from periphery to the center

Vyāna – "Outward moving", from center to periphery

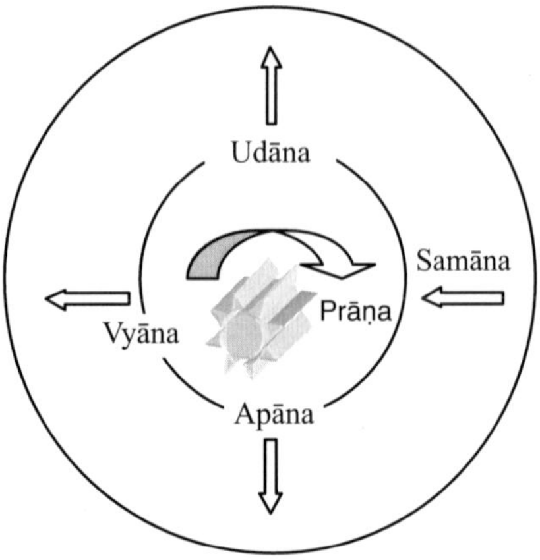

Prāṇa, literally the "forward moving *vāyū*," moves inward and governs reception of all types—from the eating of food, drinking of water, and inhalation of air, to the reception of sensory impressions and mental experiences. It is propulsive in nature, setting things in motion and guiding them. It provides the basic energy that drives us in life. *Prāṇa vāyū* governs the movement of energy from the head down to the navel, which is the *prāṇic* center in the physical body.

Apāna, literally the "*vāyū* that moves away," moves downward and outward and governs all forms of elimination and reproduction (which also has a downward movement). It governs the elimination of the stool and the urine, the expelling of semen, menstrual fluid and the fetus, and the elimination of carbon dioxide through the breath. On a deeper level it rules the elimination of negative sensory, emotional and mental experiences. It is the basis of our immune function on all levels. *Apāna vāyū* governs the movement of energy from the navel down to the root chakra.

Udāna, literally the "upward moving *vāyū*," moves upward and brings about qualitative or transformative movements of the life-energy. It governs growth of the body, the ability to stand, speech, effort, enthusiasm and will. It is our main positive energy in life through which we can develop our different bodies and evolve in consciousness. *Udāna* governs the movement of energy from the navel up to the head.

Samāna, literally the "balancing *vāyū*," moves from the periphery to the center, through a churning and discerning action. It aids in digestion on all levels. It works in the gastrointestinal tract to digest food, in the lungs to digest air or absorb oxygen, and in the mind to homogenize and digest experiences, whether sensory, emotional or mental. *Samāna vāyū* governs the movement of energy from the entire body back to the navel.

Vyāna, literally the "outward moving *vāyū*," moves from the center to the periphery. It governs circulation on all levels. It moves the food, water and oxygen throughout the body, and keeps our emotions and thoughts circulating in the mind, imparting movement and providing strength. In doing so it assists all the other *prāṇas* in their work. *Vyāna vāyū* governs the movement of energy out from the navel throughout the entire body.

Yoga practices of rhythmic breathing are aimed at restoring and strengthening the *prāṇa* metabolism and enabling the regeneration of *vāyū* into higher grades of *prāṇa.* The potency of *ākāśa* or the nucleus of each atom is thus upgraded, which brings about inner mutation. This is the safest and the most direct genetic-engineering exercise done in the lab of a human being.

Vāyū regenerate and aid spiritual progress, and their respective functions are also performed better on the astro-physical levels. *Prāṇa* directed in the area above the *viśuddhī* center refines *udāna vāyū* to the *prāṇa* state. Likewise, *Samāna vāyū* links *viśuddhī* to the *maṇipūra* centers, which will transform the symbolic flame into a roaring fire.

Through Yoga practices and breathing exercises, a *mahāyogī* learns to regenerate *vāyū* into refined, higher grades of *prāṇa*. Ordinarily, one knows only gastric gases but is not aware of *vāyū* that occupy spaces inside our flesh-bones package and carry out assigned tasks. This is what fosters inner mutation. There are five *vāyū*: *prāṇa, udāna, samāna, apāna*, and *vyāna.* Important for Yoga practice are the first three, because they have corresponding centers in the brain and along the *chakra*.

SŪTRA 5.2.9/III.40 (CONTROL OF *UDĀNA VĀYŪ*)

The sūtras in parts I to III, are instructions in practices related to various *chakras*, the psychic centers, from *mūladhāra* to *sahasrāra*. However, these are subtle centers, and the *prāṇa* rotations in them can stabilize only when there are no disturbances. *Vāyū*, the degenerated vital airs in the body, cause modifications and disturbs the *chakras*. Hence, subjugation of the *vāyū* must be explained.

Prāṇa pervades the whole body and is the principal cause of projection of the senses outward. The astral body is constituted of energy forces that use *prāṇa* as a source. Ordinarily, *prāṇa* in one's body is contaminated. Through rhythmic breathing, the air breathed in and out is synchronized with the *prāṇa* circulation, which purifies it.

When *prāṇa* intake is directed to the various force centers in the brain and along the *chakras*, their accelerated action sends impulses that rise up to the cavity of the brain. When refined *udāna vāyū* becomes potential *prāṇa*, it prevails between the nose and the top of the head covering the physical brain, the eyes, and the nose. It also covers the area around the *anāhata, viśuddhī, sahasrāra* and *bindu chakras*. When a *mahāyogī* begins *prāṇa* rotation at these *chakras*, focused attention is also directed to *udāna vāyū* so that it regenerates and helps in stabilizing the *prāṇa* practices.

When the refined *udāna* reaches the higher centers of the brain, spiritual will develops at the loop of *mūladhāra* and *swādhisthāna* for achieving perfection in Yoga. The parasympathetic system, which is more or less dormant, is fully activated, and the sympathetic system is greatly refined. The rhythmic movements activate the medulla oblongata, drive away lethargy of mind, discord, and ailments in the body, and cleanse the lower psychic nature. It becomes a dependable shield against fear and doubt, the worst enemies of humankind, by totally cleansing the *maṇipūra* chakra.

Sage Pātañjali tells us that "by subjugation of *udāna vāyū* there is liberation from drowning in water, the thorny path and *karma* (mire), and the power of ascension is gained." The powers like levitation and acting against gravity are to be taken as symbolic. From a material standpoint, they may seem dazzling, if not impossible, but at such an advanced stage on the *yogīk* path, they are insignificant. Water, thorns, and the mire are the remnants of the physical domain, and by activating and stabilizing consciousness in the higher *chakras* like *sahasrāra* and *bindu*, a *mahāyogī* is ready for "ascension" away from them into the realm of Saṃyama without seed. Now conscious out-of-body experiences are possible.

SŪTRA 5.2.10/III.41 (CONTROL OF *SAMĀNA VĀYŪ*)

A *mahāyogī* now understands how the inner subtle bodies literally illuminate and enable one to "see" and direct focused concentration to them. The illumination radiates through the whole persona, and though this real spiritual advancement is discerned only by another clairvoyant, the glow is unmistakable even to the ordinary eyes.

Samāna vāyū extends from the heart down to the solar plexus covering the *anāhata* and *maṇipūra* chakra. This ordinarily takes care of the areas of digestion and sex. Now the metabolism (food as well as thoughts) is purified, and from the biological-evolution point of view, the regenerated cells are produced all over the body. The regenerated *vāyūs* also do not stay trapped in various compartments of the body, and gradually merge.

Two sparks arise nearly simultaneously at birth, one with the first breath and the second with the divine fragment entering the physical body as the soul. They trigger a ceaseless series of sparks through the fusion and fission processes at *mūladhāra* and *swādhisthāna* chakra, respectively. With focused concentration on these chakras, as seen earlier, their energy-generating processes are purified. Refined *samāna vāyū* links *maṇipūra* to *viśuddhī* chakra. Now, with focused concentration on *samāna vāyū*, the "sparks rise up to become a flame." Sexual desire is not only sublimated, but the sex energy rises to energize the higher centers.

Now blessed with a fleeting experience of *Īśvara*, a *mahāyogī* is no longer required to see *Īśvara* symbolically as a black flame at the third eye. The final grace is just around the corner.

Phases in a Seeker's Transformation into a Yoga Master

1. A Seeker and the Thinking Process

The whole physical body is a sense organ for receiving "touch" vibrations and the astral body an electro-magnetic receptor to the environment for capturing passive vibrations of other people's thoughts. These vibrations are transmitted linearly, via brainstem, into the brain by a web of nerves, around the spinal cord forming the channels, *Idā* and *Pingalā.* While the lower part of brainstem, medulla oblongata, controls autonomous functions of heart, blood pressure and breathing, the upper part receives and organizes brain's instructions to the organs of action.

The sensory pathways pass through a valve called *taluka, to* deliver the impulses to thalamus that acts as a gatekeeper. Simultaneously, other senses reach the brain too—"sight" reaches the occipital lobe and "smell," "taste" and "sound" reach the temporal lobe. These lobes are also storehouses of long-term memory containing the individual's predispositions and tons of stored images. During the pass-by, the sense impulses tag on to those images that closely resemble them and to the associated emotional imprints. Together they create patterns congruent with our comfort zone to feed into the thoughts. This activates hypothalamus and transmits the now subtle vibrations to *mānas.*

But not everything gets handed over to *mānas*. Our predispositions consider no need for "thinking" about the most familiar patterns and pass them to cerebellum for generating a reflex response. Medulla oblongata, the expert in "automation" then relays signals to the organs of action. The remaining impulses immersed heavily in the physical aspects of things, get carried by *mānas* through the parietal lobe as the sentimental (not yet matured into emotional) imprints now build their respective component of a thought. Finally, the "thought-in-process" gets into the frontal lobe where *buddhī* churns it with reference to the pairs of opposites. Here, an "in-process" thought gets tossed to and fro memory and between the dilemma of the opposites, as cognition is reasoned out or inferred. Such highly filtered and colored cognition both results from and contributes to the "individual" reality.

This also results in our incremental learning. The "delta or variance" between the impulses and the known patterns becomes incremental knowledge that is lodged back into the long-term memory as newly known pattern. Besides the physical, emotional and intellectual composition of a thought, this delta is the fourth component. If it is too large, the thought process is abandoned resulting in no new cognition and if it is too small the thought process is substituted by a reflex response. Your ability to deal with larger delta is instrumental in expanding and deepening awareness. Later, when you explore the unknown and unseen subtle world you have to get rid of the predispositions and hoarded memory to let the learning happen.

While bulk of the thoughts are *tāmasik* and get released in a coded form from *ajna*, the charged thoughts carrying energy are delivered to the organs of action.

At this stage, the *prāṇa* sheath carries energy of the lowest, 3rd grade. *Mūlādhāra* and *swādhisthāna chakrās* are slightly active; but the energy of essence of consciousness is crude, as awareness is locked up in the physical body and the resultant will is neutral. Thoughts are predominantly *tāmasic* (sexual/ physical.)

But by the end of this phase, you would have witnessed enough signs of the "existence of spiritual Self" to become devoted to the pursuit of truth (not of mere happiness) and become a *sādhaka* (seeker.)

In the diagram, mind is represented by the predispositions and the long-term memory patterns. Thus mind invests its energy in actively driving the impulses and overloading them with sentimental baggage. The mind-driven impulse processing and thought generation take the route: 1 → 2 → 3 → 4 → 5 → 6 → 7.

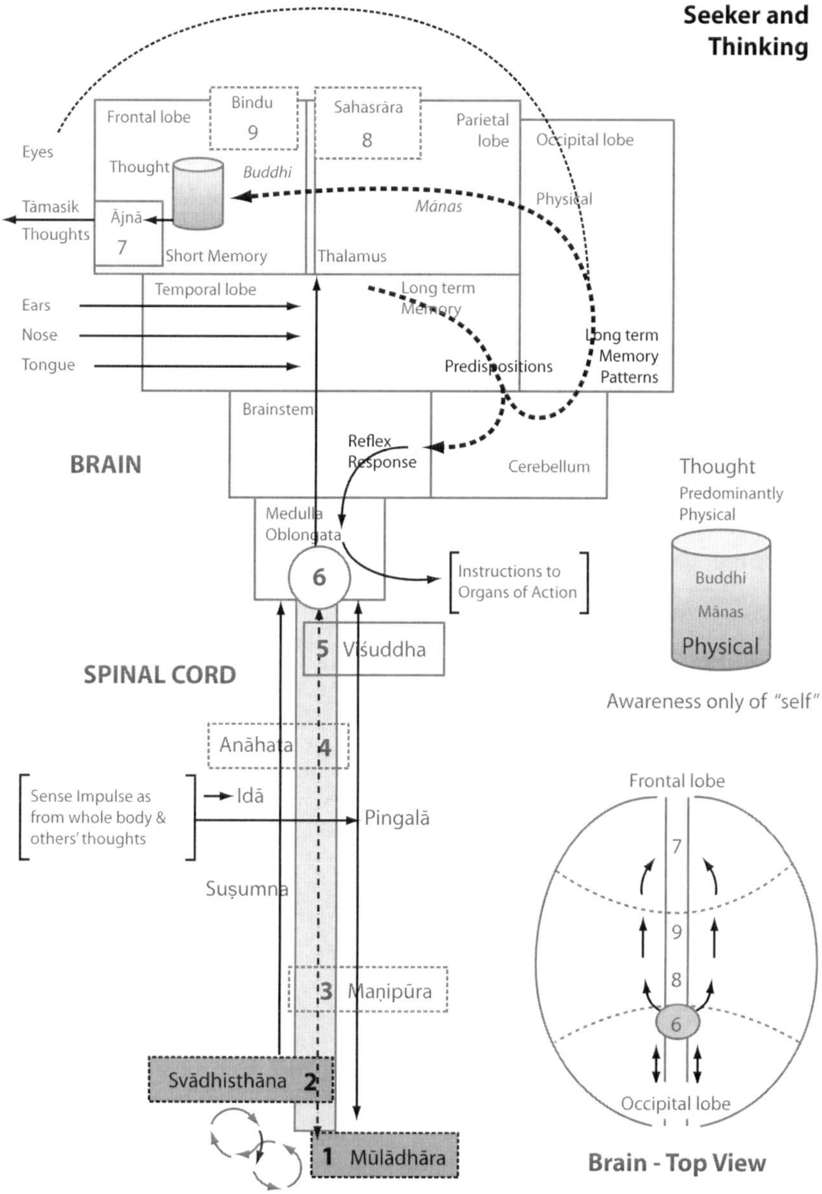
Seeker and Thinking
Eyes
Frontal lobe
Bindu
9
Sahasrāra
8
Parietal lobe
Occipital lobe
Thought
Buddhi
Tāmasik Thoughts
Ājnā
7
Mānas
Physical
Short Memory
Thalamus
Temporal lobe
Long term Memory
Ears
Nose
Tongue
Long term Memory Patterns
Predispositions
Brainstem
Reflex Response
BRAIN
Cerebellum
Medulla Oblongata
6
Instructions to Organs of Action
SPINAL CORD
5 Viśuddha
Anāhata 4
Sense Impulse as from whole body & others' thoughts
Idā
Pingalā
Suṣumna
3 Maṇipūra
Svādhisthāna 2
1 Mūlādhāra
Thought
Predominantly Physical
Buddhi
Mānas
Physical
Awareness only of "self"
Frontal lobe
7
9
8
6
Occipital lobe
Brain - Top View

2. *Disciple and a Vision*

There is no major structural change evident yet, there are a lot of qualitative changes. Nothing much changes in the flow of impulses too.

At this stage, the *prāṇa* sheath carries more purified energy of the 2nd grade. *Mūlādhāra* and *swādhisthāna,* as well as *maṇipūra* chakrās are fully active; the energy of essence of consciousness is little refined, sentiments mature into emotions upgrading awareness to emotional intelligence of the astral body and the resultant will is emotional too. Thoughts are predominantly *rājasic.*

But by the end of this phase the seeker in you has witnessed "mind as matter and as a mother of all material objects" by studying your own mind and the thought process. In fact, you have also succeeded in slowing down the thought-making to enable a gap in thoughts which is filled with vision of *Īśvara*. The vision has changed everything and you have become a committed disciple in pursuit of the ultimate truth.

The mind-driven impulse processing and thought generation still take the same route: 1 → 2 → 3 → 4 → 5 → 6 → 7.

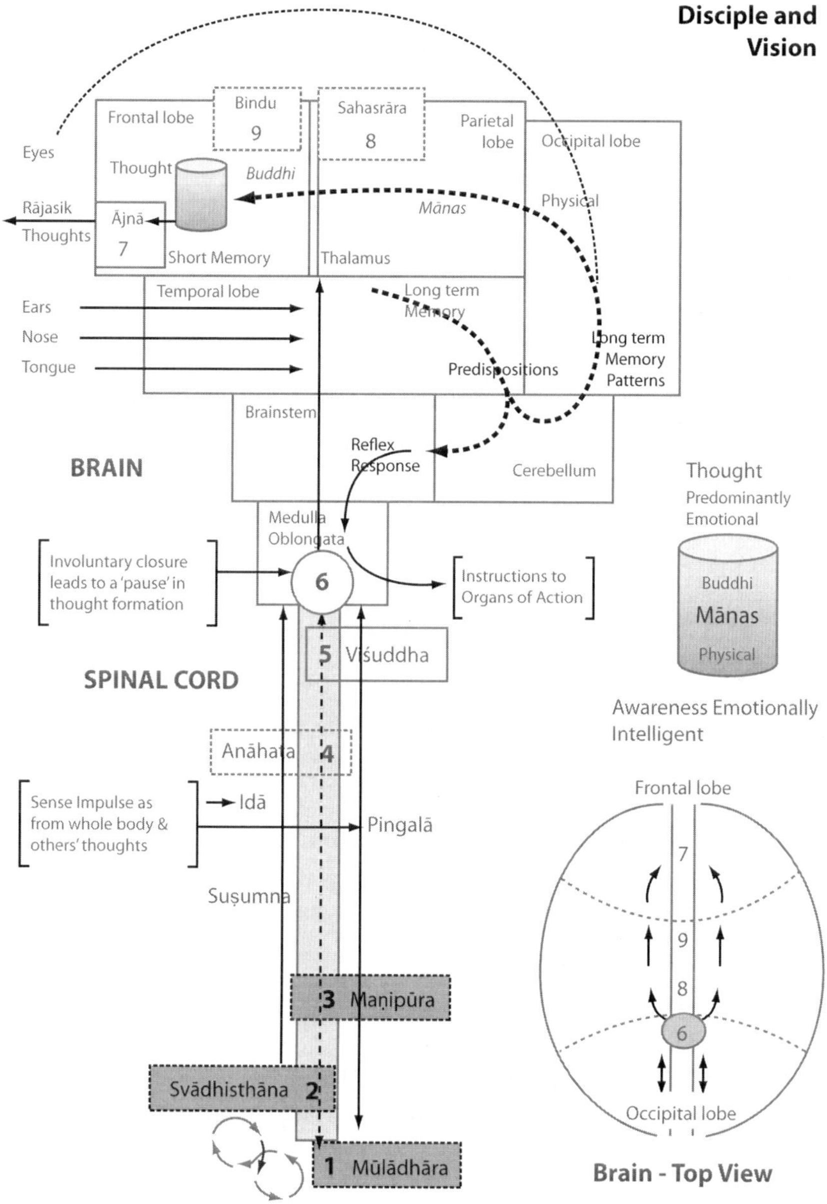
Disciple and Vision
Eyes
Frontal lobe
Bindu
9
Sahasrāra
8
Parietal lobe
Occipital lobe
Thought
Buddhi
Rājasik Thoughts
Ājnā
7
Mānas
Physical
Short Memory
Thalamus
Temporal lobe
Long term Memory
Ears
Nose
Tongue
Predispositions
Long term Memory Patterns
Brainstem
Reflex Response
Cerebellum
BRAIN
Medulla Oblongata
6
Involuntary closure leads to a 'pause' in thought formation
Instructions to Organs of Action
Thought
Predominantly Emotional
Buddhi
Mānas
Physical
5 Viśuddha
SPINAL CORD
Awareness Emotionally Intelligent
Anāhata 4
Sense Impulse as from whole body & others' thoughts
Idā
Pingalā
Frontal lobe
Suṣumna
3 Maṇipūra
Svādhisthāna 2
1 Mūlādhāra
Occipital lobe
Brain - Top View

3. Yogī *and Insight*

The qualitative improvement in the thinking process now reaches its peak as major structural changes take place. Awareness is now spiritually intelligent when the instability of emotions and their tendency to result in attachment is realized. Thought process is still the same, but the egotistic intellectualism is subjugated by the rising spiritual insight and hence, bulk of the thoughts released into the environment are now *sāttvik* in nature. Mind is not only more recognized but it stands more purified, rarified and empowered. It still remains marginally indulgent under compulsion from *karma* but readily gives in to the discriminating knowledge accruing from the spiritual experiences.

Mūlādhāra and *Swadhisthāna chakras* are fully active now, *maṇipura* is transitioning from fully negative to fully positive and the growing spiritual awareness activates *anāhata* and *viśuddhi* chakras. This energy is a combination of energies of life and awareness only but is of 1st grade now.

Though *suṣumna* is about to open it is kept consciously blocked. Both the blocks, at *taluka* and at the bottom end of *suṣumna*, open and close consciously as a two-way switch.

Now, you have developed conscious control over the vision of *Īśvara* to be able to have it at will. Having realized the "spiritual Self" a yogi can witness the same at the core of every object, from the tiniest to the massive. Thus, the third hypothesis of each object having the same multi-tiered composition has got validated and you have become a *yogi*.

The mind-driven impulse processing and thought generation take the same route: 1 → 2 → 3 → 4 → 5 → 6 → 7. However, your devoted practice of the first four means of Yoga bring you close to the break-through state of *pratyāhāra* in which you will use *suśumna* and will close the valve at *taluka* to divert the flow of impulses.

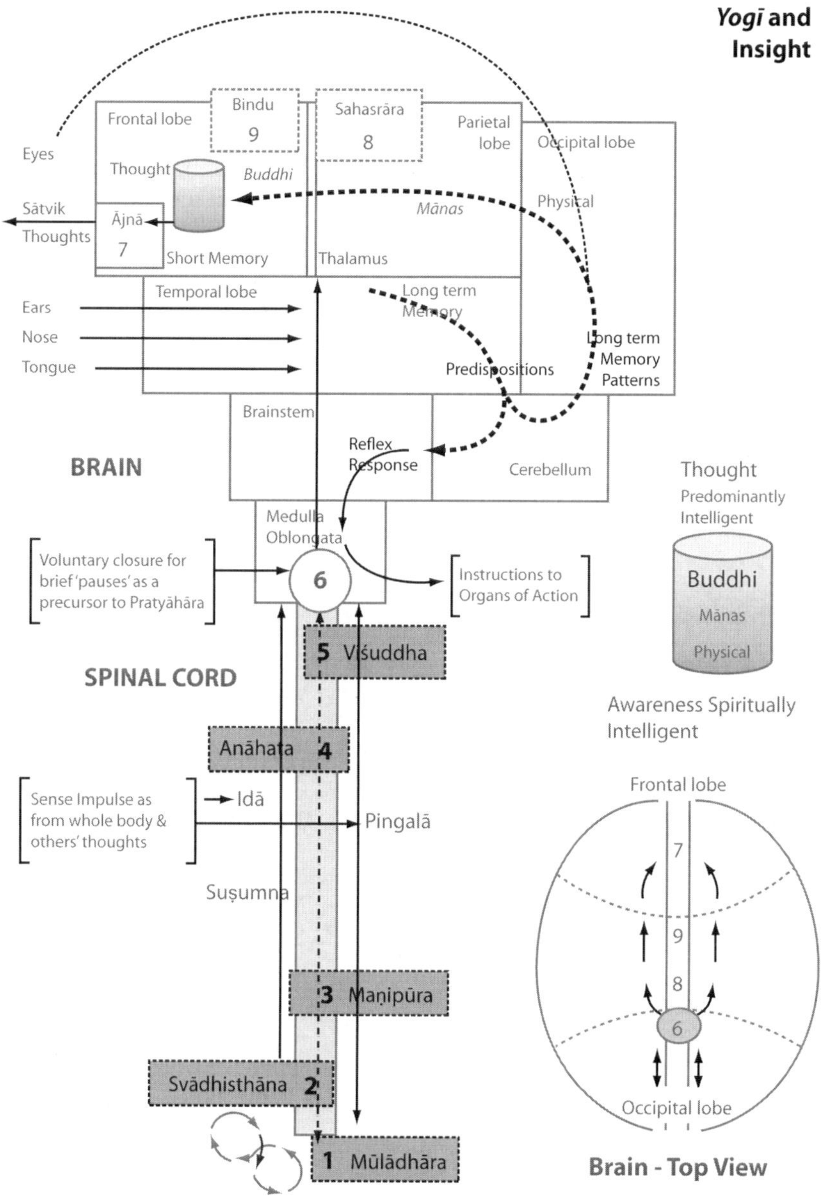
***Yogī* and Insight**
Eyes
Frontal lobe
Bindu
9
Sahasrāra
8
Parietal lobe
Occipital lobe
Thought
Buddhi
Sātvik Thoughts
Ājnā
7
Mānas
Physical
Short Memory
Thalamus
Temporal lobe
Long term Memory
Ears
Nose
Tongue
Predispositions
Long term Memory Patterns
Brainstem
Reflex Response
BRAIN
Cerebellum
Thought
Predominantly Intelligent
Medulla Oblongata
Voluntary closure for brief 'pauses' as a precursor to Pratyāhāra
6
Instructions to Organs of Action
Buddhi
Mānas
Physical
5 Viśuddha
SPINAL CORD
Awareness Spiritually Intelligent
Anāhata 4
Frontal lobe
Sense Impulse as from whole body & others' thoughts
Idā
Pingalā
Suṣumna
7
9
8
6
3 Maṇipūra
Svādhisthāna 2
Occipital lobe
1 Mūlādhāra
Brain - Top View

4. Mahāyogi *and Intuition*

This is the early stage of *pratyāhāra.* The intended bio-physical changes and purification and activation of chakras is almost complete with *bindu* and *sahasrāra* now active. *Mahāyogi* can close *taluka* to block impulses entering into the long term memory pools. Instead the impulses are diverted via the brain's side channels now opened. Stopping the impulses altogether is still dangerous to the body-mind system. But, thought-making process is put out of job with no raw material arriving and mind withholding its energy as a result of that. Unprocessed impulses now exit "as is" from *ajna*. Absence of new thoughts deprive ego of its sustenance and awareness of Self prevails.

Now with *suśumna* open, the essence of consciousness meets the energy of consciousness at *bindu*. This creates a new flow of intuitive knowledge that is not thought-based, but is rooted in the omniscient Universal Mind. This new route takes the knowledge to *sahasrāra* and then to *ājnā* where instead of exiting it reverses its course and is carried from subtle *buddhi* to the physical brain via *mānas*. This spells an end of "I" as the fulcrum of all thinking and actions.

The impulses route is shortened to 1 → 2 → 3 → 4 → 5 → 7 and an independent knowledge route emerges as 9 → 8 → 7. This stage is non-sensory and to be in this even for a short while is to be unaware of time and space. That makes you a *mahāyogi.*

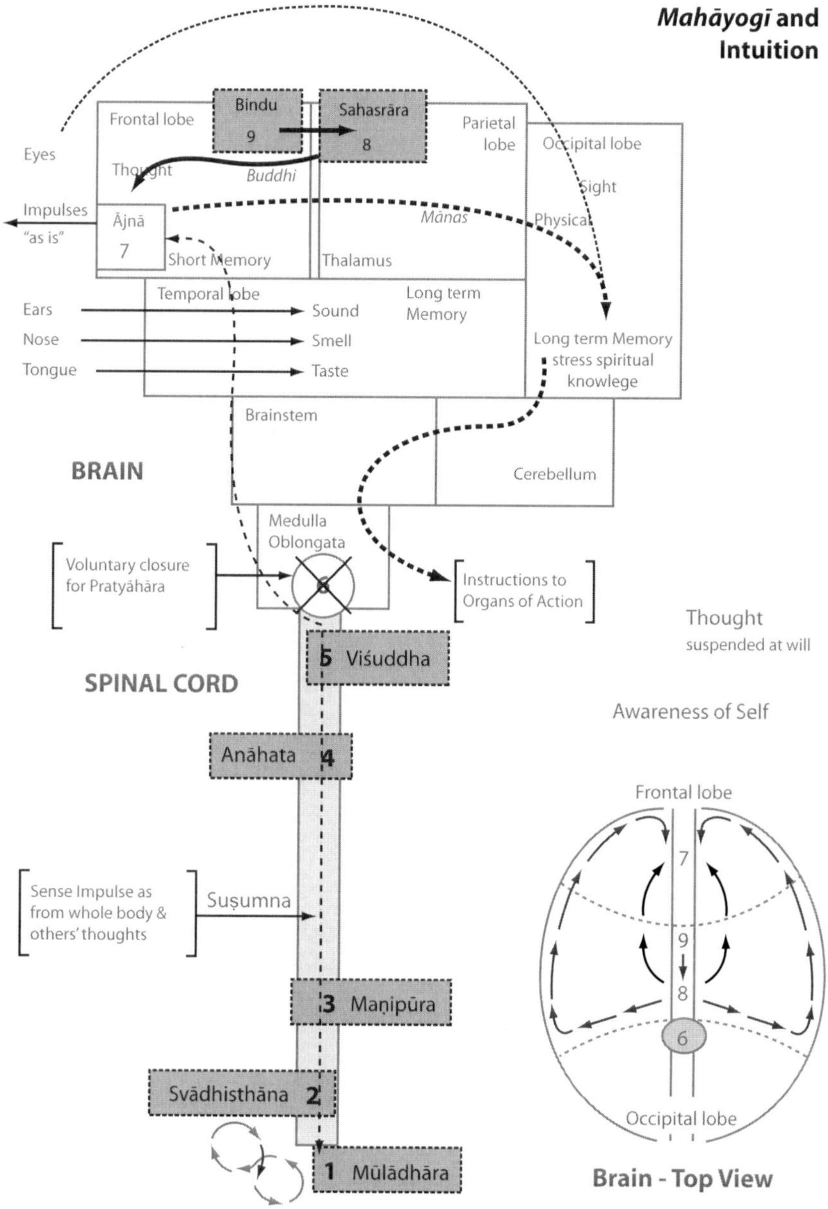
Mahāyogī and Intuition
Frontal lobe
Bindu
9
Sahasrāra
8
Parietal lobe
Occipital lobe
Eyes
Thought
Buddhi
Sight
Impulses "as is"
Ājnā
7
Mānas
Physical
Short Memory
Thalamus
Temporal lobe
Long term Memory
Ears
Sound
Nose
Smell
Tongue
Taste
Long term Memory stress spiritual knowlege
Brainstem
BRAIN
Cerebellum
Medulla Oblongata
Voluntary closure for Pratyāhāra
6
Instructions to Organs of Action
Thought
suspended at will
5 Viśuddha
SPINAL CORD
Awareness of Self
Anāhata 4
Frontal lobe
7
Sense Impulse as from whole body & others' thoughts
Suṣumna
9
8
3 Maṇipūra
6
Svādhisthāna 2
Occipital lobe
1 Mūlādhāra
Brain - Top View

5. A Master and Illumination

Absolutely no mind modifications can take place now, as there are no incoming sense impulses. Essence of Consciousness has now a permanent link with Cosmic Consciousness through *bindu*. At this stage, a master is beyond even *sāttvic* energy and has pure *prāṇa* as the only energy. A psycho-physio-biological change is now complete.

Pure *prāṇa* flows in and enters the bottom end of *suśumna*. *Taluka* remains consciously closed and *prāṇa* flows to the front brain. Pure *prāṇa* is the Universal Mind that provides all knowledge that is transcendental (and not thought-based) and in a complete reversal of roles, it is transmitted to the brain. *Bindu* and *sahasrāra* are now fully active. The *prāṇa*-flow appears to be going again as 7 → 8 → 9; but is completely different. There are no thoughts. No excretions of even *prāṇa* from ajna. Hence, on reaching 9 the flow of *prāṇa* returns 9 → 8 and all the way down to 1 ←→ 2 to form a closed circuit. This forms one *prāṇa* revolution.

An increase in the speed of *prāṇa* revolution creates a "take off" stage speed. Take-off force sufficient to send the primary body out of the physical body is 60 cycles in 60 pulse beats in *pratyāhāra* stage, 600 cycles per 60 pulse beats in *dhāraṇā* stage, 1800 cycles per 60 pulse beats in *dhyāna* stage and 3600 cycles per 60 pulse beats in *samādhī* stage.

In *dhāraṇā* and *dhyāna* stages, one can take leave to die consciously and be born again consciously; in *samādhī*, one can reach from *samādhī* with seed to *samādhī* without seed and in either of the *samādhī* stages take final leave from all physical births.

Paramayogī and Illumination

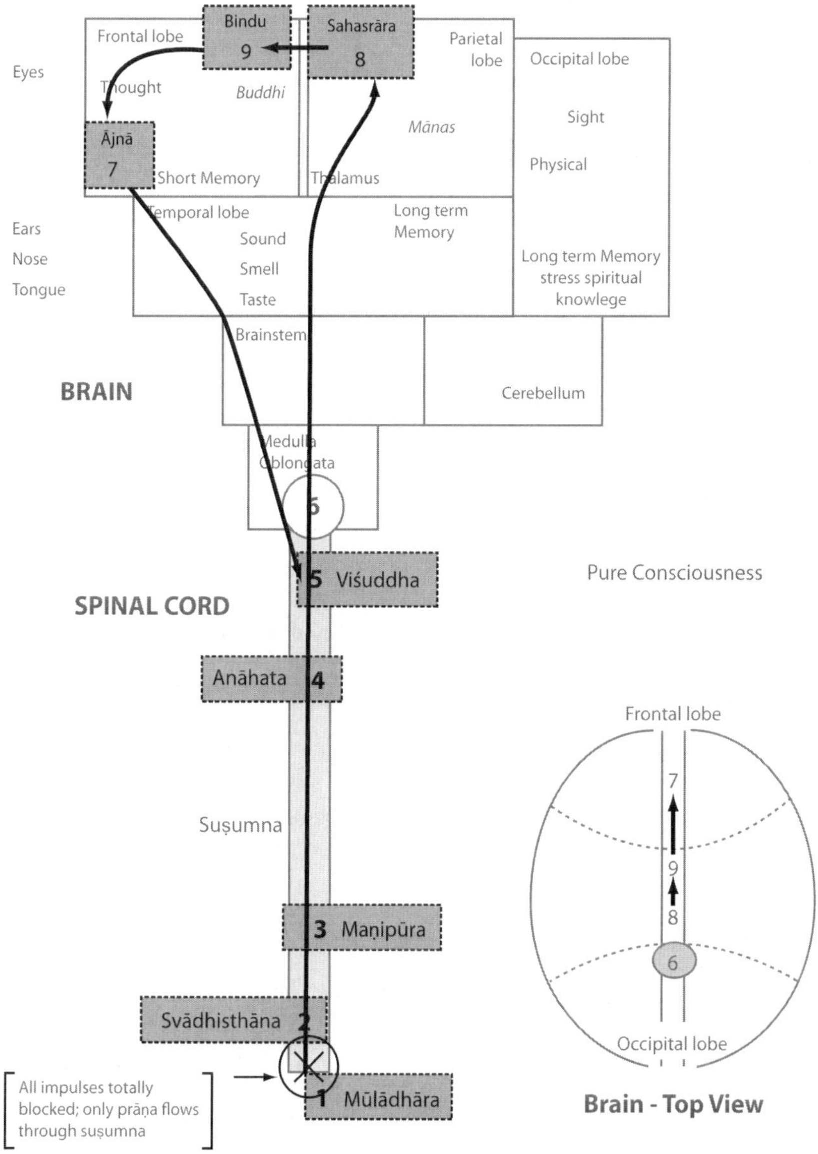

Exercises and Practices (Summary)

1. Exercises for a Sādhaka *to commence*

A. Four-fold solution for calming the mind modifications:

- Make tireless endeavor *(yatnobhyāsaḥ)*
- Value sufficiently (*satkārāsevito*) and follow methods and practices persistently (*nairantarya*)
- Non-attachment (*vairāgyam*)
- Liberate from *guṇa* (*guṇavaitṛṣṇyam)*

B. Obstacles and how they get resolved

Generic Solutions

- Do Yoga *abhyāsa* (discipline):
- Apply will intensely

Specific Solutions

- For Bodily Disability: A four-way practice: sympathy, tenderness, steadiness of purpose, and indifference with regard to happiness, misery, virtue, and vice. (Sūtra 1.20/I.33)
- For Mental Inertia: Rhythmic Breathing (Sūtra 2.1/I.34)
- For Doubt: Upgrading awareness (Sūtra 2.2/I.35).
- For Procrastination/Carelessness: Meditate on AUM (Sūtra 5.4/I.36).
- For Laziness or Lethargy: Refining exercises (Sūtra 2.3/I.37).
- For Craving/Lack of Dispassion: Meditation on Teachings in the dreams. (Sūtra 4.9/I.38).
- For Erroneous Perception: Concentration on that which is dearest to heart (Sūtra 4.10/I.39).
- For Inability to Achieve Concentration: *Dharaṇa* (Sūtra 4.19/III.2)

- For Failure to Hold the Meditative Attitude: *Samādhi* (Sūtra 4.20/III.3)

C. How to deal with hindrances

- Know them subtly
- Create an opposing mental attitude

2. *Exercises for a* Śiṣya *to add*

A. *Yama*

B. *Niyama*

C. *Āsana*

D. *Prāṇāyāma*

E. *Pratyāhāra*

F. Pause and steady spiritual perception

3. *Exercises for a* Yogī *to add*

A. Yogābhyāsa (advanced)

- How personality is acquired
- How memory sustains personality
- How structure of predispositions can be dissolved
- How all structures are fabricated in *guṇa*
- What brings *guṇa* in balance and harmony
- Why there is one mind but many forms
- Why we see what we are ourselves
- Why *Īśvara* is the *real Perceiver*

B. *Kriyā Yoga* (on medium fast-track)

C. Discerning Spiritual perception (on fast track)

4. *Exercises for a Mahāyogī to add*

A. Developing skills of:

a. Concentration
b. Meditation
c. Contemplation

B. Practice –

a. *Dhāraṇā*
b. *Dhyāna*
c. *Samādhī*

5. *Exercises for a* ParamaYogī

a. Reciting, listening to and meditating on AUM
b. Advanced *prāṇāyāma*
c. Practice *saṃyama* on –
   i. *Chakras*
   ii. *Vayūs*
d. Practice *samādhī* without seed,

Bibliography

Bailey, Alice. *The Light of the Soul, Its Science and Effect, A paraphrase of The Yogasutras of Patanjali.* New York: Lucis Publishing Company, 1927.

Hartranft, Chip. *The Yoga-Sūtra of Patañjali: a New Translation with Commentary*. Boston: Shambhala Publications, 2003.

Sri Aurobindo. *The Synthesis of Yoga*, and *The Life Divine*. Pondicherry, India: Sri Aurobindo Ashram, 1948.

Swami Vivekananda. *Raja Yoga or Conquering the Internal Nature*. Calcutta, India: Advaita Ashrama, 1998.

Tavaria, S. N. *Yoga Sutra of Sage Patanjali, Exposition and Practices*. India: S. N. Tavaria (1992)

Thakar, Vimala. *Glimpses of Raja Yoga, An Introduction to Patanjali's Yoga Sutras*. Berkeley: Rodmell Press, 2005.

Yardi, M. R. *The Yoga of Patanjali*. Pune, India: Bhandarkar Oriental Research Institute, 1979.

Recommended Reading

G. Srinivasan, Sankhya: An Ancient Philosophy Unifies Science and Religion, *http://s1.webstarts.com/Sankhyakarika/index.html* and *http://s2.webstarts.com/Sankhyakarika/index.html* (Read this for a very radical and far-reaching research work that reveals a fundamental difference between the Sanskrt words Sankhya and Samkhya, respectively belonging to the pre- and post-glacial inundation of 10-12 thousand years back, which has at times resulted in a duality of interpretations. While, Sankhya as explained in the Gita is the theoretical explanation of the dynamism of the Universe, Yoga as understood in Samkhya is its practical and consequential activity that rules all of manifestation in the Universe.)

Saraswati, Swami Satyananda. *Four Chapters on Freedom*. Bihar, India: Yoga Publications, 1976.

Sri Satya Sai Baba, *Message of the Lord, as a Practical Philosophy*. Auckland, New Zealand: Papatoetoe Printers and Stationers Ltd, 1998.

Index

I

K

M

T

U

OTHER TITLES OF INTEREST FROM HOHM PRESS

THE YOGA TRADITION
Its History, Literature, Philosophy and Practice
by Georg Feuerstein, Ph.D. Foreword by Subhash Kak, Ph.D.

A complete overview of the great Yogic traditions of: Raja-Yoga, Hatha-Yoga, Jnana-Yoga, Bhakti-Yoga, Karma-Yoga, Tantra-Yoga, Kundalini-Yoga, Mantra-Yoga and many other lesser known forms. Includes translations of over twenty famous Yoga treatises, like the *Yoga-Sutra* of Patanjali, and a first-time translation of the *Goraksha Paddhati*, an ancient Hatha Yoga text. Covers all aspects of Hindu, Buddhist, Jaina and Sikh Yoga. A necessary resource for all students and scholars of Yoga.

Paper, 520 pages, 8 ½ x 11, over 200 illustrations, $29.95
Yoga / Philosophy ISBN: 978-1-890772-18-5

• • •

YOGA MORALITY
Ancient Teachings at a Time of Global Crisis
by Georg Feuerstein, Ph.D.

This book is a hard-hitting critique of the media hype surrounding Yoga, and an exploration of Yogic philosophy and practice to discover what it *really* means to be a mature and moral person. "It is impossible to be a good yogi or yoginī without also being a morally mature individual," writes internationally-known Yoga authority and author, Georg Feuerstein. *Yoga Morality* looks at our present world situation primarily from the viewpoint of a spiritually-committed person, especially a practitioner of Yoga. It addresses the question: How are we to live consciously, responsibly, authentically, and without fear in the midst of mounting global crises?

Paper, 320 pages, 6 x 9, $19.95 ISBN: 978-1-890772-66-6

OTHER TITLES OF INTEREST FROM HOHM PRESS

MY BODY IS A TEMPLE
Yoga As a Path to Wholeness
by Christina Sell

With the freshness of a memoir, author and Yoga teacher Christina Sell draws upon her first visit to an extraordinary temple in southern India to present basic principles of Yoga. Beyond the ordinary aims of Yoga as a means of stretching and strengthening, or even for being happier or more centered, *My Body is a Temple* is an instruction manual for dedicating oneself to a life of the spirit, in and through the vehicle of the human body. The body as a temple is a common metaphor within many spiritual traditions. In this book, Christina Sell delves into the "how" and "why" of this widely accepted comparison.

Paper, 192 pages, 6 x 9, $16.95 ISBN: 978-1-935387-19-0
Yoga / Spirituality

• • •

YOGA FROM THE INSIDE OUT
Making Peace with Your Body Through Yoga
by Christina Sell

This is a book about Yoga and body image. More specifically, it is about Yoga and the issues of addiction, lack of self-love, and spiritual practice. Too many of us approach the practice of Yoga as another way to discipline the body without the inner softness necessary to be transformed by it. Author Christina Sell, a longtime student of Yoga and a master teacher, guides readers through a basic course in learning to accept *what is*, listen to the heart, and use the practice to deepen one's spiritual life.

Paper, 176 pages, 6 x 9, $14.95 ISBN: 978-890772-32-1
Yoga / Body-Mind-Spirit

About the Author

Suhas Tambe, born in India, is a Chartered Accountant and MBA (Indiana University of PA) who practices and teaches Yoga, and works in finance. In 1993, the author met his guru, a Yoga master, who had learned the practices of a well-preserved system related to Pātañjali's Sūtras. Its unique sequence seems to have been passed from master to disciple for generations. For over ten years, Suhas has studied his guru's unpublished writings, extensively researched its many unexplained concepts, and constructed a contemporary presentation for today's readers. The father of two grown married sons, he lives in Schaumburg, Illinois with his wife Vibha, an attorney and an entrepreneur.

Contact Information: suhas@suhastambe.com;
www.MakingofaYogaMaster.com

About Hohm Press

Hohm Press is committed to publishing books that provide readers with alternatives to the materialistic values of the current culture, and promote self-awareness, the recognition of interdependence, and compassion. Our subject areas include parenting, religious studies, women's studies, the arts and poetry.

Contact Information: Hohm Press, PO Box 4410, Chino Valley, Arizona, 86323; USA; 800-381-2700, or 928-636-3331;
email: *hppublisher@cableone.net*

Visit our website at *www.hohmpress.com*